Wound Care Essentials
PRACTICE PRINCIPLES

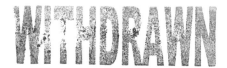

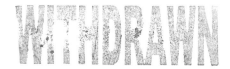

Wound Care Essentials
PRACTICE PRINCIPLES

Sharon Baranoski, MSN, RN, CWOCN, APN, FAAN
Administrative Director of Clinical Programs and Development
Administrator of Home Health
Silver Cross Hospital
Joliet, Illinois

Elizabeth A. Ayello, PhD, RN, APRN,BC, CWOCN, FAAN
Clinical Associate Professor and Director of Adult Nursing Science
Senior Adviser, The John A. Hartford Institute for Geriatric Nursing
New York University
The Steinhardt School of Education
Division of Nursing
New York

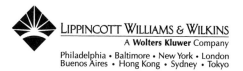

LIPPINCOTT WILLIAMS & WILKINS
A **Wolters Kluwer** Company
Philadelphia • Baltimore • New York • London
Buenos Aires • Hong Kong • Sydney • Tokyo

STAFF

Executive Publisher
Judith A. Schilling McCann, RN, MSN

Editorial Director
H. Nancy Holmes

Clinical Director
Joan M. Robinson, RN, MSN

Senior Art Director
Arlene Putterman

Editor
Jacqueline E. Mills

Clinical Project Manager
Jana L. Sciarra, RN, MSN, CRNP

Copy Editors
Kimberly Bilotta (supervisor), Heather Ditch,
Amy Furman, Dona Hightower, Catherine Kirby,
Irene Pontarelli

Designer
Susan Hopkins Rodzewich

Digital Composition Services
Diane Paluba (manager), Joyce Rossi Biletz (senior
desktop assistant), Donna S. Morris

Manufacturing
Patricia K. Dorshaw (senior manager),
Beth Janae Orr (book production coordinator)

Editorial Assistants
Megan L. Aldinger, Tara L. Carter-Bell,
Linda K. Ruhf

Librarian
Wani Z. Larsen

Indexer
Barbara E. Hodgson

Cover Photographs
Sharon Baranoski. *Top to bottom:* Necrotic,
unstageable pressure ulcer; healing ischial pressure
ulcer; tunnel wound on sacrum; trochanter ulcer
on quadriplegic patient; full-thickness pressure
ulcer

WCE010903 - 060406

Library of Congress Cataloging-in-Publication Data

Baranoski, Sharon.
Wound care essentials : practice principles — Sharon Baranoski,
Elizabeth A. Ayello.
p. ; cm.
Includes bibliographical references and index.
    1. Wounds and injuries — Patients — Care — Handbooks,
manuals, etc. 2. Wounds and injuries — Nursing — Handbooks,
manuals, etc. 3. Wound healing — Handbooks, manuals, etc. I.
Ayello, Elizabeth A. II. Title.
    [DNLM: 1. Wounds and Injuries — therapy. 2. Skin Ulcer —
therapy. 3. Wound Healing. WO 700 B225w 2003]
    RD94.B374 2003
    617.1 — dc21
ISBN 1-58255-274-6 (alk. paper)   2003013185

Contents

Contributors and consultants

Contributors

Mona Mylene Baharestani, PhD, NP,
 CWOCN, CWS
Director of Wound Healing
Division of Plastic and Reconstructive
 Surgery
Long Island Jewish Medical Center
New Hyde Park, N.Y.

Sue Bale, BA, PG Dip, RGN, NDN, RHV, Dip N
Director of Nursing Research
Wound Healing Research Unit
University of Wales, College of Medicine
Cardiff

Christine Barkauskas, BS, RN, CWOCN, APN
Wound, Ostomy and Continence
 Coordinator
Wound Healing and Treatment Center
Silver Cross Hospital
Joliet, Ill.

Joyce M. Black, PhD, RN, CPSN, CWCN
Assistant Professor
College of Nursing
University of Nebraska
Omaha

Steven B. Black, MD, FACS
Medical Director
Center for Wound Healing
Private Practice, Plastic Surgery
Omaha

Harold Brem, MD
Director, Wound Healing Program and
 Angiogenesis and Wound Healing
 Laboratory
The Mount Sinai Medical Center
New York

David M. Brienza, PhD
Associate Professor
Department of Bioengineering
Department of Rehabilitation Science
 and Technology
University of Pittsburgh

Janet Cuddigan, PhD, RN, CWCN
Assistant Professor
College of Nursing
University of Nebraska Medical Center
Omaha
Postdoctoral Nurse Fellow
Iowa City (Iowa) Veterans Affairs
 Medical Center

Linda E. Dallam, MS, APRN,BC, CWCN, GNP
Faculty
Division of Education and
 Organizational Development
Montefiore Medical Center
Bronx, N.Y.

Tami de Araujo, MD
Department of Dermatology and
 Cutaneous Surgery
University of Miami School of Medicine

Rita A. Frantz, PhD, RN, FAAN
Professor and Chair, Biobehavioral
 Nursing
College of Nursing
University of Iowa
Iowa City

Susan L. Garber, MA, OTR, FAOTA, FACRM
Associate Professor
Department of Physical Medicine and
 Rehabilitation
Baylor College of Medicine
Houston Veterans Affairs Medical Center

Sue E. Gardner, PhD, RN, CWCN
Assistant Professor
University of Iowa College of Nursing
Research Scientist
Iowa City Veteran's Affairs Medical
  Center

Mary Jo Geyer, PhD, PT, CWS, CLT
Assistant Professor
Department of Rehabilitation Science
  and Technology
University of Pittsburgh

Marc Gibber, BA
Medical Student
Wound Healing Program
The Mount Sinai Medical Center
New York

Keith Harding, MB, ChB, MRCGP, FRCS
Professor of Rehabilitative Medicine
Head of Department of Surgery
University of Wales, College of Medicine
Cardiff

Vanessa Jones, MSc, RN, NDN, RCNT, PGCE
Wound Healing Research Unit
University of Wales, College of Medicine
Cardiff

Morris D. Kerstein, MD
Chief of Staff
Veterans Administration Medical and
  Regional Office Center
Wilmington, Del.
Professor of Surgery
Jefferson Medical College
Philadelphia

Robert S. Kirsner, MD
Associate Professor
Department of Dermatology and
  Cutaneous Surgery
Department of Epidemiology and Public
  Health
University of Miami School of Medicine
Veterans Administration Medical Center

Carl A. Kirton, MA, RN, APRN,BC
Nurse Practitioner and Clinical Nurse
  Manager
AIDS Center
Mount Sinai Hospital and Medical Center
New York
Adjunct Clinical Associate Professor of
  Nursing
New York University

Ronald A. Kline, MD, FACS, FAHA
Associate Professor
Wayne State University
Department of Surgery
Program Director, Vascular Surgery
Harper University Hospital, The Detroit
  Medical Center

Steven P. Knowlton, JD, RN
Managing Attorney/Senior Trial Attorney
Law Offices of Gene Locks, PLLC
New York

Lawrence A. Lavery, DPM, MPh
Associate Professor
Department of Surgery
Texas A&M Health Science Center
Scott and White Hospital
Temple

Courtney H. Lyder, ND, GNP, FAAN
Professor
University of Virginia Medical Center
University of Virginia School of Nursing
Charlottesville

Mary Ellen Posthauer, RD, CD, LD
President
MEP Healthcare Dietary Services
Evansville, Indiana

Mary Y. Sieggreen, MSN, APRN, CS, CVN, APN
Nurse Practitioner, Vascular Surgery
Clinical Nurse Specialist in Wound Care
Harper University Hospital, The Detroit Medical Center
Assistant Clinical Professor
Wayne State University

Stephen Sprigle, PhD, PT
Associate Professor of Industrial Design and Applied Physiology
Director, Center for Assistive Technology and Environmental Access
Georgia Institute of Technology
Atlanta

David R. Thomas, MD
Professor of Internal Medicine and Geriatrics
Division of Geriatric Medicine
St. Louis University School of Medicine

Sarah Weinberger, BS, DEC
Research Assistant
Wound Healing Program
The Mount Sinai Medical Center
New York

Angela Colette Willis, RN, CWS, CDE
Staff Nurse
Wound Healing Program
The Mount Sinai Medical Center
New York

Consultants

Edna Atwater, RN
Administrative Director, Wound Management Institute
Duke University Health System
Durham, N.C.

Monica A. Beshara, RN, BSN, CWOCN
Wound Care Specialist
Decatur (Ga.) Hospital

Phyllis Bonham, RN, MSN, CWOCN
Director, Wound Care Education Program
College of Nursing
Medical University of South Carolina
Charleston

Carol Calianno, RN, MS, CWOCN
Wound, Ostomy, Continence Nurse
Abramson's Residence
North Wales, Pa.

Jo Catanzaro, RN, MSN, CWOCN
Clinical Coordinator, Comprehensive Wound Healing Center
Abington (Pa.) Memorial Hospital

Teresa A. Conner-Kerr, PhD, PT, CWS(D)
Associate Professor
Department of Physical Therapy
East Carolina University
Greenville, N.C.

Margaret C. Davis, RN, MSN
Assistant Professor
Central Florida Community College
Ocala

Judy A. Dutcher, MSN, APRN, BC, CWOCN
Consultant
Tucson, Ariz.

Barbara Pieper, PhD, RN, CS, CWOCN, FAAN
Professor/Nurse Practitioner
Wayne State University College of Nursing
Detroit

Lisa A. Salamon, RNC, MSN, ET
Clinical Nurse Specialist
Cleveland Clinic Foundation

Donna Scemons, RN, FNP, MSN, CNS, CWOCN
Private Practice
Healthcare Systems, Inc.
Panorama City, Calif.

Janice Stanbury, RN, MScN, GNC (C)
Assistant Professor
Okanagan University College School of
 Nursing
Kelowna, B.C., Canada

Cynthia A. Worley, RN, BSN, CWCN, CDCN
Wound, Ostomy, Continence Nurse
University of Texas M.D. Anderson
 Cancer Center
Houston

Karen Zulkowski, RN, DNS, CWS
Assistant Professor
Montana State University
Billings

Foreword

When asked to write the foreword for this book, I was reluctant but assented as a favor to my friends, Elizabeth Ayello and Sharon Baranoski. My reluctance stemmed from a belief that several very good books were already available on the general topic of wound care, and I wondered if I could muster enthusiasm for a book that might not add to the discussion, a book that might not stand apart from the others.

However, Sharon and Elizabeth have succeeded brilliantly! After browsing through the chapters, I am in love with this book and recommend it to every professional who is involved in wound care!

Wound Care Essentials: Practice Principles is unique in many ways. First, it pays attention to both the state of the science and the state of the art. To concentrate solely on the state of the science is to diminish the usefulness of the book to practitioners. The *science* of wound care remains at a somewhat primitive stage, despite an unprecedented level of interest in research in this area. However, the need for good wound care can't wait for science to answer our questions. Practitioners must cope with wound care problems, using the best research, expert opinion, and theoretical reasoning available; this is the *art* that the book serves up.

It goes without saying that this book covers the basic concerns of every professional who cares for patients with wounds. There are chapters on wound assessment, treatment, and care. Even then, there's often a new twist. For example, it's typical to find content on wound infection, but here we find a chapter on wound bioburden, which represents a broader and more recent view of wound care. It's also typical to find a chapter on support surfaces, but unusual to find a chapter that covers seating support as well; and it's usual to see content related to the mechanics of the various support surfaces, but very unusual to see a thorough treatment of biomechanics of the skin and underlying tissues.

Immediately apparent is the fact that *Wound Care Essentials: Practice Principles* also reflects our modern concerns. Ten years ago it would have been unusual to find more than passing reference to legal aspects and regulatory issues in a wound care textbook. Yet today, these are crucial issues in the daily practice of those caring for persons with wounds. Similarly, the research on quality of life for people and the experience of pain for people with wounds is relatively recent and the practical concerns that arise from this knowledge are more often discussed among experts than written about for consumption by practitioners. These topics are given whole chapters for exploration of both theoretical issues and practical applications.

Most wound care books have a general emphasis on pressure ulcers, vascular ulcers and, sometimes, diabetic ulcers. This book goes beyond the ordinary in its coverage of a wide variety of wounds. Included is substantial information on sickle cell wounds as well as additional content on complex wounds and atypical wounds. Finally, an entire chapter devoted to special populations covers such

such topics as risk factors in critical care, special problems of skin integrity in spinal cord injury, and skin manifestations common to people with HIV and AIDS.

Wound Care Essentials: Practice Principles has aspects at once practical and esoteric. Its content should appeal to both the novice and the expert. It is interdisciplinary in both authorship and utility. In short, *Wound Care Essentials: Practice Principles* has great information for anyone who's involved in caring for patients with or at risk for wounds.

Barbara Braden, PhD, RN, FAAN
Dean, Graduate School and University College
Creighton University
Omaha

Preface

"Wisdom is the power to put our time and our knowledge to the proper use."
Thomas J. Watson, IBM Founder

In answer to our colleagues, we finally wrote the book you all were asking us to do. We thought about writing a book that contained the essential elements of wound care that we had learned over our nursing careers, information that wasn't available to us in any one book as we began our practice in the wonderful world of wounds so many years ago.

The result is *Wound Care Essentials: Practice Principles*. Our book is the culmination of a long-standing friendship, partnership, educational bond, and need to share what we learned in the trenches of patient care. It's the marriage of practice and education done by two friends with the same dream: our interest in educating others about wounds because we hold dearly the belief that excellence in practice depends upon excellence in education. It combines all that we have learned from our patients, colleagues, research, literature, industry, seminars, and educational programs into one concise wound care source.

Have fun with our book. That's important to us because learning should be enjoyable. It's a guide, but it isn't a cookbook. Neither is it all-inclusive. In our book as in wound care, we had to make choices as to what can realistically be done.

We had a great group of writers! Thank you to our authors! As we were limited to book size, the hardest part for us was to decide among the vast number of our colleagues who would contribute to this first edition. We have saved some of them for the next edition. Imagine our pleasure when Barbara Braden agreed to write our foreword! We were delighted with the interest, support, excitement, and enthusiasm that all our writers showed when invited to be part of this book. Without their willingness to share their time, knowledge, and expertise, this book wouldn't be a reality.

Teamwork is important, whether it's in wound care or publishing. A special thank you to Roberta Abruzzesse who was instrumental in guiding us in our early writing careers. The diligent editing, meticulous attention to detail, understanding, and flexibility from our crew at Lippincott Williams & Wilkins made it a much less tenacious and threatening experience. We are grateful to the Lippincott staff who worked behind the scenes on our behalf. We may not know all of you personally, but your efforts are very known and appreciated. Thank you, Judy McCann, Joan Robinson, Jana Sciarra, and Nancy Holmes, for your guidance and support in making this book possible. It seems unbelievable to us that together it took only 1 year to write this book.

To our readers, we hope the pages will be tattered and torn from use — that our book doesn't sit on your shelf. For we both believe the old adage, "Teachers can open the door of learning, but you must enter it yourself."

Sharon and Elizabeth

Dedication

To my wonderfully unique husband, Jim, I thank you for the love, laughter, and fun you've brought into my life. There is no greater hero in my life than you. Thank you for helping me be all that I can be.

To my four fabulous children, Jim Jr., Deborah, Jeff, and J.R., thanks for tolerating the many years of TV dinners, missed events, and looking at wound pictures you couldn't begin to understand or stomach. I am filled with pride and joy as I look at the young adults you've all become. Thanks for letting me be your Mom.

To my parents, Virginia and John, thanks for planting the seeds of enthusiasm, hard work ethics, and determination in me.

To my colleagues Andrea, Chris, and Linda, thanks for always supporting and holding up my wings. To Courtney and Rita, thank you for believing in me.

And finally to my co-editor, Elizabeth A. Ayello, I would not have fulfilled my dream of writing this book if it hadn't been for your friendship, love, support, and respect. I can't think of a better person to share my dream with than YOU. We did it!

Sharon

"Family is everything."

To my parents, Phyllis and Tony, my brothers Bob and Ron and their families, and Florence and Bert, whose love and support have nurtured me throughout all my educational endeavors.

To my nursing colleagues Katie, Carl, Teddy, Sheila, Joanne, Courtney, and Janet for always "being there" for me. Your presence in my life has made a difference.

To Sharon, the best book partner. Sharing our work and passion for wounds and education has been a great experience.

To the sunshines of my life, my daughters Wendy and Sarah, you are my dreams made reality.

To my husband, A. Scott, with love, for making all my dreams come true. Now the music's begun, let's dance!

E.A.A.

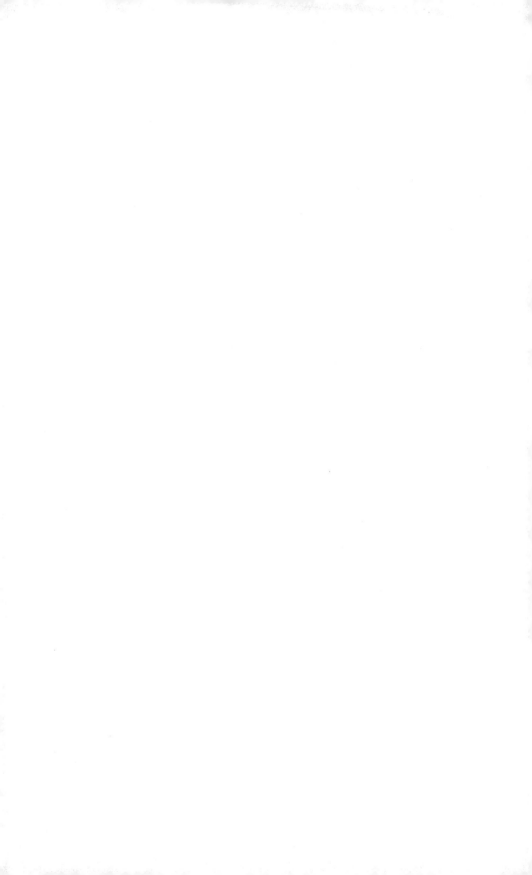

Part One

Wound care concepts

CHAPTER 1

Quality of life and ethical issues

Mona Mylene Baharestani, PhD, NP, CWOCN, CWS

OBJECTIVES

After completing this chapter, you'll be able to:

- describe how wounds and those afflicted by wounds are viewed

- identify quality of life impact on patients with wounds and their caregivers

- describe ethical dilemmas confronted in wound care

- identify issues and challenges faced by caregivers of patients with wounds

- describe strategies aimed at meeting the needs of patients with wounds and their caregivers.

Treating the patient as well as the wound

The practice of wound healing is undergoing revolutionary change as research unlocks the mysteries of the complex processes of tissue degradation, regeneration, and repair. Research has also given birth to many new wound-healing technologies: Living skin equivalents, matrix metalloproteinase modulation, topical growth factors, negative pressure, normothermia, and slow-release antimicrobial therapies are now all within the armamentarium of wound-care practitioners, making possible the healing of previously recalcitrant wounds.

But faster, more efficient healing is only one element of providing advanced wound care — wounds affect patients on many levels. Wounds bring financial, psychological, and social implications that we must also address. Yet, in our fast-paced, stressful clinical practices, do we encourage the patient to disavow his wounds?[1] Do we acknowledge the profound life changes and day-to-day challenges faced by chronic wound sufferers?[2] Or do we perpetuate patients' fear, shame, and isolation?[1] Do we give patients and their families and caregivers the impression that "wound care is a dehumanizing and reductionist special-ty"?[3]

Assessing the meaning and significance of the wound to the patient and his care-giver should be as routine as assessing wound size and the percentage of granu-lation and necrotic tissue, but is it? Hyland et al.[4] report that patients spend an average of 1.5 to 2 hours per day thinking about their leg ulcers. Do we know what the patient is thinking? Do we ever ask? The answer to the question "What impact has your wound had on your quality of life?" posed by a caring and concerned practitioner provides valuable insight into the patient's experi-ence and needs, while setting the stage for mutual goal identification and treat-ment planning.

Beyond possession of knowledge in ba-sic science, anatomy, pathophysiology, wound-care dressings, drugs, and tech-nologies, advanced wound-care practition-ers must be able to deliver care in a com-passionate manner, sensitive to the unique impact wounds have on quality of life.

How are wounds viewed?

A wound is defined as a disruption of the integrity and function of tissues in the body. The state of having a wound infers an imperfection, an insult resulting in a physical and emotional vulnerability.[5] Wounds and their management are de-scribed within a variety of personal, philo-sophical, and socioeconomic paradigms. (See *Emotional impact of wounds.*)

How are patients with wounds viewed?

Given the negative image by which wounds are viewed, it isn't surprising that patients with wounds are sometimes considered unattractive, imperfect, vul-nerable, a nuisance to others and, in some cases, even repulsive.[5-8] Health

---

Emotional impact of wounds

In addition to the dangers associated with wounds and the physical discomfort they often bring, wounds have an emo-tional effect on the patient, caregivers, family and friends, and strangers he may encounter. Even health care profession-als aren't immune to an emotional re-sponse to a patient's wound.

Wounds are typically perceived as:
- unpleasant, uncomfortable
- nuisance, time-consuming, costly
- smelly
- appalling, disgusting, repulsive
- haunting, scary, associated with hor-ror movies
- a betrayal of one's own body.

The patient's own perception of his wound may include such feelings as:
- embarrassment, humiliation
- guilt, shame
- needing bandages to "hide the evi-dence" (that is, of imperfection).

---

care professionals, in particular, often blame patients and caregivers for the de-velopment and recalcitrance of pressure ulcers and venous ulcers, as the follow-ing comments reveal.

"When I have a pressure ulcer, health care professionals ask, 'What hap-pened?' This makes me feel ashamed be-cause I was unable to prevent the pres-sure ulcer. Why is it that other complica-tions of quadriplegia don't carry this type of stigma? Nobody makes me feel guilty when I have a urinary tract infec-tion."[1]

A 79-year-old caregiver for her bedrid-den, paralyzed 83-year-old spouse states, "I thought it was nothing." (Referring to nine pressure ulcers.) "The plastic surgeon was quite angry about the sores, asking why I waited so long to bring him to the hospital. I was just dumbfounded. I felt so bad, I said, I just thought it was a sore that would just heal up. I feel so guilty that I didn't do the right thing."[9]

Wounds on the face, neck, and hands are obviously the most difficult to conceal, not only from others, but also from the patient's own view. The emotional trauma experienced by facial disfigurement requires long periods of adjustment.[10] In fact, one study reports that 30% to 40% of adult burn patients with facial scarring experienced severe psychological problems up to 2 years after discharge from rehabilitation.[11]

For those with visible wounds, the teasing, name-calling, looks of pity, stares, and insensitive comments can make even a walk down the street a daunting experience.[12] According to Partridge,[12] disfiguring wounds on the face create a painful double bind of "extreme self-consciousness and self-imposed social isolation." Bernstein[13] describes a "social death" among facially disfigured patients. Social death occurs as the patient's self-consciousness about being in public increases, ties with family and friends are severed and, ultimately, all social interactions cease. Without positive social reinforcement, the patient's self-esteem vanishes and self-confidence ebbs away.[13]

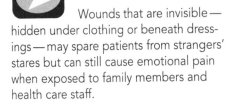

PRACTICE POINT

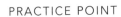

Wounds that are invisible — hidden under clothing or beneath dressings — may spare patients from strangers' stares but can still cause emotional pain when exposed to family members and health care staff.

Feelings of shame, embarrassment, powerlessness, and fear can be overpowering for patients as they lie undressed during examinations by health care professionals. As health care practitioners, we must be aware of the way we touch and dress wounds as well as our posturing and distance from the patient.[12] Partridge[12] emphasizes that we must pay particular attention to the unspoken word conveyed by our communication triangle (from the eyes to the chin).

Quality of life

Unquestionably, wounds have varying effects on the quality of life of those afflicted and on their caregivers. To explore the impact further requires a definition of this complex, multifactorial construct.

Quality of life is a vague and ethereal construct that reflects a patient's perspective on life satisfaction in a variety of situations.[14,15] In an attempt to narrow down the all-encompassing term "quality of life," the term "health-related quality of life" (HRqol) was first used in the late 1980s.[16] In Price's[16] view, "health-related quality of life is defined as the impact of disease and treatment on disability and daily living, or as a patient-based focus on the impact of a perceived health state on the ability to lead a fulfilling life."

Franks and Moffatt[17] add, "The state of ill health may be defined as feelings of pain and discomfort or change in usual functioning and feeling. This is key to the concept of health-related quality of life since it's the patient's own sense of well-being which is important, not the clinician's opinion of [the patient's] clinical status."

The four domains of quality of life, as described by Schipper et al.,[18] are physical and occupational function, psychological state, social interaction, and somatic sensation, with some investigators adding a financial component.

Physical and occupational function

In Brod's[19] pilot study examining the impact of lower extremity ulcers on patients with diabetes, the participants reported feeling drained and fatigued due to sleep disturbances and the high energy expenditure required for mobility. Additionally, antibiotic-related adverse effects of nausea, fatigue, and general malaise were considerable. In Brod's[19] sample, 50% of patients (N = 14) had to retire early or lost their jobs because of an ulcer. Even patients who were still employed experienced decreased productivity, lost time from work due to health care appointments, and lost career opportunities.[19]

Marked restrictions in activities of daily living (ADLs) among those with leg ulcers are reported in many studies, including those by Hyland et al.,[4] Brod,[19] Phillips et al.,[20] and Walshe.[21] Another study, consisting of 88 patients with chronic leg ulcers, reported that 75% had difficulty performing basic housework.[22] The study by Hyland et al.,[4] consisting of 50 patients with leg ulcers, demonstrated that 50% of the participants had problems getting on and off a bus and 30% always had trouble climbing steps.

Pain, leg edema, fatigue, and bulky dressings can make simple acts of changing one's clothing and bathing frustrating, if not impossible.[19,21,22] In personal interviews of 73 patients with leg ulcers by Phillips et al.,[20] 81% described their mobility as adversely affected by their ulcer, and edema was felt to be the dominant factor.

In another study, 42% of patients identified the leg ulcer as a key factor in their decision to stop working.[20] All patients interviewed felt that the leg ulcer limited their work capacity and 50% added that their jobs required standing most of their shift.[20] For younger patients, leg ulceration was correlated with time lost from work, job loss, and adverse effects on finances.[20]

Factors affecting patient response to wounds

Factors that shape a patient's emotional response to his wound include:
- etiology
- preparedness
- visibility
- response of others
- pain
- odor, leakage
- healing outcomes
  - expectation of healing
  - time to healing
  - acute versus chronic
- meaning, significance
- impact on activities of daily living
- coping patterns
- spirituality
- social supports
- age
- gender.

Psychological function

Multiple factors affect the psychological response to having a wound or caring for a loved one with a wound. (See *Factors affecting patient response to wounds.*)

Etiology

According to Magnan,[23] an individual's psychological response to a wound may be closely related to the mechanism of wounding. Imagine the terrifying flashbacks and the flurry of emotions and fears elicited when patients and family caregivers view open amputation wounds sustained after motor vehicle accidents, burn wounds exposed during whirlpool treatments, gangrenous limbs from peripheral vascular disease, and necrotic pressure ulcers with bone exposed.

PRACTICE POINT

Each dressing change draws attention to the wounded body part and its associated pain, but it also serves as a reminder of the circumstance or disease that resulted in the injury and engenders fears about the future.[23]

Preparedness

From the onset of hospital, rehabilitation, and home care admission, health care professionals plan for a patient's discharge by preparing patients and caregivers for independence. But are we sensitive to the patient's psychological and emotional readiness to deal with his wound? To deal with the initial wounding, the patient and his family may need to relinquish control to the health care provider.[1] The reality is that some patients may be unable to deal with their physical wounds because they're simultaneously struggling with deep, emotionally stirred wounds. This point is illustrated by patients' remarks: "It took everything I had to deal with the reality of having to spend the rest of my life as a quadriplegic" ... "When I have an ulcer (referring to a pressure ulcer), I don't want to see it. I feel like I am in hell and to survive I must separate myself from the wound." ... "I fear the sight of the ulcer."[1]

Visibility

As discussed previously, the visibility, severity, and circumstances under which wounding occurred can dramatically affect the patient's assimilation of the wound into his changed body image.

Response of others

Acceptance, pity, dismay, fear, repulsion, and avoidance are the gamut of responses displayed by others to wounds and to those who have been wounded. This can dramatically affect a patient's emotional response to his wound and his self-esteem.

Pain

Physical pain associated with wounds is one of the areas in which health care professionals are least attentive. Pain, as described by Krasner[24] "is one of those experiences of being that often confounds our understanding, sometimes we may actually flee from facing it." Yet pain is a major factor affecting the HRqol of those with wounds, as we'll see in the section discussing somatic sensation, page 10.

Odor and leakage

The impact of odor from a fungating breast wound, a necrotic pressure ulcer, or a draining and infected venous leg ulcer can be emotionally and psychologically devastating. A patient may try in vain to mask wound odor with perfumes and colognes. His self-image can be crushed by feelings of shame, disgust, and embarrassment. He may say that the wound's odor makes him feel dirty, and may apologize to others about the odor. Some patients feel isolated by an odorous wound and limit their social encounters due to fear of offending others. Friends and family members may add to these feelings of isolation by avoiding the patient because of the wound's odor. Increased anxiety and depression scores, lower life satisfaction, and decreased social contacts among those with malodorous leg ulcers are reported by Roe et al.[22]

Healing outcomes

In clinical practice, the three questions most frequently posed by patients and caregivers are:

- Will this wound heal?
- How long will it take to heal?
- Will the treatment cause pain?

For patients and their caregivers, just hearing that there's hope of healing, that improvement is occurring, and that the pain, odor, and restrictions will one day be gone or lessened can make the situation easier to bear.[6,21]

Among patients with chronic leg ulcers and high recurrence rates, healing potential is often viewed with pessimism.[21] In interviews of 73 patients with leg ulcers by Phillips et al.,[20] only 3% felt their ulcers would ever heal. This uncertainty toward healing is often mirrored by health care professionals.[21]

Time to healing

Lack of a known time scale for healing is a common complaint, leading to increased frustration, depression, and restricted ADLs by those with leg ulcers,[4,21] pressure ulcers,[25] and other types of wounds. In Krasner's[26] phenomenological study examining the impact of painful venous ulcers on HRqol, one of the major themes identified is that of frustration. Frustration in this sample of 14 patients suffering with leg ulcers from 2 months through 7 years stemmed from slow healing rates, lower limb swelling, infection, and the formation of new ulcers.[26] Other frustrations were related to years of multiple unsuccessful treatments, inadequate health care professionals, or self-blame for the lack of healing.[26]

While it's obvious that most patients desire wound healing, we would be remiss to not ask our patients about their specific goals in relation to their wounds. Wientjes[27] identifies four common behavioral attitudes exhibited by patients whose wounds heal:

- sets attainable goals (for example, to return to work, attend child's wedding)
- receptive to learning
- compliant with treatment
- curious; willingness to see the wound and actively participate in care.

According to Myss,[28] "assuming that everyone wants to heal is both misleading and potentially dangerous. Illness can, for instance, become a powerful way to get attention a patient might not otherwise receive." For some, there can be a manipulative value to keeping a wound, a figurative "street value or social currency." Defining oneself by the wound is an attitude described by Myss as "woundology."[28] For these patients, staying wounded provides benefits, such as continued nursing visits, Meals On Wheels,[22] home health aide services, an excuse to remain unemployed, and continued attention by family and health care professionals.[27]

Acute versus chronic

Some wounds heal quickly and uneventfully, while others are present for years or even a lifetime. Yet are these wounds similarly perceived by those afflicted? Do coping styles vary based on wound chronicity?

Expanding on the works of Parsons,[29] O'Flynn[30] postulates that following an acute minor wounding event, the wound and its treatment become the main focus of the patient and his family. Viewing his wound as deviant, the patient is eclipsed by the wound and readily assumes the role of "sick person." Individual roles and responsibilities are overshadowed by pain and incapacity.[30] During the healing and coping phase the individual remains a patient. Once healing is achieved, however, the individual reemerges; normality is regained as good health and quality of life are restored.[30]

Trauma patients experience a flurry of emotions and employ various defense mechanisms, such as suppression, regression, denial, distraction, magical thinking, or rationalization.[31] According to Lenehan,[32] the severe injuries endured may open floodgates of intense emotions and disturbed images of self. As a result, the patient may present with a rather shallow or blunted affect or "ego constriction" in an attempt to conserve psychological energy.[32] An inner battle occurs between anger, depression, and fear as the patient asks himself, "Will I be treated differently?" and "Will anyone care for me in light of disability and disfigurement?"[32]

Conversely, Phillips et al.,[20] Price and Harding,[33] and Walshe[21] report that patients with chronic wounds cope with the impaired mobility, pain, and sleep disturbances by the process of normalization. Coping with chronic wounds, according to Dewar and Morse,[34] is accomplished by adaptation, or the untenable process of silent acceptance. Interestingly, Price and Harding[33] found that those with venous leg ulcers of greater than 24 months duration rated themselves as having less pain and better general health than those with ulcers of less than 24 months duration.

In a phenomenological study of 10 patients with chronic nonhealing wounds by Neil and Munjas,[2] two patterns and six themes emerged. The two identified patterns are: Contending with the wound and staying home or staying back.

Contending with the wound includes four themes:
• noticing; that is, the first time the patient noticed the wound wasn't improving, and other people noticing and caring for the wound
• contending with exudate and odor—issues that can cause significant distress, social isolation, and embarrassment

• losing sleep
• being in pain.

The second constitutive pattern, staying home or staying back, includes themes of isolation and trouble walking. Isolation stemmed from the patient's fear of going out and acquiring infection and being housebound secondary to immobility (for example, having to stay in bed or with the affected leg elevated). Trouble walking was due to pain or loss of function secondary to the wound. For these participants "the wound becomes the focus of their lives as it makes them immobile or makes walking difficult."[2]

Contrary to other authors who described feelings of normalization among those with chronic wounds, Neil and Munjas[2] found that "chronic wound participants 'became their wound.' The wound is all encompassing. The participant constantly hopes that their wound will get better so that they can resume their former wound-free life. With each passing year, or with worsening of the wound despite therapy, hope, and compliance may fade."

Meaning, significance

To gain understanding into how a patient's HRqol is affected, what his goals are, and how we can best assist him, we must acquire insight into the meaning and significance that his wound holds for him. As one patient aptly states, "True understanding doesn't occur unless we share our strengths, fears, and weakness."[1]

Painful venous ulcers have been described as "the literal breakdown of the skin and the figurative breakdown of the embodied self."[35] Pressure ulcer formation has been described by family caregivers as a normal thing to happen to the bedridden[9] and as "truly the worst thing that can happen" by those directly afflicted.[1]

Impact on activities of daily living

Physical, somatic, financial, and medical restrictions can result in limitations on a patient's ability to engage in ADLs. Restrictions in ADLs can further impact and be impacted by the psychological and emotional ramifications of the wound experience.

Coping patterns

Breaches in the skin, as with other types of loss, can illicit the process of grieving. While most patients transcend the continuum from denial, depression, anger, and bargaining to ultimate acceptance, some may become frozen at a certain point or even exhibit regressional behavior. Walshe's[21] phenomenological study examining what it's like to live with a venous leg ulcer from the patient's perspective identifies four major coping strategies.

• Coping by comparison — by comparing himself to others with ulcerations, the patient experiences normalization; by comparing himself to patients with other illnesses (such as stroke), the patient feels more fortunate.

• Feeling healthy — despite the leg ulcerations and the associated debilitating symptoms and restrictions, most participants felt otherwise healthy.

• Altered expectation — as all of the participants were elderly, they reported having reached a point of acceptance, viewing the ulcer as a part of the aging process.

• Being positive — most participants described themselves as lucky and dismissed the symptoms as "not bad at all."[21]

Spirituality

The power of prayer, hope, and support of a patient's religious beliefs can't be underestimated in providing emotional strength.

Social supports

Many patients with wounds see a shrinking of the social circle as pain, fears, and physical restrictions increase. The patient with a wound may experience guilt about friends having to change their activities to accommodate his limitations, and may therefore further limit social interaction.[19] As discussed earlier, odor, leakage, and wound visibility may also result in decreased social contact. For some patients, overdependence for physical, emotional, and psychological strength may fall on a single caregiver, usually a spouse.

Age

In a study by Phillips et al.,[20] younger patients exhibited greater negative emotions related to their leg ulcers and greater problems with mobility ($p < 0.001$) than older patients. Older patients proved more effective in coping with or adapting to their limitations and disability.[20] Similar findings are reported by Franks and Moffatt.[36] In a cross-sectional study using the Nottingham Health Profile (NHP) and age- and sex-matched normal scores of 758 patients with leg ulcers, younger males were found to experience the greatest negative impact on HRqol.[36] Among those with diabetes and lower extremity ulcers, Brod[19] reports that older patients were less effected in the social, employment, and familial arenas. Conversely, in a study measuring HRqol in 63 patients with chronic leg ulcers by Price and Harding, age wasn't statistically significant.[33]

Gender

The impact of gender on HRqol in those with wounds is met with debate in the literature. Lindholm et al.[37] report that males have significantly poorer HRqol than females in the areas of pain and physical mobility. Additionally, when compared to the normative scores for males in the areas of sleep disturbance, emotional reaction, and social isolation, males with leg ulcers exhibited increased scores.[37] Price and Harding[33] found poorer HRqol scores in women in the domains of vitality and physical and social functioning. A database of 758 patients with leg ulcers similarly reports women to have a poorer HRqol than males.[17] But as Franks and Moffatt[36] point out, in studies of the general population, women score worse on HRqol than males, especially in older age groups. Therefore, the poorer scores among women with leg ulcers may not be directly related to the ulcer, but rather to generally poorer HRqol scores among women.

Social interaction

Limitations in social interactions among those with wounds may stem from the following:
• impaired mobility secondary to pain, causing many patients to become essentially housebound[4,21,22]
• treatment restrictions, such as the need to stay on bed rest for pressure ulcer management; leg elevation for edema control, and the need to be homebound to receive skilled home care nursing services
• avoidance of social activities where crowds, children, or pets might be encountered, out of fear of injuring the wound site or creating new ulcers[4,21]
• fatigue from disrupted sleep and adverse effects of antibiotics[22,25]
• embarrassment from odor, leakage, and wound visibility
• need to rely on others and assistive devices[19]
• additional time required to perform dressing changes[4,19]

• difficulty maintaining appearance because shoes and clothing may not fit over bulky dressings.[4,22]

Patients with wounds may be forced to make significant life changes and find satisfaction in new activities.[35] The ability to enjoy a sauna, bicycling, running, swimming, or tennis is eliminated because of bulky dressings and compression wraps.

Although health care professionals encourage and recognize the value of social interaction to a patient's psychological and emotional function, don't we simultaneously blame patients or label them as noncompliant when they come to our offices with worsening of their edema and deterioration of their leg and foot ulcers secondary to being out with friends, trying to enjoy life?

PRACTICE POINT

As health care professionals, we must not only acknowledge, but also creatively work with the patient in the challenge of balancing physical wound healing with psychological and emotional healing.

Listen to the words of a patient describing the difficulties of maintaining bed rest to heal his pressure ulcer: "I can remember lying in the hospital ... looking at the paint on the wall. And I could tell you how many little bubbles were in that particular spot. I memorized them to keep from going mad."[25]

Somatic sensation

According to Schipper et al.,[18] the domain of somatic sensation "encompasses unpleasant physical feelings that may detract from someone's quality of life (such as pain)."

The devastating impact on all aspects of HRqol among those with wounds has recently received attention in numerous studies,[2,17,20,21,25,26,35,39] although incorporation of findings into clinical practice has been slow to follow.

Patients have described pain as the worst thing about having a leg ulcer,[21,39,40] with the "first daily act of weight bearing as the most severe pain they experience."[40] The unrelenting nature of the pain frequently makes patients feel like they aren't in control of their lives.[21] Leg elevation often makes the pain worse, sleep is frequently disrupted by pain,[40] and pain medication is often ineffective.[21] Among those with venous ulcers, pain is often described in three distinct locations: within the ulcer, around the ulcer, and elsewhere in the leg.[40]

Krasner's[35] qualitative phenomenological study of 14 patients with painful venous ulcers identifies 8 key themes. (See *Painful venous leg ulcers: Key themes.*)

Participants in Krasner's[35] study vividly described the pain as "the worst thing I have ever gone through in my life" … "like someone is sticking pins in you all the time" … "absolute murder." Pain was described as worse when the leg was more edematous and during infection. Interestingly, patients considered pain a normal or expected occurrence with having a leg ulcer. Pain during and after debridement was considered the most intense pain experienced by patients, bringing on a cycle of pain and fear that left many depressed. Yet, despite the pain, suffering, and limitations brought on by these ulcers, patients tried to maintain a positive attitude and to "carry on despite the pain."[35]

Similar reports of pain are described in studies of those with pressure ulcers. In a phenomenological study by Langemo et al.,[25] pain is described as "getting a knife and really digging in there good and hard" and "stinging."

Painful venous leg ulcers: Key themes

Krasner[35] identifies eight key themes in patients with painful venous leg ulcers:
- Expecting pain with the ulcer
- Feeling frustrated
- Experiencing pain caused by swelling
- Being unable to stand
- Interfering with the job
- Starting the pain all over again with painful debridements
- Having to make life changes
- Trying to find satisfaction in new activities

The duration of pain is described as an issue most of the time, even being a problem after healing.[25] In a sample of 32 patients with stage III and IV pressure ulcers, Szor and Bourguignon[43] found that 88% experienced pain with dressing changes, although dressings used were consistent with principles of moist healing. Furthermore, 84% of the participants reported pain at rest, and 18% described the pain as horrible or excruciating.[43]

Despite the prevalence and intensity of pain among those with wounds, Roe et al.[42] found that 55% of community nurses don't include pain as a part of their assessment. Walshe[21] reports that patients' descriptions of pain are often devalued. In studies by Hollinworth[44] and Dallam et al.,[38] pain medications were seldom administered to manage pain associated with dressing changes. Similarly, Szor and Bourguignon[43] reported a mere 6% of patients receiving medication for pressure ulcer pain.

In an attempt to capture nurses' stories about coping with patients' pressure ulcer pain, Krasner[24] conducted a phenomenological study of 42 nurses, identifying three patterns and eight themes:

- Nursing expertly includes the ability to recognize, validate, attend to, acknowledge, and caringly empathize with the patient in pain.
- Denying the pain includes assuming it doesn't exist or failing to hear the patient's complaints or cries. This was described as an effective coping mechanism for the health care professional, assisting them in avoiding feelings of failure but obviously at severe detriment to the patient.
- Confronting the challenge of pain occurs when the health care professional must come to terms with his own feelings of frustration. Negative feelings associated with wound care include anger, helplessness, hopelessness, being upset about performing a procedure that will cause pain, and experiencing pain along with the patient. Perhaps we must, as Krasner[24] states, "take a step back and make a special effort to understand the nearness of the near." By "being with" the patient we may gain insight into the meaning that the pain experience holds for the patient.[24]

In examinations of the impact of leg ulcer clinics on HRqol, a study of 57 patients found 88% with pain at baseline; after 8 weeks of 4-layer compression therapy this fell to 60%.[41] Even more significantly, 78% of another sample, consisting of 185 patients, reported pain prior to entering a community leg ulcer clinic; after 12 weeks of 4-layer compression therapy this dropped to 22%.[45]

Financial impact

Time lost from work, missed career opportunities, decreased productivity on the job secondary to pain, early retirement, and loss of a job are just a few of the financial stressors affecting the HRqol of the patient with a wound. Too often, patients are faced with having to choose between compliance with medical management (such as keeping one's leg elevated or remaining nonweight bearing) and keeping their job. How does a truck driver, a cashier, or a health care professional keep his leg elevated and still perform his job? How do wound patients pay their mortgages, pay the bills, and feed their families? What happens when a wound patient loses his health care coverage after losing his job?

Beyond occupational stressors and dilemmas, patients may also incur additional out-of-pocket expenses for transportation, parking, and telephone bills for medical follow-up, home health aide services, dressing supplies not covered by insurance, and drug costs if they have no prescription plan. Those who have no insurance but don't qualify for public assistance may be forced to tap into their savings or refinance their homes. To illustrate this point, listen to the words of wives caring for their bedridden husbands with full-thickness pressure ulcers.

"...all these medical supplies you need to treat these bedsores. I think in the past 2 months, I've spent close to $300 out of my pocket and you're on a fixed income." ... "Thirty-five dollars per month for the hospital bed and $10 for the chair. I paid with our Social Security checks and his pension. Also there were bills and food...not much was left...He had a pension and I used to put that aside and we had to live on my Social Security which was $302."[46]

Additional expenses may also be incurred for home modifications such as wheelchair ramps.

Approaches to pain management

Krasner[35] offers the following recommendations to address pain management:

• Allow patients to remove their own dressings when possible.
• Allow patients to call "time out" during dressing changes.
• Develop standing protocols to address procedural pain (such as topical or local anesthetic agents prior to debridement) and pain medication prior to dressing changes.
• Provide adjunctive medication to improve sleep and reduce anxiety.
• Offer referrals to pain management specialists.
• Cover wound pain management in the health care professional curricula.

Additional recommendations include:
• Separate the patient from the wound.
• Assist patients and families in venting.[8]
• Explain procedures before performing them.
• Provide positive reinforcement.
• Discuss care options and give choices.
• Ask patients and caregivers if they have specific questions regarding the wound or its appearance.[23]
• Provide simple, concrete, truthful answers in a caring, reassuring manner.[23] When patients and families feel cared for, they cope better and can more easily adapt and make life changes.[26]
• Be aware of body language and the communication triangle.[12]
• Provide hope; reflection on even the slightest improvement offers a sense of hope and progress to patients and families dealing with chronic convalescence.[2,47] The simple act of sharing photos of wound care progress can be beneficial to patients and their caregivers.[26]

• Allow caregivers to stay during examinations and procedures if this is acceptable to the patient.
• Explain what has happened and what to expect with the wound.
• Discuss the prognosis for healing.
• If a worsening condition is expected, prepare the patient and family in a gentle, kind, and calm manner.
• Make referrals to comprehensive specialty wound care programs.
• Assist in accessing supplies and available resources.
• Recognize depression and make appropriate referrals.
• Advocate for the patient and family.
• Give permission for redirection to resume other activities.
• Reassure the caregiver that they aren't the cause of the patient's anger.[23]
• Avoid urgency toward patient and family acceptance of the wound; avoid unfair attacks on their self-protection.[23]

Ethical dilemmas in wound care

No other wound type is fraught with as much ethical dispute as pressure ulcers. Despite major technological breakthroughs in wound healing, the area of pressure ulceration continues to be the "scarlet letter of poor care."[9] Pressure ulcers are considered an individual and institutional embarrassment, a point of frustration, failure, and a marker of inferior care rendered. Great expense is incurred in "hiding the ulcer." As Moss and La Puma[48] state, "to hide ugly aesthetics and to unknowingly deny the conditions that contribute to pressure ulcer development, our clinical response may be to cover up or remove the sore, using dressings, skin grafts, myocutaneous flaps, disarticulations, amputations, and hemicorporectomies." But what right do we have as health care providers to make such decisions? What gives us the right to exhaust our patients' finances and subject them and their families to spending their lives undergoing aggressive procedures? Decisions for care, and the degree of aggressiveness or lack thereof, must be consistent with the patient's overall physiological status, as well as the patient's and family's "goals of restoration, of function, prolongation of life, or only provision of comfort."[49]

It's important to remember that HRqol is the *patient's* perception of well-being, not your opinion of his clinical status.[17] Acknowledging this, clinicians must partner with patients and their families in making short- and long-term treatment decisions regardless of wound etiology.

Issues and challenges for caregivers

The only prerequisite to becoming a caregiver to a family member with a wound is a willingness to take on the role. Most often, family members are untrained and unprepared for this role.[9] Along with the patient, family caregivers have to deal with their own varying levels of grief. Caregivers' grief work is further affected by the patient's overall status, the circumstance leading to the wounded state, and the patient's response to the wound.

Caregivers often experience feelings of helplessness compounded by guilt. They struggle with the increased stress and strain of family tension and receive the brunt of the patient's anger and frustration.[19] When no clear end-point to illness is seen, anger may then be displaced on health care providers.[19]

As the patient struggles with fears of burdening others, social isolation, loss of control and independence, possible disfigurement, and rejection, the caregiver also struggles. Fears commonly voiced by caregivers include damaging the wound from a lack of knowledge; development of new wounds; wound recurrence; need for amputation, rehospitalization, ER visits, or surgery; disfigurement; reaction of others; possible disability; and fear that the wound may never heal. Additional fears, related to performing dressing changes, include harming the wound or doing something wrong, causing pain, packing the wound improperly, and dealing with both their own and the patient's emotional conflicts.

A recurring fear among caregivers is that they themselves might become ill or disabled and unable to provide care.[9,19] Family caregivers are often dealing with disrupted sleep secondary to worrying about the patient and responding to the patient's restlessness.[9,19] A general lack of attention to their own health, progressive fatigue, decreased appetite, and decreased nutritional intake may occur as all attention is focused on the patient.[9,19]

Caregivers often find their social circle decreasing as they spend increased time providing care.[19] Even time taken for respite may be fraught with feelings of guilt. Emotionally, caregivers may experience deep feelings of fear and loss — fear of losing their loved one, fear of losing the relationship to death — as they witness a loved one's bedridden or increasingly debilitated state. Reminiscing about how things used to be may be all that some caregivers have to pull them through. Elderly caregiving spouses usually pursue nursing home placement only as a last resort, holding true to their vows of "till death do us part."[9]

Family caregivers also experience financial struggles owing to increased out-of-pocket expenses, decreased productivity in the workplace, unpaid days off due to used vacation and personal time, forced early retirement, and potential job loss.[19] Among elderly caregivers, frustration and confusion regarding reimbursement for needed wound care supplies and drugs and the inability to afford private help in the home are compounded by their meager funds from Social Security and pension checks.[19]

Summary

Having a wound or caring for a loved one with a wound can affect multiple facets of a patient's life, possibly unleashing unprecedented fears and vulnerabilities.

PRACTICE POINT

If we as health care professionals are to help our patients with wounds and their family caregivers, we need to "...stay connected with our patients; listen, attend ("be with") and comfort; and use a gentler hand."[24]

In each patient and family caregiver encounter, we as health care professionals should ask ourselves "Do we care enough about the patient's perspective to bear the costs involved to ensure that each person feels that they are being treated as a person?"[50] Do our actions show that we care? For it's caring that's quintessential to all that we do and all that we are.

Show what you know

1. Those afflicted with wounds are often viewed as:

A. pleasant and comfortable.
B. pain-free.
C. appalling and repulsive.
D. attractive.

ANSWER: C. Those with wounds are often viewed as appalling and repulsive.

2. Which of the following is one of the four domains of quality of life as identified by Schipper et al.[18]?

A. Pain-free
B. Financial freedom
C. Religious expression
D. Somatic sensation

ANSWER: D. In addition to physical and occupation function, psychological state, and social interaction, somatic sensation is identified as a domain of quality of life.

3. Wound assessment is commonly lacking in the area of:

A. size.
B. odor.
C. drainage.
D. pain.

ANSWER: D. Assessment of pain is commonly lacking in wound assessment; size, odor, and drainage are usually assessed.

4. Quality of life treatment decisions should be based on the:

A. patient's perception of well-being.
B. nurses' perceptions of well-being.
C. family's perception of well-being.
D. physicians' perceptions of well-being.

ANSWER: A. The patient's perceptions of well-being should direct quality of life treatment decisions.

5. Which one of the following strategies in caring for a patient with a wound would be LEAST effective?

A. Be aware of body language when communicating with the patient.
B. Explain what the aspects of the treatment plan will be.
C. Avoid telling the patient that the wound looks worse.
D. Provide simple, truthful answers to patient questions.

ANSWER: C. It's important to always tell the patient the truth. If the wound is deteriorating, the patient needs to be told in a gentle, compassionate way.

6. Krasner [35] recommends all of the following strategies to manage pain except:

A. allowing patients to remove their own dressings.
B. proceeding through dressing changes without breaks for the patient.
C. providing adjunctive medication to improve sleep and reduce anxiety.
D. offering referrals to pain management specialists.

ANSWER: B. The patient should always have the opportunity to call "time out" and take a break during dressing changes.

References

1. van Rijswijk, L., and Gottlieb, D. "Like a Terrorist," *Ostomy/Wound Management* 46(5):25-26, May 2000.
2. Neil, J.A., and Munjas, B.A. "Living with a Chronic Wound: The Voices of Sufferers," *Ostomy/Wound Management* 46(5):28-38, May 2000.
3. Harding, K. "Complete Patient Care," *Journal of Wound Care* 4(6):253, June 1995.
4. Hyland, M.E., et al. "Quality of Life of Leg Ulcer Patients: Questionnaire and Preliminary Findings," *Journal of Wound Care* 3(6):294-298, June 1994.
5. van Rijswijk, L. "The Language of Wounds," in *Chronic Wound Care: A Clinical Sourcebook for Health Care Professionals,* 3rd ed. Edited by Krasner, D.L., et al. Wayne, Pa.: HMP Communications, 2001.
6. Anderson, R.C., and Maksud, D.P. "Psychological Adjustments to Reconstructive Surgery," *Nursing Clinics of North America* 29(4):711-24, December 1994.
7. Faugier, J. "On Being Wounded," *Senior Nurse* 8(1):18, January 1988.
8. Hopkins, S. "Psychological Aspect of Wound Healing," *Nursing Times Plus* 97(48):57-58, 2001.
9. Baharestani, M.M. "The Lived Experience of Wives Caring for their Frail, Homebound, Elderly Husbands with Pressure Ulcers," *Advances in Wound Care* 7(3):40-52, May 1994.
10. Knudson-Cooper, M. "Adjustment to Visible Stigma: The Case of the Severely Burned," *Social Science Medicine* 15B:31, 1981.
11. Wallace, L., and Lees, J. "A Psychological Follow-up Study of Adult Patients Discharged from a British Burns Unit," *Burns* 14:39, 1988.
12. Partridge, J. "The Psychological Effects of Facial Disfigurement," *Journal of Wound Care* 2:168-71, May 1993.
13. Bernstein, N. *Emotional Care of the Facially Disfigured.* Boston: Little, Brown & Co., 1976.
14. Campbell, A., et al. *The Quality of American Life: Perceptions, Evaluations and Satisfaction.* New York: Russell Sage, 1976.
15. Price, P. "Quality of Life," in *Chronic Wound Care: A Clinical Source Book for Health Care Professionals,* 3rd ed. Edited by Krasner, D.L., et al. Wayne, Pa.: HMP Communications, 2001.
16. Price, P. "Defining and Measuring Quality of Life," *Journal of Wound Care* 5(3):139-40, March 1996.
17. Franks, P.J., and Moffatt, C.J. "Quality of Life Issues in Patients with Chronic Wounds," *Wounds* 10(suppl E):1E-11E, September-October 1998.
18. Schipper, H., et al. "Quality of Life Studies: Definitions and Conceptual Issues," in *Quality of life and Pharmacoeconomics in Clinical Trials,* 2nd ed. Edited by Spilker, B. Philadelphia: Lippincott-Raven, 1996.

19. Brod, M. "Quality of Life Issues in Patients with Diabetes and Lower Extremity Ulcers: Patients and Caregivers," *Quality of Life Research* 7(4):365-72, May 1998.

20. Phillips, T., et al. "A Study of the Impact of Leg Ulcers on Quality of Life: Financial, Social and Psychological Implications," *Journal of American Academy of Dermatology* 31(1):49-53, July 1994.

21. Walshe, C. "Living with a Venous Leg Ulcer: A Descriptive Study of Patients' Experiences," *Journal of Advanced Nursing* 22(6):1092-100, December 1995.

22. Roe, B., et al. "Patient's Perceptions of Chronic Leg Ulcers," in *Leg Ulcers: Nursing Management: A Research Based Guide*. Edited by Cullum, N., and Roe, B. Harrow, U.K.: Scutari Press, 1995.

23. Magnan, M.A. "Psychological Considerations for Patients with Acute Wounds," *Critical Care Nursing Clinics of North America* 8(2):183-93, June 1996.

24. Krasner, D. "Using a Gentler Hand: Reflections on Patients with Pressure Ulcers who Experience Pain," *Ostomy/Wound Management* 42(3):20-29, April 1996.

25. Langemo, D.K., et al. "The Lived Experience of Having a Pressure Ulcer: A Qualitative Analysis," *Advances in Skin & Wound Care* 13(5):225-35, September/October 2000.

26. Krasner, D. "Painful Venous Ulcers: Themes and Stories about their Impact on Quality of Life," *Ostomy/Wound Management* 44(9):38-49, September 1998.

27. Wientjes, K.A. "Mind-body Techniques in Wound Healing," *Ostomy/Wound Management* 48(11):62-67, November 2002.

28. Myss, C. *Why People Don't Heal and How They Can*. New York: Three Rivers Press, 1997.

29. Parsons, T. "The Sick Role and the Role of the Physician Reconsidered," *MMFQ/ Health & Society* 53(3):257-78, Summer 1975.

30. O'Flynn, L. "The Impact of Minor Acute Wounds on Quality of Life," *Journal of Wound Care* 9(7):337-40, July 2000.

31. Schnaper, N. "The Psychological Implications of Severe Trauma: Emotional Sequelae to Unconsciousness," *Journal of Trauma* 15(2):94-98, February 1975.

32. Lenehan, G.P. "Emotional Impact of Trauma," *Nursing Clinics of North America* 21(4):729-40, December 1986.

33. Price, P., and Harding, K. "Measuring Health-related Quality of Life in Patients with Chronic Leg Ulcers," *Wounds* 8(3):91-94, May-June 1996.

34. Dewar, A.L., and Morse, J.M. "Unbearable Incidents: Failure to Endure the Experience of Illness," *Journal of Advanced Nursing* 22(5):957-64, November 1995.

35. Krasner, D. "Painful Venous Ulcers: Themes and Stories about Living with the Pain and Suffering," *Journal of Wound, Ostomy, and Continence Nursing* 25(3):158-68, May 1998.

36. Franks, P.J., and Moffatt, C.J. "Who Suffers Most from Leg Ulceration?" *Journal of Wound Care* 7(8):383-85, September 1998.

37. Lindholm, C., et al. "Quality of Life in Chronic Leg Ulcer Patients," *Acta Dermato-Venereologica* 73(6):440-43, December 1993.

38. Dallam, L, et al. "Pressure Ulcer Pain: Assessment and Quantification," *Journal of Wound, Ostomy, and Continence Nursing* 22(5):211-18, September 1995.

39. Hamer, C., and Cullum, N.A. "Patients' Perceptions of Chronic Leg Ulcers," *Journal of Wound Care* 3(2):99-101, February 1994.

40. Hofman, D., et al. "Pain in Venous Ulcers," *Journal of Wound Care* 6(5):222-24, May 1997.

41. Liew, I.H., et al. "Do Leg Ulcer Clinics Improve Patients' Quality of Life?" *Journal of Wound Care* 9(9):423-26, October 2000.

42. Roe, B.H., et al. "Assessment, Prevention and Treatment of Chronic Leg Ulcers in the Community: Report of a Survey," *Journal of Clinical Nursing* 2(5):299-306, September 1993.

43. Szor, J.K., and Bourguignon, C. "Description of Pressure Ulcer Pain at Rest and at Dressing Change," *Journal of Wound, Ostomy, and Continence Nursing* 26(3):115-20, May 1999.

44. Hollinworth, H. "Nurses' Assessment and Management of Pain at Wound Dressing Changes," *Journal of Wound Care* 4(2):77-83, February 1995.

45. Franks, P.J., et al. "Community Leg Ulcer Clinics: Effects on Quality of Life," *Phlebology* 9:83-86, 1994.

46. Baharestani, M.M. "The Lived Experience of Wives Caring for their Homebound Elderly Husbands with Pressure Ulcers: A Phenomenological Investigation" (doctoral dissertation, Adelphi University, 1993). Dissertation Abstracts International (No. 9416018), 1993.

47. Benner, P., and Wrubel, J. *The Primacy of Caring: Stress and Coping in Health and Illness.* Menlo Park, Calif.: Addison-Wesley-Longman Publishing Co., 1989.

48. Moss, R.J., and La Puma, J. "The Ethics of Pressure Sore Prevention and Treatment in the Elderly: A Practical Approach," *Journal of the American Geriatric Society* 39(9):905-08, September 1991.

49. La Puma, J. "The Ethics of Pressure Ulcers," *Decubitus* 4(2):43-44, May 1991.

50. Price, P. "Health-related Quality of Life and the Patient's Perspective," *Journal of Wound Care* 7(7):365-66, July 1998.

CHAPTER 2

Legal aspects of wound care

Steven P. Knowlton, JD, RN

OBJECTIVES

After completing this chapter, you'll be able to:

- identify and describe the major litigation players and their roles in a lawsuit

- identify and define the four elements of a malpractice claim

- describe the general rules for proper charting

- identify and describe the ways the medical record can be used in a malpractice case

- identify and describe the ways a standard or guideline can be used in a malpractice case

- define negligence *per se*.

The current climate

In recent years, the concept of patients as "consumers of health care" has risen to the forefront. Rather than blindly trusting clinicians, the consumer-patients of today, better educated and more aware of health care issues, are more willing to make use of legal resources when treatment goes awry. Although wound care generates no more litigation than many areas of health care practice, and arguably less than some others, the threat of litigation affects the way clinicians approach the delivery of care.

Clinicians need to protect themselves while ensuring evidence-based, high-quality care to their consumer-patients. This chapter sets forth basic legal principles and suggests practice strategies that protect clinicians *and* advance patient care.

Litigation

Over the course of human history, it became apparent that some nonviolent means of settling disputes must be developed. The law and the legal process, including litigation, were and continue to be one of civilized society's experiments at achieving nonviolent resolutions to disputes. The success of this experiment is itself the source of much dispute, to which no resolution (nonviolent or otherwise) is currently in sight.

Contrary to television and movie portrayals, real-life litigation process is arduous and time-consuming. While television and movie lawsuits resolve in a matter of weeks or months, usually ending with a dramatic trial resulting in a stunning jury verdict, most real-life cases take years to get through the system. In some jurisdictions with crowded dockets, matters can take as long as 4 or 5 years to resolve. Those that require appeals can take considerably more time before all issues are finally put to rest. Trials (dramatic or not) are few and far between, as nearly all lawsuits are settled before trial. When trials do happen, they're usually slow-moving, uninteresting affairs that tax the patience and attention of jurors. Litigants expecting "Perry Mason" moments from their attorneys are sure to be disappointed and, as anyone who has ever served jury duty knows, closing arguments by attorneys are never, ever over in the five minutes before the final commercial.

Despite the difficulties and drawbacks, the litigation process does afford citizens an impartial forum for dispute resolution grounded in the law. And the law, as Plato has said, is "a pledge that citizens of a state will do justice to one another."

The discussion in this chapter is limited to *civil litigation;* that is, litigation in which citizens have a dispute with each other — rather than *criminal litigation,* in which the state or a government seeks to prosecute a party for the violation of law. There are significant differences between the two forms of litigation (standards of proof, for example). The remedy sought in civil litigation is monetary damages. In contrast, only the prosecuting state or government may seek to deprive the alleged lawbreaker of his liberty by incarceration.

How is a medical malpractice lawsuit born?

Litigation begins the moment a person believes he has been wronged by another and seeks the advice and counsel of an attorney in an effort to "right the wrong" or "get justice." During the initial interview between the prospective client and the attorney, the attorney makes a number of preliminary judgments usually based almost solely on the client's presentation:

• Is this the type of case the attorney is capable of handling? Does it fall within his expertise and practice experience? Does the attorney have the time to handle the matter?
• Is the client's story credible?
• Will the client make a good witness?
• Are the damages, if proven, sufficient to warrant entering into the litigation process?
• Is there a party responsible (liable) for the client's injuries?
• How likely is it that both liability and damages can be proven?
• Are there any glaring problems or difficulties with the case?

If the answers to these questions are satisfactory and the client wishes to retain the attorney, a lawsuit has then been conceived.

Before filing the legal papers that start the litigation process in a medical malpractice case, most attorneys perform an intensive investigation in order to definitively answer questions concerning liability and damages. Medical records and other information must be obtained and examined by an expert to determine whether a malpractice claim can be made, information related to the identities of potential defendants must be analyzed, and strategic legal issues related to jurisdiction (which court can the case be brought in) must be thought through. If

Players in the litigation process

The litigation process is initiated and enacted by people with a dispute to resolve and those whose task is to aid in resolving that dispute.

The parties

The principal parties involved in litigation are the litigants—the individuals on either side of the dispute. The *plaintiff* is the person who initiates the lawsuit and who claims he has suffered injury due to the actions of another. A lawsuit may be filed by multiple plaintiffs.

The plaintiff sues the defendant—the person or organization alleged to have injured the plaintiff by his or its actions. In most cases the parties are individuals, but parties can be corporations, companies, partnerships, government agencies or, in some cases, governments themselves.

The judge

The judge is an individual, usually an attorney, who has been appointed or elected to oversee lawsuits on behalf of the state or government under whose jurisdiction the lawsuit is brought. The judge acts as referee during the pretrial phase of the case and decides legal issues that arise as the lawsuit progresses toward trial. In a trial, the judge's responsibility is *to interpret the law*.

The jury

The *jury* is a panel of citizens chosen by the attorneys for the litigants to hear evidence in the case and render a decision or verdict. The jury's responsibility is *to determine the facts* in a trial. It's up to the jury to decide whether the plaintiff and his attorney proved their case, thereby rendering a decision about the defendant's liability and the amount of damages the defendant should pay to the plaintiff.

---

after this investigation the attorney still believes the case has merit, legal papers starting the actual lawsuit will be filed, and a lawsuit will be born. (See *Players in the litigation process*.)

The pretrial litigation process

The pretrial litigation process consists of several steps: complaint and answer, discovery, and motion practice.

Complaint and answer

The initial legal paper that gives rise to a lawsuit is called the *complaint*. While procedural requirements vary between jurisdictions, generally the complaint is a paper that sets out the claims made by the plaintiff against the defendant, sets forth the basis of the jurisdiction of the court, sets out the legal theories under which the plaintiff is making the claims, and in some jurisdictions, may set forth the amount of damages claimed.

The defendant must then file an *answer* within the permitted time that responds on a count-by-count basis to the plaintiff's complaint and which, depending again on jurisdictional rules, may also include claims against the plaintiff. These two basic *pleadings* initiate the formal lawsuit.

Discovery

Discovery is the process by which the parties find out the facts about each other, and about the incidents that have given rise to the claims of malpractice alleged by the plaintiff, and the defenses to those claims asserted by the defendant. In order to obtain discovery, the law has provided discovery devices — procedural mechanisms by which the parties ask for and receive information. Demands are routinely made for documents and other tangible items related to the claims in the lawsuit, statements made by the parties to others, and witnesses to the incidents. Pretrial testimony (*deposition*) is taken of the parties to the lawsuit. This testimony, while out of court, is sworn testimony transcribed by a certified court reporter and can be used for any purpose in the lawsuit, including for purposes of *impeachment* — the demonstrating of prior untruthful or inaccurate testimony, or a challenge to the credibility of a witness — at trial.

Finally, *expert discovery* — information about the opinions of experts retained by the parties — is usually permitted in this phase of the proceedings. Experts are individuals accepted by the Court to assist the finder of fact — the jury — in understanding issues that commonly fall outside of the experience of the typical juror. In medical malpractice cases, as we will see later, the plaintiff must prove that there was a deviation from the standard of care that resulted in an injury. Expert testimony related to the field of medicine, treatments, and standard of care at issue in the case is usually essential to successfully meet proof requirements for each element of a malpractice claim brought by a plaintiff. Likewise, the defense of such claims nearly always mandates opposing expert testimony — in essence, an explanation by a credentialed individual supporting the actions taken by the defendant from which the claim of malpractice stems.

Motion practice

Disputes over discovery often arise in the context of a lawsuit and those disputes that can't be resolved by the parties require court intervention. Formal resolution of these disputes usually requires an application to the court — a *motion* — setting forth the dispute and the position of the party making the application (the moving party, or *movant*) and requesting certain *relief* or results to be *ordered* by the court. Naturally, this requires a response from the other party — the *opposition* — that sets out the reasons why the court shouldn't grant the relief requested.

Some motions can be decided by the court *on the papers*, that is, without a formal oral presentation (*oral argument*) by the parties before the judge is assigned. More complicated motions, especially those seeking to eliminate or modify legal claims, almost always require argument before the presiding judge or court.

The trial

While the vast majority of lawsuits settle sometime before trial ("out-of-court settlements"), some cases do proceed to trial. Medical malpractice trials are almost without exception jury trials. Once it's determined that settlement isn't an option, a trial date is set and the attorneys begin to prepare for the trial. In federal jurisdictions and many state courts, litigants are required to prepare pretrial statements and submissions. They also disclose exhibit lists (materials and documents the attorneys anticipate they will use at trial). Furthermore, they designate deposition testimony to be read or, if the testimony was videotaped, to be shown at trial. The pretrial submission and disclosure process helps to ensure that the trial is as fair as possible and eliminates the possibility of "trial by ambush" — thus, the "Perry Mason" moments of television and movie renown are relatively few and far between.

On the day of the trial, the attorneys for the parties proceed with jury selection. Each attorney tries to select jurors that he believes will decide in favor of (*find for*) his client. (See *How attorneys select jurors.*) Procedurally, the jury selection process varies widely by jurisdiction. In some courts, the trial judge will take an active role by questioning the jurors. The fight over selection is then left to the attorneys. Other jurisdictions permit the attorneys to question jurors directly without court supervision and the trial judge becomes involved only when a dispute arises. As you can imagine, jury selection in a jurisdiction with strong judicial control is a much briefer process than in those jurisdictions where the attorneys are left to their own devices. No matter what the individual procedure, once the jury is chosen (*empanelled*), the trial begins.

At trial, the parties each give opening statements, one of the two times in the entire trial that the attorneys are permitted to speak directly to the jurors. After opening statements, the plaintiff's attorney states the plaintiff's case. Because the burden of proof is on the plaintiff, the plaintiff's attorney goes first. After the plaintiff's direct case is finished, the plaintiff "rests," and the defendant's attorney presents the defendant's case. The *direct case* consists of factual testimony from witnesses (the plaintiff and others) as well as expert testimony, deposition testimony, and demonstrative evidence such as charts, medical records, graphs, photographs, and drawings.

The opposing party has the right to cross-examine each witness after the direct examination, and then redirect examination and recross-examination may follow as necessary. After all the evidence has been presented by both sides, the parties make closing statements—

How attorneys select jurors

Volumes have been written on the art and science of jury selection. Litigation-support service firms run countless seminars each year on how to pick jurors, and jury consultants—individuals with backgrounds in psychology, sociology, and other human sciences—provide their services at substantial fees to lawyers. Each attorney has his own methods and beliefs about selecting jurors. All methods require the attorneys to elicit information from the prospective jurors to gain insight into how a juror thinks, what he thinks about the case, and how likely he is to find in favor of the attorney's client.

the closing statement (*summation*) being the last time the attorneys are permitted to speak directly to the jurors.

Once summations are completed, the judge then instructs the jurors on the appropriate law that they're to apply to the facts of the case. Remember that the jury is the *finder of fact*—it determines what happened, when it happened, who did it, where it happened, and how it happened—and the judge is the *interpreter of the law*. After the jurors receive the judge's instructions, they leave the courtroom and begin deliberations.

Every trial attorney hopes to be lucky enough to serve on a jury that goes to deliberations. For trial lawyers, understanding what happens inside the jury room during deliberations is the holy grail of trial practice. In jurisdictions that permit attorneys to interview jurors after verdict, attorneys often spend many hours with the jurors who are willing to discuss the case in order to determine what did — and what didn't — work during the trial. It's often surprising to find that what the lawyer thought was of prime importance wasn't so important to the jury. The jury room in our system of jurisprudence is sacrosanct, but no matter how it happens, the jury will eventually arrive at a verdict that will be delivered to the parties in open court. Once the verdict is read and the jury excused, the trial is over.

Appeals

Each jurisdiction has an appellate process that the litigants may avail themselves of. Depending on the jurisdiction, appeals may add years (and many dollars) to the resolution of claims and lawsuits.

Legal elements of a malpractice claim

A medical malpractice claim is made up of four distinct elements, each of which must be proven to the applicable standard of proof in the jurisdiction in which the case is brought. The usual standard of proof for civil cases is a *preponderance of the evidence*. The preponderance standard is best described by thinking of scales representing the plaintiff on one side and the defendant on the other, evenly balanced at the start. In a trial, the one who wins is the one whose scale dips lower at the end. In other words, in order to prevail, plaintiffs need to show by only 50.0000001% — just a bit more than one-half — that they've proven each of the elements that make up a malpractice claim.

The four general elements that make up the claim are:
• existence of a duty owed to the plaintiff by the defendant
• breach of that duty

• injury that's causally related to that breach of duty
• damages recognized as law.

Duty

In general, there's no duty to protect a person endangered by the actions or omissions of another if there's no special relationship between the two persons. The patient-physician relationship is the basis for the claim of duty between the plaintiff-patient and the defendant-health care professional in medical malpractice cases since that relationship permits the patient to rely upon the physician's knowledge, expertise, and skill in treatment. Thus, the allegations of medical negligence arise within the course of that professional relationship. Translating that definition into health care terms, some examples of a duty may be the obligation of a health care practitioner to give patients care that's:
• consistent with level of experience, education, and training
• permitted under the applicable state practice act
• permitted or authorized under the policies and procedures of the institution that are applicable to the position.

 PRACTICE POINT

Duty: In negligence cases, *duty* may be defined as obligation, to which the law will give recognition and effect, to conform to particular standard of conduct toward another. The word *duty* is used throughout the Restatement of Torts to denote the fact that the actor is required to conduct himself in a particular manner at the risk that if he doesn't do so, he becomes subject to liability to another to whom the duty is owed for any injury sustained by such other, of which that actor's conduct is a legal cause. (Restatement, Second, Torts, Section 4.[1])

Breach of duty

In addition to proving the existence of a duty, the plaintiff must also prove the defendant breached that duty. Breach of duty can be by either commission, omission, or both. Most often, to establish this element of the claim, the plaintiff in a medical malpractice case must also show that the defendant health care practitioner deviated from an accepted standard of care or treatment. The practitioner isn't required to provide the highest degree of care, but only the level and type of care rendered by the average practitioner. What the standard of care is, and whether and how it was deviated from, must be established for the jury, and this is most often the province of expert testimony.

Breach of duty in the health care setting may be illustrated in the following ways:
- the failure to give care within the applicable practice act
- the failure to perform professional duties with the degree of skill mandated by the applicable practice act
- the failure to provide care for which the circumstance of the patient's condition warrants.

PRACTICE POINT

Breach: The failure to meet an obligation to another person that's owed to that person; the breaking or violating of a law, right, obligation, engagement, or duty by either commission, omission, or both.[1]

Injury causally related to a breach of duty

Proximate cause: In a medical malpractice case, proof of an injury isn't enough unless that injury can be causally linked to a breach of duty by a health care practitioner. That breach of duty is then considered the proximate cause. Without the breach of duty, the injury wouldn't

---

Proving proximate cause

While standards of proof related to proximate cause may vary among jurisdictions, one of two questions is almost always used to determine this issue:
- Was the health care practitioner's negligent conduct a "substantial factor" in causing the injury?
- Would the injury not have happened if the health care practitioner hadn't been negligent?

---

have occurred. (See *Proving proximate cause*.)

PRACTICE POINT

Proximate cause: That which, in a natural and continuous sequence, unbroken by any efficient intervening cause, produces injury, and without which the result wouldn't have occurred and without which the accident couldn't have happened, if the injury be one which might be reasonable anticipated or foreseen as a natural consequence of the wrongful act.[1]

Proximate cause in the health care setting can be illustrated by the following examples:
- fractured hip due to a fall because of failure to raise the siderails of the bed
- decreased total protein due to failure to provide nutrition (either failure to provide actual nourishment or failure to call consult)
- osteomyelitis resulting in limb amputation for failure to call infectious disease consult and provide antibiotic therapy.

Damages

A health care practitioner may be held liable for damages when the jury finds that the practitioner deviated from the applicable standard of care in treating the plaintiff-patient and as a result, caused injury resulting in legally recognized damages. In most jurisdictions, a plaintiff may recover for proven monetary losses (lost wages and unreimbursed medical expenses) and for pain and suffering that result from the injury proven. As noted above, it's the jury — the finder of fact — that sets the monetary award to the plaintiff.

PRACTICE POINT

Damage: Loss, injury, or deterioration caused by the negligence, design, or accident of one person or another, in respect of the latter's person or property.

Damages: A pecuniary compensation or indemnity, which may be recovered in the courts by any person who has suffered loss, detriment, or injury, whether to his person, property, or rights, through the unlawful act or omission or negligence of another.[1]

As we have shown, in order for a plaintiff to prevail in a medical malpractice claim they must satisfy all four of the elements discussed above. Three of four won't do. They must score perfectly on all four to prevail before a jury.

The medical record in litigation

The medical record is arguably the single most important piece of evidence in a medical malpractice case. It's also a crucial tool for the delivery of science-based care. It's:

- a legal document
- a communication tool
- the supporting basis for treatment decisions and modifications
- one of the primary tools for the evaluation of treatment modalities.

At one time or another in the education of a health care practitioner, whatever the specialty or discipline, the following directive is taught: "If it wasn't written down, it didn't happen." Nowhere does this ring more true than in a medical malpractice case, as we shall see. But before we consider the role documentation plays in the medical-legal world, let's consider for a moment just how important the medical record is in the care and treatment of patients.

Communication tool

The medical record is the primary method of communication between members of the health care team. Oral report and rounding are essential communication devices, but it's impractical and unrealistic to expect that every member of the health care team be present during report or rounds. Such disciplines as physical therapy, occupational therapy, and respiratory therapy are rarely present for report or rounds. The myriad of medical specialists available to the primary physician (infectious disease consultants, for example) are also rarely present during rounds, yet it's imperative for the delivery of good science-based care that every member of the health care team have the most current and up-to-date information related to the patient. The medical record is the only way to accomplish this. It's available 24 hours per day to any practitioner who can utilize it to stay informed about the patient's progress.

PRACTICE POINT
General documentation guidelines

Listed below are some general rules for documentation that serves your patient's needs and can help in the defense of a lawsuit.

- Be thorough — record the date and time for each entry.
- Be accurate — use units of measure instead of estimates (for example, "patient had a 6-oz cup of ice chips" instead of "patient had some ice chips."
- Be factual — think of yourself as a newspaper reporter and answer the following questions: who, what, when, where, and why.
- Be objective — record only the facts. Remember that you're communicating information that others will rely on. If your patient is to benefit from your professional training, judgment, and observational skills, your colleagues must have objective, factual information to rely on.

- Write legibly — print if necessary.
- Use approved abbreviations.
- Make contemporaneous entries — finish your documentation before you leave work for the day. Don't add notations days later unless your facility permits such additions — and even then, adhere strictly to your facility's policy governing such additions.
- Be truthful — don't fake, misrepresent, exaggerate, or misstate the facts in the medical record.
- Most importantly, don't assign blame. While it's important to relate the facts completely and accurately, assigning blame in the medical record is fodder for malpractice actions and does nothing to advance the care of your patients.

Treatment evaluation and support

Documentation of patient outcomes and responses to treatments in the medical record is a key method for evaluating treatment modalities and therapies. The typical patient with pressure ulcers will undergo an extended course of treatment that will change and be modified over the course of time. In order to establish a basis for treatments and modifications, there must be well-documented observations and evaluations of the patient. Upon initiation of treatment, careful observation and documentation of the patient's condition is critical in order to establish both a baseline to measure treatment against and to establish the basis for the initial treatment and care. Without a carefully documented record, treatment,

evaluation, patient outcomes, and treatment modifications are impossible to justify — in court or at the bedside.

PRACTICE POINT

Accurate and complete patient outcomes and responses to treatment and care must be documented in the record, as they're the basis for care decisions and legal defense.

What's good documentation?

While there's no one true answer to this question, there are concepts that can be generally applied to the issue of charting and documentation. (See *General documentation guidelines*.)

Red flags in documentation

Certain elements in a medical record can serve as red flags that catch the attention of the plaintiff's attorney. When documenting information about the patient with a wound, try to avoid the following errors.

Things that don't add up

Make sure the information you're documenting is as accurate as possible. Questions may be raised if the assessment findings don't logically support the resulting diagnosis. The list below shows assessment findings that were documented for a patient with a stage III pressure ulcer on his coccyx; note that they don't lead one to believe that a stage III pressure ulcer should have developed.

- Braden score = 17 (mild risk)
- Ambulates well
- Bed-to-chair transfer with assistance
- Continent when on a toileting schedule
- Fair appetite
- Medical diagnoses: diet-controlled diabetes, hypertension, arthritis, benign prostatic hyperplasia

Things that are too good to be true

The second entry in the sample chart below shows a dramatic, yet highly unlikely, improvement in the patient's ulcer, especially considering his rapid decompensation 5 days later. Describe wounds as accurately as possible. Read the previous notes so that you can precisely chart how the wound is progressing.

6/5/03 *Stage IV pressure ulcer to sacrum, 6 × 7 cm, 3 cm deep, 4 cm tunneling at 8 o'clock, 65% necrotic tissue in base, foul-smelling gray drainage, alginate dressing QOD.*

6/9/03 *Sacrum ulcer improved, 2 × 2 × 1 cm, 100% granulation tissue, minimal serous drainage.*

6/14/03 *Unresponsive, BP 60/40, HR 156, Temp 102.4°F, MD called, Sent to ER.*

Inconsistencies within the record

Documentation within the medical record should provide a consistent picture of the patient. As the example below illustrates, three different forms in the record give three different pictures of the patient. Which is a jury to believe?

Monthly summary: *Skin remains intact. Turned Q 2 hours while in bed. Up in chair for 1 hour Q day. Eating 75% to 100% of meals. Fed by staff. Hydration maintained.*

Flow sheets: *Turned every 4 to 6 hours. Eating 25% of meals. 7-lb weight loss in last month. Intake 500 to 700 cc per 24 hours.*

Nurse's notes: *Stage III ulcer on coccyx. Hydrocolloid intact. In chair 0900 to 1500 daily.*

Courtesy of J. Cuddigan, PHD, RN, CWCN

Health care practitioners must be intimately familiar with the policy and procedures related to documentation in the facility in which they work and must follow them. This is to ensure that colleagues will be able to utilize notations to their best advantage in making treatment decisions. A well-documented entry in a medical record that follows facility guidelines shows care and professionalism — key aspects in the defense of a medical malpractice action. (See *Red flags in documentation.*)

Completeness and thoroughness are absolutely essential components of good charting and documentation. In order for the medical record to be used as a health care tool, all pertinent and relevant information must be included. In order for the medical record to be a defensive aid in a malpractice action, it must be absolutely complete. In the usual course, a facility's risk management department will get notice of a filed lawsuit and a chart review will begin. Often, the staff involved in the plaintiff's care will be interviewed to determine whether any additional information can be gleaned from them. More likely than not, the staff who treated the plaintiff will have little or no independent memory or recollection of the plaintiff, the specific days, or shifts at issue in the suit. This isn't surprising or of concern; most lawsuits are filed years after the incident in question. During the intervening time, a health care professional could have cared for hundreds of other patients. A complete, thorough medical record thus serves the important defense task of acting to refresh the memory of those who treated the plaintiff. If the record is complete, an individual can make notes to assist in remembering the facts of the treatment in order to be able to testify at either deposition or trial. Incomplete charting precludes this. (See *Effects of incomplete charting.*)

A well-documented, complete, and thorough medical record is first and foremost a critical tool for the delivery of good science-based care. It's secondarily a tool for preparing defense witnesses (refreshing memory) and a support for treatment modalities. At its worst, a poorly documented, incomplete chart is a potent weapon for the attorney bringing a claim.

Standards of care and practice guidelines in litigation

Like the medical record, standards of care, practice guidelines, state practice acts governing the various professional health care specialties, and facility poli-

---

Effects of incomplete charting

What happens when charting is incomplete? In addition to providing a poor record of the facts of a patient's care to jog the practitioner's memory in case of a lawsuit, it can create other problems. Competent attorneys can create havoc when gaps exist in the record. Nothing makes proving the plaintiff's case easier than such gaps, especially near or around the time of the alleged malpractice if the claim revolves around a single incident. If the claim concerns a continuous or extended course of treatment, the absence of documentation related to treatment outcomes, observations, and the basis for the treatment is strong evidence of negligence. Where the record contains gaps, you can be certain that the plaintiff's attorney will be happy to suggest to a jury what happened during those times, and those suggestions won't be of benefit to the health care facility or the individual practitioner.

---

cies and procedures play a role in both the delivery of care and litigation related to allegations of practitioner negligence. And like the medical record, they can be either sword or shield, yield benefit or be a detriment.

Standards of care and practice guidelines set out what the reasonably prudent health care provider would do in the same or similar situation. Nursing staff is held to standards that relate to nursing. Other health care providers are held to the clinical standards of those who have the same education, training, and experience. Any health care practitioner can be held to standards of care or practice guidelines developed at the national, state, local, or institutional level.

It's axiomatic that standards of care and practice guidelines that are based on validated scientific principles and reviewed and updated regularly are valuable tools in the delivery of good health care. Such guidelines provide a template for the delivery of care, permit the evaluation of treatment modalities, provide for the observation, recording, and analysis of patient outcomes, and act as a foundation for research.

State practice acts are laws that regulate the activities of health care professionals and others and define and limit the practice of such people. The laws are an effort by state legislatures to standardize the scope of the various professions and licensure in an effort to ensure that practitioners meet minimum educational requirements. Violation of these laws may result in sanction, license suspension, or license revocation.

Facility policies and procedures, while often incorporating practice guidelines and standards of care stand on their own in importance — especially as they govern documentation, chain-of-command issues, and reporting requirements. Taken together, when each category of these documents are thoughtfully drafted, regularly evaluated, modified as needed, and rigorously followed, they act in concert to assist both health care institution and individual provider to give the best, science-based care possible.

PRACTICE POINT

Annually review (date and sign) and revise if necessary all policies and procedures based on current evidence.

In litigation, each of these documents can be used to support a patient's claim of malpractice or defend against such a claim. If an attorney wishes to utilize one or more of these documents, he can ask the court (judge) to take "judicial notice" of these documents. The practical legal effect of the granting of such a request is that the document so recognized becomes, in legal terms, "the law of the case." This is important because a proven violation of the contents of the document (for example a standard of care or practice guideline) can result in an instruction to the jury that such violation is evidence of negligence *per se* or "by itself." This is a valuable "short cut" for the attorney bringing the claim. A brief discussion of the uses of each follows.

Standards of care and practice guidelines

As mentioned earlier, the attorney bringing a malpractice claim must show that there was a deviation in the standard of care and that deviation caused the injury alleged. Expert testimony is the primary tool in showing a deviation from the standard, but just as effective is showing the jury that a health care practitioner deviated from a written standard of care or practice guideline developed and utilized by the institution at which the health care provider practices. Any attorney bringing a claim will request copies of the applicable standards of care related to the treatment or conditions at issue in the case. If the institution has none, generally accepted standards will apply and the litigation experts of both parties will testify concerning this. If the standards do exist, the plaintiff's attorney will generally perform an analysis (with the assistance of an expert) in order to determine:

• whether the defendants had violated the standards or guidelines
• whether the guidelines themselves sufficiently reflect science and research based methods of care — in other words, whether the standards or guidelines reflect good care.

A positive response to the first or a negative response to the second will advance the plaintiff's claims and naturally, the reverse will bolster the defense. Any standard or guideline used by a facility or health care provider must reflect care that's science- and research-based, and should be regularly reviewed for sufficiency, especially in the face of new or advancing research. Thus, standards and guidelines can cut both ways.

State practice acts

A violation of a state practice act isn't only a serious offense that can lead to license suspension, revocation, or censure, it's also evidence or negligence *per se* that may likely result in a jury instruction to that effect, or may even cause the judge to grant a finding of liability against the defendant responsible for such a violation. When a judge takes the very unusual step of making a finding of liability, the trial proceeds with only the question of damages (how much should be awarded) going to the jury. Such a ruling is devastating to the defendant's case.

Facility policies and procedures

Each practitioner should know exactly where the facility policy and procedure manual referable to their practice area, unit, or group is located and what it contains. This reference tool must be available to all. As with standards and guidelines, policies and procedures should be regularly reviewed and amended as necessary. Additionally, any changes should be brought to the attention of personnel via memorandum or notice; staff training programs should be considered for new procedures if required. A violation or deviation from policies and procedures if proven can serve the plaintiff's attorney in a number of ways—it can challenge the credibility of the defendant by reflecting either ignorance of the policy or outright disre-

gard for it. If the deviation was the cause of the injury, it can also serve as evidence of negligence.

Legal outcomes of wound care cases

To place this chapter in context, short descriptions of a small number of wound care cases that have gone through the trial process follow.

Texas, April 25, 2002

While at a senior living center, the plaintiff, a 71-year-old man, developed a pressure ulcer that became infected with an antibiotic-resistant organism. He developed osteomyelitis and subsequently fatal pneumonia. Allegations against the nursing home included failure to treat the ulcer for 19 days and failure of the nursing staff to notify physicians about the ulcer in a timely fashion. The defense countered that the ulcer was unpreventable, that physicians were notified in a timely fashion, and that the plaintiff's death wasn't caused by the infection. The nursing home was found liable for more than $3.8 million for improper treatment.[2]

Missouri, September 23, 1996

The plaintiff was an unmarried, 45-year-old paraplegic male at the time of the (nonjury) trial. He alleged that the care he received for pressure ulcers on his hips and buttocks at two hospitals was negligent and resulted in the need for complete surgical disarticulation of both legs at the hip. The pressure ulcers initially were formed as a result of the plaintiff's own negligence in not properly utilizing equipment given to him for such prevention. This contributory negligence was taken into consideration by the court in arriving at its findings. The

plaintiff successfully brought forward proof at trial that the two hospitals were negligent in the following ways:
• permitting the development of a perirectal abscess
• failure to order and provide timely surgical consultations
• failure to prevent the advancement of existing pressure ulcers
• failure to document and treat osteomyelitis
• insufficient "monitoring" of treatments and outcomes.

Taking these proofs into account, and also taking into account the plaintiff's own negligence, the judge made the following awards:
• Lost wages: $501,774
• Pain and suffering: $288,750
• Future medical costs: $2,082,625
• Total award: $2,873,149[3]

Florida, September 25, 1995

The plaintiff was an 88-year-old male suffering from Alzheimer's disease and the complications of a subdural hematoma at the time of his death. He had been admitted to a nursing home in October 1989 following acute medical management of his neurological condition, and while a patient there he was frequently restrained in a "geri-chair." While there, he developed pressure ulcers that eventually became necrotic, requiring three hospital admissions until his death in October 1990.

The plaintiff's attorney called two expert witnesses, one a medical director of a long-term-care facility who testified that a review of the medical records revealed numerous violations and deprivations of the plaintiff's rights as a patient. Among the findings were the following:
• patient falls resulting from inadequate supervision
• improper and inappropriate restraint policies and procedures
• improper documentation and falsification of records (one entry related to nutrition and self-feeding when the plaintiff was clearly unable to feed himself)
• failure to institute a team care plan
• failure to evaluate the need for and to provide comfort measures, including pain relief
• development of contractures
• nursing abuse.

The second expert opined that the treatment for the pressure ulcers, when given and documented, was improper and incorrect. The expert said that the charting, when done, was inadequate, and that from the charting that was attempted, it was impossible to follow the assessments offered. At trial, it was also determined that the nursing home had instructed employees to fill in gaps in the charting, even if those employees had not cared for the patient. Additional deficiencies found were inadequate nursing staff and improper and inappropriate delegation of nursing duties and responsibilities to nursing assistants.

The jury found the nursing home liable and returned the following verdicts:
• Compensatory damages: $719,064
• Punitive damages: $2,000,000

The nursing home's appeals were denied.[4]

Alabama, June 29, 1990

The plaintiff had been a resident of a nursing home since her admission in February 1985 for organic mental syndrome, heart failure, osteoarthritis, and hypertension. The first notation of a pressure ulcer in the medical record was made approximately 2 weeks after admission. No ulcerations or alterations in skin integrity were noted in the admitting physical examination. In August 1985, the plaintiff was admitted to a hospital for surgical debridement and management of multiple pressure ulcers of the left hip, left thigh, and left heel. In February 1986, the plaintiff was again admitted to the hospital for surgical debridement of a pressure ulcer of her right hip. Ulcers were also noted on her left hip, back, and legs on that admission. The plaintiff died in the hospital in March 1986, following unsuccessful management of her advanced ulcers.

At trial evidence of the following deficiencies was presented to the jury:
- inadequate documentation of treatments given for ulcers
- dressings and treatments not given or changed as ordered
- inadequate documentation concerning the plaintiff's condition, progress, and reactions to treatments
- ineffective policies and procedures
- lack of nursing assessments
- incomplete or missing patient care plans
- incomplete or missing documentation concerning nutrition.

The jury found the nursing home liable for the plaintiff's injuries and death and awarded the plaintiff's family $2 million.[5]

Summary

The patient's chart is an important legal document as it provides the written record of the care provided. It also serves as a means of communication among health care professionals about the patient's care and responses to that care. Completeness and accuracy of documentation is essential not only for good patient care but as a basis for mounting a defense in the event of legal action. Make your entries in the patient's record legible, thorough, professional, and factual. Make sure all information is correct and accurate.

Show what you know

1. In a medical malpractice trial, what's the role of the jury and the judge?

   A. Interpreter of the law; finder of fact
   B. Finder of fact; finder of fact and interpreter of the law
   C. Finder of fact; interpreter of the law
   D. Both judge and jury find fact and interpret the law

ANSWER: C. The jury determines who, what, when, why, and where — in other words, what happened. The judge interprets the law by instructing the jury about the law to be applied to the facts as it has determined them.

2. At trial, how many of the four elements of a medical malpractice claim must a defendant convince a jury that the plaintiff has failed to prove in order to successfully defend against a claim of medical malpractice?

   A. One
   B. Two
   C. Three
   D. Four

ANSWER: D. Plaintiff must prove all four elements in order to prevail at trial.

3. The medical record is:

   A. a communication tool.
   B. destroyed after 1 year.
   C. a tool to communicate opinions related to a patient's care.
   D. optional part of health care.

ANSWER A. Opinions related to patient care aren't proper entries in a medical record. The medical record is a communication tool between practitioners, and is best used for the transmittal of factual information.

4. Which one of the following statements about Standards of Care, Practice Guidelines, and policies and procedures is FALSE?

A. Should be reviewed at regular intervals but never amended

B. Should be reviewed at regular intervals and amended to reflect new information and research

C. Should be based on research and practice experience

D. Should be patient-outcome oriented and quantifiable

ANSWER: A. Standards must be reviewed and amended to reflect the latest research and practice experience in a treatment area. Standards based on practice experience only and not supported by research may not survive judicial scrutiny at trial, and don't offer the patient the best care.

References

1. *Black's Law Dictionary*, 5th ed. New York: West Publishing Company, 1979.
2. *Smith v. Senior Living Properties*, LLC, No. 017-184243-00 (Tarrant Co., Texas District Court, 2002)
3. *Wyatt v. United States of America*, 939 F. Supp. 1402, 1996
4. *Spilman v. Beverly Enterprises-Florida, Inc.*, 661 So. 2d 867; (Ct. App. Fla. 5th Dist. 1995)
5. *Montgomery Health Care Facility, Inc. v. Ballard*, 565 So.2d 221 Alabama, June 29, 1990.

CHAPTER 3

Regulation and wound care

Courtney H. Lyder, ND, GNP, FAAN

OBJECTIVES

After completing this chapter, you'll be able to:

- discuss the significance of the U.S. Centers for Medicare and Medicaid Services

- discuss reimbursement issues related to hospitals, skilled nursing facilities, and home health agencies

- describe essential wound documentation required for reimbursement.

Importance of regulation

The important association between regulatory agencies and quality wound care can't be underestimated. Quite often, regulation and what's reimbursed determines the level of wound care that's delivered. Clinicians can become frustrated when regulations and the level of reimbursement don't match the care planned for a specific patient. However, as financial resources become tight, astute wound clinicians know that they must increasingly become knowledgeable about the regulations that guide reimbursement in their practice setting if they're to provide optimum wound care.

Several key questions underpin optimum wound care. They are:
- Is the product required for wound care reimbursed in the specific clinical setting?
- Is the service needed reimbursed for the specific clinical setting?
- Is the reimbursement appropriate to sustain the financial health of the clinical setting?

Key to any level of reimbursement is good documentation on the need of the product or service to heal the wound, level of patient adherence with care plan, and the outcomes achieved that support the need for such service or products.

Medicare and Medicaid

The Centers for Medicare and Medicaid Services (CMS) is a federal agency within the U.S. Department of Health and Human Services. Prior to July 1, 2001, it was called the Health Care Financing Administration (HCFA). CMS administers the Medicare and Medicaid programs—two national health care programs that benefit about 75 million Americans. CMS also regulates all laboratory testing (except research) performed on humans in the United States. CMS spends over $360 billion a year buying health care services for beneficiaries of Medicare and Medicaid.

Both the Medicare and Medicaid programs are administered through federal statutes that determine beneficiary requirements, what's covered, payment fees and schedules, and survey processes of clinical settings (such as skilled nursing facilities or home health agencies). Both programs have a wide variance on coverage, eligibility, and payment fees and schedules. Thus, it's important for the clinician to know what's covered and the level of reimbursement prior to developing a treatment plan with the patient. Since CMS remains the largest health insurance agency, many private insurance companies will provide coverage at similar levels.

Medicare

The Medicare program was developed in 1965 by the federal government.[1] In order to qualify for Medicare benefits, a person must be age 65 or older, have approved disabilities under age 65, or have end-stage renal disease.

Medicare has two components: Part A (hospital insurance) and Part B (medical insurance). People with Medicare Part A have no premiums. Medicare Part A covers care in hospitals as an inpatient, critical access hospitals (small facilities that give limited outpatient and inpatient services to people in rural areas), skilled nursing facilities, hospice care, and some home health care services. Medicare Part B assists with physician services, outpatient hospital care, and some other medical services that Medicare Part A doesn't cover, such as the services of advanced practice nurses, physical and occupational therapists, and some home health care. There is a premium associated with Medicare Part B. Currently, the premium for Medicare Part B is $58.70 per month.[2] However, in some cases this amount may be higher if the person doesn't choose Medicare Part B when they first become eligible at age 65.

The Medicare + Choice program was authorized by the Balanced Budget Act of 1997.[3] In this program, the beneficiary has the traditional Medicare Part A and Part B, but they may also select Medicare managed care plans (such as HMOs or PPOs) or Medicare Private Fee-for-Service plans. Medicare + Choice plans provide care under contract to Medicare. They may provide benefits like coordination of care or reducing out-of-pocket expenses. Some plans may offer additional benefits, such as prescription drugs.

Medicaid

The Medicaid program was developed in 1965 as a jointly funded cooperative venture between the federal and state governments to assist states in the provision of adequate medical care to eligible needy people.[4] Medicaid is the largest program providing medical and health-related services to America's poorest people. Within broad national guidelines provided by the federal government, each of the states:

• establishes its own eligibility standards

- determines the type, amount, duration, and scope of services
- sets the rate of payment for services
- administers its own program.

Thus, the Medicaid program varies considerably from state to state, as well as within each state over time. This wide variance also affects what's covered in wound care depending on the state.

Implementation of the Medicare program (for instance, eligibility requirements and payments) is handled by numerous insurance companies that are subcontracted by CMS. The processing of Medicare claims is handled by fiscal intermediaries (Medicare Part A only) and carriers (Medicare Part B only). The other major functions of fiscal intermediaries and carriers include controlling over-utilization of services and communicating with beneficiaries and the health community. Durable Medical Equipment (DME) Regional Carriers are also contracted by CMS. These carriers have the primary responsibility of processing durable medical equipment, prosthetic, orthotic, and supply claims. It should be noted that Medicare benefits don't vary across states. However, coverage and reimbursement often vary dependent on the fiscal intermediaries and carriers.

Reimbursement across health settings

Reimbursement directly impacts how clinicians deliver care. Increasingly, third-party payer sources (Medicare, Medicaid, health maintenance organizations) are examining where their money is going and whether they're getting the most from providers on behalf of their beneficiaries. Thus, third-party payers are requiring more documentation regarding patient outcomes to justify payment. Clinicians who can document comprehensive and accurate assessments of wounds and outcomes of their interventions are in a stronger position to obtain and maintain coverage.

Wound care that's evidence-based should always be the goal of clinicians. However, they're increasingly being challenged to provide optimum wound care dependent on health care setting and third-party payer. This section reviews various health care settings and how wound care products and services are reimbursed by CMS.

Hospitals

Hospitals are paid at a predetermined rate for each discharge under the prospective payment system (PPS). Hence, the PPS is a method of reimbursement based on a predetermined, fixed amount. The payment amount for a particular service is derived based on the classification system of that service. For hospitals, wound care products, devices, and support surfaces are included in the payment amount. Because the PPS payment is based on an adjusted average payment rate, some cases will receive payments in excess of cost (less than the billed charges) while other cases will receive payment that's less than cost.[5] The system is designed to give hospitals the incentive to manage operations more efficiently by evaluating those areas in which increased efficiencies can be instituted without affecting the quality of care and by treating a mix of patients to balance cost and payments.

Rehabilitation hospitals and units and long-term-care facilities (defined as those with an average length of stay of at least 25 days) are excluded from PPS. Instead, they're paid on a reasonable-cost basis, subject to per-discharge limits.[5] They're also paid depending on hospital-specific contracts and different payer sources. Note that CMS doesn't recognized suba-

Coverage under the surgical dressings benefit

To have the cost of dressings reimbursed under the Medicare/Medicaid surgical dressings benefit, the following criteria must be met:

- The dressings are medically necessary for the treatment of a wound caused by, or treated by, a surgical procedure.
- The dressings are medically necessary when debridement of a wound is medically necessary.

In certain situations, dressings aren't covered under the surgical dressings benefit, including those for:

- drainage from a cutaneous fistula which has not been caused by or treated by a surgical procedure
- stage I pressure ulcer
- first-degree burn
- wounds caused by trauma that don't require surgical closure or debridement (such as skin tears and abrasions)
- venipuncture or arterial puncture site other than the site of an indwelling catheter or needle.

Examples of dressing classifications that are covered under the surgical dressing benefit include foam dressings, gauze, nonimpregnated and impregnated dressings, hydrocolloids, alginates, composites, hydrogels, and transparent films. Tape is reimbursed when it's needed to hold a wound cover in place; however, it isn't reimbursed if an adhesive border is used.

Hospital outpatient centers

The Balanced Budget Act of 1997 provided authority for CMS to develop a PPS under Medicare for hospital outpatient services. The new outpatient PPS took effect in August 2000.[6] All services paid under this PPS are called Ambulatory Payment Classifications (APCs). A payment rate is established for each APC, depending on the services provided. Services in each APC are similar clinically and in terms of the resources they require. Currently, there are approximately 500 APCs. Hospitals may be paid for more than one APC per encounter. A coinsurance amount is initially calculated for each APC based on 20% of the national median charge for services in the APCs. The coinsurance amount for an APC doesn't change until the amount becomes 20% of the total APC payment. It should be noted that the total APC payment and the portion paid as coinsurance amounts are adjusted to reflect geographic wage variations using the hospital wage index and assuming that the portion of the payment/coinsurance that's attributable to labor is 60%.

The surgical dressings benefit covers primary and secondary dressings in outpatient acute care clinic settings (for example, a hospital outpatient wound center) and physician offices.[7] (See *Coverage under the surgical dressings benefit.*)

Skilled nursing facilities

A patient who is Medicare eligible will receive Medicare Part A for up to 100 days per benefit period in a skilled nursing facility (SNF).[8] The patient must satisfy specific rules in order to qualify for this benefit. These rules include the following:

- Beneficiary must have been in a hospital receiving inpatient hospital services for at least 3 consecutive days (counting

cute status; rather, subacute facilities are governed by the skilled nursing facility regulations.

the day of admission, but not the day of discharge)
• Skilled services are required for the same or related health problem that resulted in the hospitalization
• Beneficiary is admitted to SNF or to the SNF level of care in a swing-bed hospital within 30 days after the date of hospital discharge
• Beneficiary requires skilled nursing care by or under the supervision of a registered nurse; or requires physical, occupational, or speech therapy that could only be provided in an inpatient setting
• Services are needed on a daily basis.

After the SNF accepts a patient with Medicare Part A, all routine, ancillary, and capital-related costs are covered in the PPS. Thus, wound care supplies, therapies, and support surfaces are included in the PPS per diem rate. The Balanced Budget Act (BBA) of 1997 modified how payments were made for Medicare SNF services.[8] After July 1, 1998, SNFs were no longer paid on a reasonable cost basis or through low volume prospectively determined rates, but rather on the basis of a PPS. The PPS payment rates are adjusted for case mix and geographic variation (urban versus rural) in wages. It also covers all costs of furnishing covered SNF services. The SNF isn't permitted to bill under Medicare Part B until the 100 days are in effect.[8]

Resident Assessment Instrument

After a person is admitted to the SNF, an assessment using the Resident Assessment Instrument (RAI) must be completed. The RAI includes the Minimum Data Set (MDS 2.0), Resident Assessment Protocols (RAPs), and utilization guidelines. The MDS is a 400-item assessment form that attempts to identify functional capacity of residents in SNFs.[9] Based on the MDS section, further assessments are triggered by RAPs. The RAPs assess common clinical problems found in SNFs, such as pressure ulcers and urinary incontinence. RAPs also have utilization guidelines that assist the health care team in planning the overall care of the resident. The comprehensive RAI is completed annually, with quarterly MDS assessment (less comprehensive) completed between the annual date. The SNF is required to do another RAI if the resident's health status changes significantly. Only pressure and stasis ulcers are clearly delineated on the MDS 2.0 version; all other ulcers are grouped in the "other" category. This section of the MDS is currently under revision to address the above inadequacies.

The RAI is a very useful instrument to plan the care of SNF residents. It's also linked to payment. All Medicare Part A is linked to the RAI and, in some states, Medicaid payments are solely based on completion of the MDS. Since 1998, SNFs are required to complete and transmit MDS data to the designated state agency for all residents as a condition of participation in the Medicare and Medicaid programs.

Resource utilization groups

Based on the MDS, each resident is assigned to one of 44 resource utilization groups (RUGs).[10] RUGs are clusters of nursing home residents based on resident characteristics that explain resource use.[11] RUG rates are computed separately for urban and rural areas, and a portion of the total rate is adjusted to reflect labor market conditions in each SNF's location. The daily rate for each RUG is calculated using the sum of three components:
• a fixed amount for routine services (such as room and board, linens, and administrative services)
• a variable amount reflecting the intensity of nursing care patients are expected to require

Qualifying for home health benefits

A patient who is Medicare-eligible can also receive Medicare home health services. To qualify for this benefit, the patient must satisfy specific rules:

- The patient's physician must determine that medical care is needed in the home and must then generate a care plan.
- The patient must need at least one of the following:
  - intermittent skilled nursing care
  - intermittent physical therapy
  - intermittent speech/language pathology.
- The patient must be classified as homebound according to the condition for participation in Medicare.

- a variable amount for the expected intensity of therapy services.

Because of RUGs, it's essential for the SNF to complete the MDS correctly. The SNF must pay close attention to all health problems of the resident because the more intensive the care required, the higher the daily rate. Moreover, completing the MDS accurately and timely will help to ensure correct payments. If a SNF doesn't complete the MDS in a timely manner, they receive a default payment, which is usually significantly lower, or they may not receive payment at all.

The majority of SNFs accept the Medicaid program as the major payer for residents. Like Medicare, most state Medicaid programs pay a per diem rate for SNF services. If Medicaid is paying for SNF services and the resident has Medicare Part B, some wound products (such as dressings and negative pressure wound therapy) may be covered.

Federal oversight

The state Survey Agency (SA) is required to conduct annual unannounced surveys at SNFs to determine compliance with federal regulations. The SA can also conduct an abbreviated standard survey to follow up a resident complaint, change in SNF ownership, or change in administrator or director of nursing.

A major focus for many survey teams is the determination of avoidable versus unavoidable pressure ulcers. Federal Tag 314 is the federal regulation that specifically addresses pressure ulcer prevention and treatment in SNFs.[12] Thus, clear, comprehensive documentation on interventions used to heal pressure ulcers, or programs in place to them, is critical to the successful outcome of a survey. Both financial and civil penalties can result from a poor survey on pressure ulcers.[13]

Home health agencies

The Balanced Budget Act of 1997 called for the development and implementation of a PPS for Medicare home health services. In October 1, 2000, home health PPS was implemented.[14] (See *Qualifying for home health benefits*.)

OASIS

The process of quality wound management begins on admission. Suggested components of a quality program are: assessment (including risk assessment and intervention), documentation and wound measurement, case manager report and collaboration, protocols and physician orders, ulcer care, management of tissue loads, nutrition, and outcomes tracking.[15]

When a Medicare patient is accepted to receive home health services, the Outcome and Assessment Information Set (OASIS) must be completed. OASIS is a group of comprehensive assessments that form the basis for delivering care to the patient, as well as for measuring patient outcomes for purposes of outcome-based quality improvement. Revisions to the OASIS tool were introduced in late 2002. These changes have reduced the dataset questions by 25%. The new tool drops 45 items from follow-up assessments, establishes a patient data tracking sheet, and eliminates two collection time-points. Additional changes are pending approval by CMS.

Major items on the OASIS include: sociodemographic, environmental, support system, health status, and functional status. Based on these assessments, a care plan can be generated. The OASIS document specifically classifies stasis ulcers, surgical wounds, and pressure ulcers.[16]

Payment for home health services is directly linked to the completion of OASIS. A case-mix is also applied to calculate reimbursement. Hence, the case mix involves 20 data points to assess three factors within the case-mix: clinical severity, functional status, and service utilization. The system has created 80 home health resource groups (HHRGs).[17] Patients are grouped into the HHRGs based on the OASIS.

Medicare pays home health agencies for each covered 60-day episode of care.[14] A patient can receive an unlimited number of medically necessary episodes of care. Payments cover skilled nursing and home-health aide visits, covered therapy, medical social services, and routine and nonroutine supplies. For each 60-day episode, the payment system can range from about $1,100 to $5,900, depending on the HHRG, with adjustments to reflect area wage differences.[17]

Home health agencies are required to electronically transmit OASIS data to the State system. Improper completion of OASIS can lead to significantly low payments or no payments at all. Thus, accurate assessments and charting is essential for recouping payments. Clinicians may find the Wound, Ostomy, and Continence Nurses (WOCN) Society guidance on OASIS skin and wound status helpful in completing this form. (See *WOCN wound classification guidelines*, pages 42 to 44.) Educating clinicians about how to complete and use OASIS is a challenge. Some authors[15,18,19,20] have described innovative ways of teaching staff and assuring their competency in completing OASIS.

PRACTICE POINT

Accurate completion of OASIS by clinicians is essential. If you don't answer the questions appropriately, accurately, and completely, your facility won't receive the money and will lose reimbursement.

Durable medical equipment carriers

In 1993, CMS contracted with four carriers to process claims for durable medical equipment, prosthetics, orthotics, and supplies (DMEPOS) under Medicare Part B.[21] CMS divided the country into four regions, with each region having its own DME regional carrier (DMERC). The Healthcare Common Procedure Coding System (HCPCS), an alpha-numeric code used to identify coding categories not included in the American Medical Association's CPT-4 codes are usually used with DMEPOS.[22]

DMERCs clearly define medical coverage policies. The beneficiary usually pays the first $100.00 for covered medical services annually. Once that has been met, the beneficiary pays 20% of the Medicare approved amount for services or supplies. If services weren't provided on assignment, then the beneficiary pays for more the Medicare coinsurance plus certain charges above the Medicare-approved amount.

(Text continues on page 44.)

WOCN wound classification guidelines

If a patient is to receive reimbursement for home health care services and treatments, his wound status must be described accurately. The system for wound classification uses terms such as "nonhealing," "partially granulating," and "fully granulating," but these terms have long been open to individual interpretation, making precise classification for reimbursement purposes difficult. To standardize the definitions of terms used to describe wounds, the Wound, Ostomy, and Continence Nurses (WOCN) Society convened a panel of experts to develop the following guidelines for filling out the OASIS tool.

Classifications

- MO 445: Presence of a pressure ulcer
- MO 450: Current number of pressure ulcers at each stage
- MO 460: Stage of most problematic (observable) pressure ulcer
  - 1 Stage I
  - 2 Stage II
  - 3 Stage III
  - 4 Stage IV
  - NA No observable pressure ulcer
- MO 464: Status of most problematic (observable) pressure ulcer
  - 1 Fully granulating
  - 2 Early/partial granulation
  - 3 Not healing
  - NA No observable pressure ulcer
- MO 468: Does the patient have a stasis ulcer?
- MO 470: Current number of observable stasis ulcer(s)
- MO 474: Does this patient have at least one stasis ulcer that can't be observed?
- MO 476: Status of the most problematic (observable) stasis ulcer
  - 1 Fully granulating
  - 2 Early/partial granulation
  - 3 Not healing
  - NA No observable stasis ulcer
- MO 482: Does the patient have a surgical wound?
- MO 484: Current number of (observable) surgical wounds
- MO 486: Does the patient have at least one surgical wound that can't be observed due to the presence of a nonremovable dressing?
- MO 488: Status of the most problematic (observable) surgical wound
  - 1 Fully granulating
  - 2 Early/partial granulation
  - 3 Not healing
  - NA No observable surgical wound

Definitions

Avascular: Lacking in blood supply; synonyms include dead, devitalized, necrotic, and nonviable. Specific types include slough and eschar.

Clean wound: Wound free of devitalized tissue, purulent drainage, foreign material, or debris.

Closed wound: Edges of the top layers of epidermis have rolled down to cover the wound.

Dead space: A defect or cavity.

Dehisced (dehiscence): A separation of the surgical incision or loss of approximation of the wound edges.

Early or partial granulation: At least 25% of the wound bed covered with granulation tissue; minimal avascular tissue (that is, less than 25% of the wound bed covered with avascular tissue); the wound may have dead space; no signs or symptoms of infection present; the wound edges are open.

Edges: Lower edge of epidermis, including basement membrane, so that epithelial cells can't migrate from wound edges; also described as epibole; presents clinically as

WOCN wound classification guidelines (continued)

sealed edge of mature epithelium; may be hard/thickened; may be discolored (for example, yellowish, gray, or white).

Epidermis: Outermost layer of the skin.

Epithelialization: Regeneration of the epidermis across a wound surface.

Eschar: Black or brown necrotic, devitalized tissue; tissue can be loose or firmly adherent, hard, soft, or soggy.

Full thickness: Tissue damage involving total loss of epidermis and dermis and extending into the subcutaneous tissue and possibly into the muscle or bone.

Fully granulating: Wound bed filled with granulation tissue to the level of the surrounding skin or new epithelium; no dead space, no avascular tissue; no signs or symptoms of infection; wound edges are open.

Granulation tissue: The pink or red, moist tissue comprised of new blood vessels, connective tissue, fibroblasts, and inflammatory cells, which fills an open wound when it starts to heal; typically appears deep pink or red with an irregular, "berry-like" surface.

Healing: A dynamic process involving synthesis of new tissue for repair of skin and soft tissue defects.

Healing by primary intention: Approximated incisions are wounds that heal by primary intention. These wounds may exhibit full granulation, early or partial granulation, or be nonhealing.

Healing by secondary intention: Wounds healing by secondary intention are dehisced wounds healing by granulation, contraction, and epithelialization. These wounds may exhibit full granulation, early or partial granulation, or be nonhealing.

Healing ridge: Palpatory finding indicative of new collagen synthesis. Palpation reveals induration beneath the skin that extends to approximately 1 cm on each side of the wound. Becomes evident between 5 and 9 days after wounding; typically persists till about 15 days post-wounding. This is an expected positive sign.

Hyperkeratosis: Hard, white or gray tissue surrounding the wound.

Infection: The presence of bacteria or other microorganisms in sufficient quantity to damage tissue or impair healing; wounds can be classified as infected when the wound tissue contains 10^5 (100,000) or greater microorganisms per gram of tissue. Typical signs and symptoms of infection include purulent exudate, odor, erythema, warmth, tenderness, edema, pain, fever, and elevated white cell count. However, clinical signs of infection may not be present, especially in the immunocompromised patient or the patient with poor perfusion.

Necrotic tissue: See avascular.

Nongranulating: Absence of granulation tissue; wound surface appears smooth as opposed to granular. For example, in a wound that is clean but nongranulating, the wound surface appears smooth and red as opposed to berry-like.

Nonhealing: Wound with more than 25% avascular tissue OR signs/symptoms of infection OR clean but non-granulating wound bed OR closed/hyperkeratotic wound edges OR persistent failure to improve despite appropriate comprehensive wound management.

Nonobservable: Wound is unable to be visualized due to an orthopedic device, dressing, etc. A pressure ulcer can't be accurately staged until the deepest viable tissue layer is visible; *this means that wounds covered with eschar or slough can't be staged, and should be documented as nonobservable.*

Partial thickness: Confined to the skin layers; damage does not penetrate below the dermis and may be limited to the epidermal layers only.

(continued)

WOCN wound classification guidelines (continued)

Pressure ulcer: Any lesion caused by unrelieved pressure that results in damage of the underlying tissue. Pressure ulcers are usually located over bony prominences and are classified by stage according to the degree of tissue damage observed.

Sinus tract: Course or path of tissue destruction occurring in any direction from the surface or edge of the wound; results in dead space with potential for abscess formation. Also sometimes called "tunneling". (Can be distinguished from undermining by fact that sinus tract involves a small portion of the wound edge whereas undermining involves a significant portion of the wound edge.)

Slough: Soft moist avascular (devitalized) tissue; may be white, yellow, tan, or green; may be loose or firmly adherent.

Stage I: Nonblanchable erythema of intact skin, the heralding lesion of skin ulceration. In individuals with darker skin, discoloration of the skin, warmth, edema, induration, or hardness may also be indicators.

Stage II: Partial thickness skin loss involving epidermis, dermis, or both. The ulcer is superficial and presents as an abrasion, blister, or shallow crater.

Stage III: Full thickness skin loss involving damage to or necrosis of subcutaneous tissue that may extend down to, but not through, underlying fascia. The ulcer presents clinically as a deep crater with or without undermining of adjacent tissue.

Stage IV: Full thickness skin loss with extensive destruction, tissue necrosis, or damage to muscle, bone, or supporting structures (for example, tendon or joint capsule). Undermining and sinus tracts may also be associated with stage IV pressure ulcers.

Tunneling: See sinus tract.

Undermining: Area of tissue destruction extending under intact skin along the periphery of a wound; commonly seen in shear injuries. Can be distinguished from sinus tract by fact that undermining involves a significant portion of the wound edge, whereas sinus tract involves only a small portion of the wound edge.

Adapted from "WOCN Guidance on OASIS Skin and Wound Status M0 Items," Wisconsin Department of Health and Family Services. Available at www.dhfs.state.wi.us/rl_DSL/HHAs/HHAs01-036b.htm

Medicare Part B also provides coverage for negative pressure wound therapy (NPWT) pumps.[23] In order for a NPWT pump and supplies to be covered, the patient must have a chronic stage III or IV pressure ulcer, neuropathic ulcer, venous or arterial insufficiency ulcer, or a chronic (at least 30 days) ulcer of mixed etiology. Extensive documentation is required prior to a DMERC approving coverage for NPWT. Thus, it's important to review the coverage policy prior to applying for coverage.

Support surfaces are covered under Medicare Part B.[24-26] The CMS has divided support surfaces into three categories for reimbursement purposes. Group 1 devices are those support surfaces that are static and don't require electricity. Static devices include air, foam (convoluted and solid), gel, and water overlay or mattresses. Group 2 devices are powered by electricity or pump and are considered dynamic in nature. These devices include alternating and low-air-loss mattresses. Group 3 devices are also considered dynamic in nature.

This classification comprises only air-fluid beds. Specific criteria must be met before Medicare will reimburse for support surfaces. It's essential to review the policy before applying for coverage.

Documentation

Comprehensive documentation is critical for reimbursement of services and products. Moreover, good documentation justifies the medical necessity of services and products. Regulatory agencies, independent of health care setting, set forth the requisite documentation for reimbursement, and their requirements for documentation should always be reviewed prior to applying for coverage. In general, good documentation should reflect the need for the service or products. Moreover, good documentation should reflect the care required in the prevention or treatment of wounds. (See *Essential wound documentation.*)

Summary

Regulatory agencies play a major role in wound care. With the increasing need to evaluate the cost-effectiveness of wound care, regulatory agencies will most likely impose further regulations. Increasing regulation will lead to greater complexity in obtaining and maintaining reimbursements. Thus, the key to providing optimum wound care will depend on good documentation that clearly articulates the need for services and products. Moreover, good documentation will clearly identify assessment of the patient, interventions instituted, and outcomes achieved. When this is accomplished, the patient, provider, and regulatory agency benefit.

Essential wound documentation

For essential wound care documentation, include the following:
- Regular assessment and reassessment of the wound (such as daily or weekly)
- Characteristics of the wound, including:
  - length
  - width
  - depth
  - exudate amount
  - tissue type
  - pain.
- Repositioning and turning schedules
- Pressure-reducing support surfaces (both bed and chair)
- Local wound care
- Routine skin assessment and care
- Moisture management
- Nutritional status
- Change in clinical status or wound healing progress
- Education of patient and caregivers
- Minimum Data Set (MDS 2.0) per schedule in the skilled nursing facility
- Outcome and Assessment Information Set (OASIS) per schedule in home health care.

Show what you know

1. Medicare Part B is a federal program that:

A. supports state programs to provide services and products to the poor.
B. reimburses hospitals for wound care services.
C. reimburses for selected wound services and products in skilled nursing facilities and home health agencies.
D. doesn't require copayment from beneficiary.

ANSWER: C. A is incorrect because it refers to the Medicaid program, which is a collaboration between the federal and state governments to deliver care. B is incorrect because Medicare Part A is for inpatient hospital costs. D is incorrect because Medicare Part B requires the beneficiary to pay a 20% copayment.

2. For which one of the following health care settings is completion of OASIS required?

   A. Hospitals
   B. Home health agencies
   C. Hospital outpatient centers
   D. Skilled nursing facilities

ANSWER: B. OASIS is only used by home health agencies to assess patients and determine reimbursement.

3. Which one of the following criteria must a patient with a wound meet in order to qualify for skilled nursing facility care?

   A. Skilled services must be required for the same or related health problem that resulted in the hospitalization.
   B. Beneficiary must be in the hospital for 2 consecutive days.
   C. Services are needed once per week.
   D. Beneficiary must be admitted to the SNF within 90 days of admission to the hospital.

ANSWER: A. B is incorrect because the beneficiary must spend 3 consecutive days in the hospital. C is incorrect because skilled nursing services must be needed on a daily basis. D is incorrect because the beneficiary must be admitted within 30 days of hospitalization.

References

1. *www.medicare.gov/Coverage/Home.asp*
2. *www.medicare.gov/Basics/Amounts2003.asp*
3. *www.medicare.gov/Choices/Overview.asp*
4. *www.cms.hhs.gov/medicaid*
5. *www.cms.hhs.gov/providers/hipps/default.asp*
6. *www.cms.hhs.gov/regulation/hopps*
7. *www.umd.nycpic.com/rev21_ch17-1_dressings_psc.html*
8. *www.cms.hhs.gov/providers/snfpp/default.asp*
9. *www.cms.hhs.gov/medicaid/mds20/default.asp*
10. Fries, B.E., et al. "Refining a Case-mix Measure for Nursing Homes: Resource Utilization Groups (RUG-III)," *Medical Care* 32(7):668-85, July 1994.
11. Rantz, M.J., et al. "The Minimum Data Set: No Longer just for Clinical Assessment," *Annals of Long Term Care* 7(9):354-60, September 1999.
12. Health Care Financing Administration, *Investigative Protocol, Guidance to Surveyors-Long Term Care Facilities*, Rev 274. U.S. Department of Health and Human Services; June 2000.
13. *www.access.gpo.gov/nara/cfr/waisidx_99/42cfr484_99.html*
14. *www.cms.hhs.gov/providers/hhapps/default.asp*
15. Johnston, P.J. "Wound Competencies and OASIS- One Organization's Plan," *The Remington Report* 10(3), 5-10, May-June, 2002.
16. *www.cms.hhs.gov/oasis/hhoview.asp*
17. *cms.hhs.gov/medlearn/hh0201b1v2.pdf*
18. Wright, K., and Powell, L. "Wound Competencies and OASIS- One Organization's Plan," *Caring Magazine* XXI(6):10-13, June 2002.
19. Cullen, B., and Parry, G. "Wound Competencies and OASIS- One Organization's Plan," *Caring Magazine* XXI(6):14-16, June 2002.
20. Everman, R., and Ferrell, J. "Wound Care Case Management Influences Better Patient Outcomes," *The Remington Report* 10(3):36-37, May-June 2002.
21. *www.umd.nycpic.com/aboutdme.html*
22. *www.tricenturion.com/content/hcpcs.cfm*
23. *www.umd.nycpic.com/rev22_ch14-31_negative_pressure_psc.html*
24. *www.umd.nycpic.com/rev22_ch14-22_group1_psc.html*
25. *www.umd.nycpic.com/rev22_ch14-23_group2_psc.html*
26. *www.umd.nycpic.com/ch14-24_group3_psc.html*

CHAPTER 4

Skin: An essential organ

Sharon Baranoski, MSN, RN, CWOCN, APN, FAAN
Elizabeth A. Ayello, PhD, RN, APRN,BC, CWOCN, FAAN

OBJECTIVES

After completing this chapter, you'll be able to:

- discuss the different layers of the skin

- state the functions of the skin

- list skin changes associated with the aging process

- differentiate between a skin and wound assessment

- describe risk factors for skin tears

- identify and classify skin tears

- develop a care plan to prevent or treat skin tears.

Skin anatomy and physiology

Human skin is composed of two distinct layers: the epidermis, the outermost layer; and the dermis, the innermost layer. (See *Layers of the skin*, page 48.) The dermal-epidermal junction, commonly referred to as the basement membrane zone (BMZ), separates the two layers. Under the dermis lies a layer of loose connective tissue, called subcutaneous tissue, or hypodermis. (See *Skin layer functions*, page 49.)

The epidermis is a thin, avascular layer that regenerates itself every 4 to 6 weeks. It's divided into five layers or strata (presented in order from the outermost layer inward):

- Stratum corneum: consists of keratinocyte cells; flakes and sheds; is easily removed during bathing activities
- Stratum lucidum: packed translucent line of cells; not seen in thin skin; found only on the palms and soles
- Stratum granulosum: contains Langerhans cells
- Stratum spinosum: contains Langerhans cells
- Stratum basale or germinativum: single layer of cells; contains melanocytes; can regenerate. (See *Layers of the epidermis*, page 50.)

The epidermis is composed of hard, horny keratinocyte cells that migrate up

Layers of the skin

Two distinct layers of skin, the epidermis and dermis, lie above a layer of subcutaneous fatty tissue (also called the hypodermis). The dermal-epidermal junction (also called the basement membrane zone) lies between the dermis and epidermis.

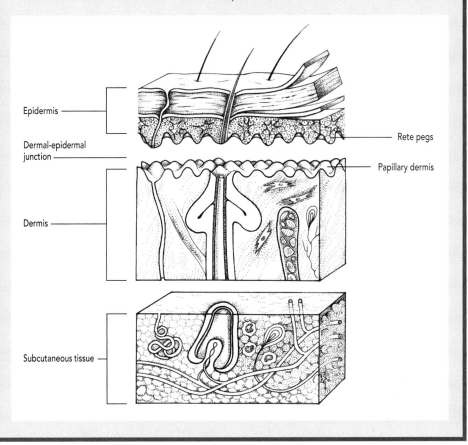

from the bottom single layer of cells to the stratum corneum. This cellular migration usually takes 28 days and is affected by aging and chemotherapy. The primary functions of the epidermis are protection from epidermal water loss, and maintaining skin integrity against physical barriers, such as shear, friction, and toxic irritants.

The BMZ divides the epidermis from the dermis. It contains fibronectin (an adhesive glycoprotein), type IV collagen (a nonfiber forming collagen), heparin sulfate proteoglycan, and glycosaminoglycan.[1] The BMZ has an irregular surface—called rete ridges or pegs—projecting downward from the epidermis that interlocks with the upward projections of the dermis. The two interlocking sides resemble the two sides of a waffle iron coming together. This structure anchors the epidermis to the dermis, preventing it from sliding back and forth. As skin ages, the basement membrane

Skin layer functions

The chart below shows characteristics and general functions of each layer of the skin.

Skin layer	Characteristics	General function
Epidermis	• Outer layer of skin • Consists of five layers (or strata): corneum, lucidum, granulosum, spinosum, and basale (or germinativum) • Repairs and regenerates itself every 28 days	• Protective barrier • Organization of cell content • Synthesis of vitamin D and cytokines • Division and mobilization of cells • Maintaining contact with dermis • Pigmentation (contains melanocytes) • Allergen recognition (contains Langerhans cells) • Differentiates into hair, nails, sweat glands, and sebaceous glands
Dermis	• Consists of two layers—papillary dermis and reticular dermis—composed of collagen, reticulum, and elastin fibers • Contains a network of nerve endings, blood vessels, lymphatics, capillaries, sweat and sebaceous glands, and hair follicles	• Supports structure • Mechanical strength • Supplies nutrition • Resists shearing forces • Inflammatory response
Subcutaneous tissue (hypodermis)	• Composed of adipose and connective tissue • Contains major blood vessels, nerves, and lymphatic vessels	• Attaches to underlying structure • Thermal insulation • Storage of calories (energy) • Controls body shape • Mechanical "shock absorber"

flattens and the area of contact between the epidermis and dermis is decreased by 50%, thus increasing the risk of skin injury by traumatic, accidental separation of the epidermis from the dermis. (See *Effects of aging on the BMZ,* page 51.)

The dermis is the most important part of the skin and is commonly referred to as the "true skin."[2] As the second layer, it's the thickest layer and is composed of many cells. The major proteins found in this layer are collagen and elastin, which are synthesized and secreted by fibroblasts. Collagen forms up to 30% of the volume or 70% of the dry weight of the dermis.[1] This dermal layer is a matrix supporting the epidermis and can be divided into two areas, the papillary dermis and the reticular dermis.[1,2]

• The papillary dermis is composed of collagen and reticular fibers. Its distinct, unique pattern allows fingerprint identification for each individual. It contains capillaries for skin nourishment and pain touch receptors (pacinian corpuscles and Meissner's corpuscles).

• The reticular dermis is composed of collagen bundles that anchor the skin to the subcutaneous tissue. Sweat glands, hair follicles, nerves, and blood vessels can be found in this layer.

The main function of the dermis is to provide tensile strength, support, moisture retention, and blood and oxygen to

Layers of the epidermis

The epidermis consists of five layers, as illustrated below.

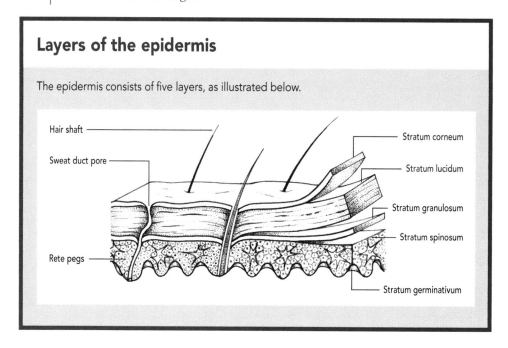

Hair shaft

Sweat duct pore

Rete pegs

Stratum corneum

Stratum lucidum

Stratum granulosum

Stratum spinosum

Stratum germinativum

the skin.[1,2] It protects the underlying muscles, bones, and organs.[1] The dermis also contains the sebaceous glands, which secrete sebum, a substance rich in oil that lubricates the skin.

The subcutaneous tissue or hypodermis attaches the dermis to underlying structures. Its function is to promote an ongoing blood supply to the dermis for regeneration. It's primarily adipose tissue, which provides a cushion between skin layers, muscles, and bones. It promotes skin mobility, molds body contours, and insulates the body.[2]

Skin function

Skin is an important organ whose diverse functions aren't always appreciated. (See *Skin functions*, page 52.) The largest external organ, in adults the skin weighs between 6 and 8 lb (2.7 to 3.6 kg) and covers over 20 ft² (1.9 m²). Skin thickness varies from 0.5 mm to 6 mm according to its location on the body; for example, skin can be as thin as

$\frac{1}{50}''$ on the eyelids and as thick as ⅛″ on the palms and soles, where greater protection is needed. The normal range of skin pH is 4.5 to 6.[3] This "acid mantle" has a protective advantage and helps to maintain a normal skin flora. The skin receives one-third of the body's circulating blood volume — an oversupply of blood compared to its metabolic needs.

The skin's major functions are protection, sensation, thermoregulation, excretion, metabolism, and communication.[1] Skin protects the body by serving as a barrier from invasion by organisms such as bacteria. Because staphylococcal species (such as *Staphylococcus aureus* or *Staphylococcus epidermis*) tolerate salt, they are present in large numbers as resident bacteria on the skin.[3] Another organism found on the skin is yeast, which is commonly found on the trunk and ear, and as fungus between the toes.[3]

Sensation is a well-known and key function of the skin. Areas that are most sensitive to touch have a greater number of nerve endings. [3] These include the

Effects of aging on the BMZ

The illustrations below show the effects of aging on the basement membrane zone (BMZ). Specifically, the basement membrane flattens, reducing the area of contact between the epidermis and the dermis by 50%.

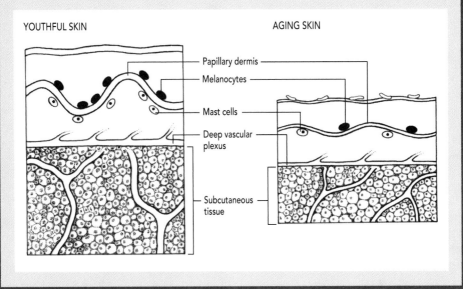

YOUTHFUL SKIN

AGING SKIN

Papillary dermis

Melanocytes

Mast cells

Deep vascular plexus

Subcutaneous tissue

lips, nipples, and fingertips. In humans, the fingertips are the most sensitive touch organ and enable us to correctly identify objects by touch (stereognosis) rather than sight. Many tactile corpuscles lie at the base of hair follicles, and shaving reduces the tactile sensibility of that skin area. In hairless body regions, the tactile corpuscles are called Meissner's corpuscles. [3] Pleasurable, firm touching sensations, such as from a massage or hugs of affection, are transmitted via the skin as they generate nerve transmissions through these tactile corpuscles.

Somatic pain (from the outer body surfaces and framework) is also communicated through the skin. Superficial (acute) pain to a local area is usually transmitted by very rapid nerve impulses by A-delta fibers. [3] It tends to be sharp and ceases when the pain stimulus stops.

Deep (chronic) pain impulses are transmitted slowly over the smaller, thinly myelinated C fibers. In contrast, this type of pain tends to be felt over a more diffuse area, lasts for longer periods of time, and remains even after the pain stimulus is gone.[3] As a sign of possible skin injury, pressure also serves as a protective warning sensation.

Temperature regulation and fluid and electrolyte balance are achieved in part by the skin. Thermoregulation is controlled by the hypothalamus in response to internal core body temperature. Peripheral temperature receptors in the skin assist in this process of temperature homeostasis. By sweating and insensible loss of water through the skin, lungs, and buccal mucosa, homeostasis of body temperature is maintained. Skin temperature is controlled by the dilatation or

Skin functions

Functions of the skin include:
- protection from:
  - fluid and electrolyte loss
  - mechanical injury
  - ultraviolet injury
  - pathogens
- temperature regulation
- fluid and electrolyte balance
- metabolism
- sensation
- synthesis
- communication.

The skin also aids in the excretion of end products of cell metabolism and prevents excessive loss of fluid. Other important functions of the skin include its manufacturing ability and immune functions. When exposed to ultraviolet light, the skin can synthesize vitamin D. While the skin's hypersensitivity responses in allergic reactions are commonly seen, the skin's role in immune function isn't always fully appreciated. Present in the skin are Langerhans cells and tissue macrophages, which play an important role in digesting bacteria, as well as mast cells, which are needed to provide proper immune system functioning.[1,4]

constriction of skin blood vessels. When body core temperature rises, the body will attempt to reduce temperature by releasing heat from the skin. This is accomplished by sending a chemical signal to increase blood flow in the skin from vasodilation, which will raise skin temperature.

PRACTICE POINT

Increased temperature → Skin blood vessel vasodilation → Heat loss from epidermis → Body maintains temperature homeostasis

In contrast, the opposite occurs when body core temperature is reduced; the chemical signal causes decreased blood flow from vasoconstriction to lower skin temperature.[3,4]

PRACTICE POINT

Decreased temperature → Skin blood vessel vasoconstriction → Heat conservation → Body maintains temperature homeostasis

Skin integrity and pathology

Alteration in skin integrity is a clinical practice issue in every continuum of care. Because normal skin changes occur with aging, elderly people are especially vulnerable to alterations in skin integrity. (See *Effects of normal aging on the skin*.) As skin ages, the epidermis gradually thins. The dermal-epidermal junction flattens and dermal papillae and epidermal rete pegs are effaced, making the skin more susceptible to mild mechanical trauma.[5,6] Decreases in the number of sweat glands and their output explains some of the dry skin seen in elderly people.[5] The ability to retain moisture is decreased in aging skin due to diminished amounts of dermal proteins, which causes oncotic pressure shifts and diminished fluid homeostasis,[3] thereby putting elderly patients at risk for dehydration. Since soap increases skin pH to an alkaline level, using emollient soap and bathing every other day instead of every day can decrease the incidence of skin injury, such as skin tears, in elderly patients.[6]

An elderly person's skin is more easily stretched due to a decrease in elastin fibers.[6] The skin becomes a less-effective barrier against water loss, bruising, and infection, accompanied by impaired thermal regulation, decreased tactile sensitivity, and decreased pain perception.[7] Due to a decreased amount of dermal proteins, the blood vessels become thinner and more fragile, thereby leading to a type of hemorrhaging known as senile purpura. According to Malone and colleagues,[8] skin tears commonly occur at the site of senile purpura.

Age-related changes in the dermis are numerous, but the most striking is the approximately 20% loss in dermal thickness that probably accounts for the paper-thin appearance of aging skin.[5] This decrease in dermal cells, blood vessels, nerve endings, and collagen leads to altered or reduced sensation, thermoregulation, rigidity, moisture retention, and sagging skin. The decrease of epidermal cell migration upward to the stratum corneum in aging skin is believed to account in part for the longer wound healing rates in elderly people.[5]

The subcutaneous fat below the dermis consists primarily of adipose tissue and provides mechanical protection and insulation. Its loss during aging results in parallel reductions in these protective functions.[5] Subcutaneous tissue undergoes site-specific atrophy in such areas as the face, dorsal aspect of the hands, shins, and plantar aspects of the foot, increasing the energy absorbed by the skin when trauma occurs to these areas. A decrease in pain perception may make elderly people more vulnerable to traumatic environmental insults.[8] Aging skin is less able to manufacture vitamin D when exposed to ultraviolet sunlight.[4,5] The decline in the number of Langerhans cells and mast cells in aging skin translates into diminished immune functioning of the skin.[5]

Effects of normal aging on the skin

The following changes in skin can occur due to the normal aging process.
Decreased:
- Dermal thickness, causing thinning of the skin (especially over the legs and forearms)
- Fatty layers (leaving the bony prominences less protected)
- Collagen and elastin fibers (leaving the elastin unable to recoil)
- Size of rete ridges (making the basement membrane flatter, which allows the epidermis and dermis to separate more easily, increasing the risk for injury such as a skin tear)
- Sensation and metabolism
- Sweat glands (leading to dry skin)
- Subcutaneous tissue (leading to less padding protection over bony prominences)
- Circulation (leaving the elderly patient more prone to heat stroke)
Increased:
- Time for epidermal regeneration (leading to slower healing)
- Damage to skin from the sun

Medications also have adverse affects on the skin. Steroids cause a thinning of the epidermis and suppress the skin's immune system.

Skin assessment vs. wound assessment

A skin assessment differs from a wound assessment in that skin assessment should include an actual observation of the patient's entire body, not just areas with wounds. No consensus as to what constitutes a minimal skin assessment

Elements of a basic skin assessment

To perform a basic skin assessment you must, at a minimum, assess its temperature, color, moisture, turgor, and integrity.

Temperature
- Normally warm to the touch
- Warmer than normal could signal inflammation
- Cooler than normal could signal poor vascularization

Color
- Intensity: paleness may be an indicator of poor circulation
- Normal color tones: light ivory to deep brown, yellow to olive, or light pink to dark, ruddy pink
- Hyperpigmentation or hypopigmentation reflect variations in melanin deposits or blood flow

Moisture
- Dry or moist to touch
- Hyperkeratosis (flaking, scales)
- Eczema (endogenous or exogenous?)
- Dermatitis, psoriasis, rashes
- Edema

Turgor
- Normally quickly returns to its original state
- Slow return to its original shape (dehydration or effect of aging)

Integrity
- No open areas
- Type of skin injury (Use the appropriate classification system to identify and record injury type.)

exists in the literature. The usual practice includes a minimum of the following five parameters: temperature, color, moisture, turgor, and intact skin or presence of open areas.[9] (See *Elements of a basic skin assessment.*) Some patients may require a more thorough skin assessment, which includes looking for and documenting any lesions, scars, bruising, or hemosiderin deposits. (See *Elements of a comprehensive skin assessment.*)

Once skin integrity is lost and the epidermis is no longer intact, a thorough wound assessment with documentation is required. (See chapter 6, Wound assessment, for more information.) The first step is to identify the type or etiology of the wounded skin — for example, differentiate a skin tear from a pressure ulcer. Next, a wound assessment should minimally describe the following characteristics: location, size, exudate, depth, and type of tissue. Remember the phrase frequently heard in wound care, "Look at the whole patient, not just the hole in the patient."

Implications for practice

Maintaining skin integrity in patients who have frail skin is a challenge. The friction and shear that may occur with turning or lifting can injure the skin. In many instances, simply moving an elderly patient can cause a skin tear. Ambulating or transferring patients can present a problem when they bump into objects, such as chairs, beds, or tables. Removing adhesive dressings or tape can tear delicate skin. Despite the frequency with which skin tears — defined as a traumatic wound resulting from separation of the epidermis from the dermis[8] — are seen in practice, the literature contains limited information about these wounds.

Elements of a comprehensive skin assessment

Consider the following criteria when performing a comprehensive skin assessment.

Inspection
- Normally smooth, slightly moist, and same general tone throughout
- Tone depends on patient's melanocytes—skin pigmentation continuum can vary from light ivory, deep brown, black, yellow to olive, light pink to dark ruddy pink, or red
- Pigmentation can exhibit:
  - pallor: mucosa, conjunctivae
  - cyanosis: nail beds, conjunctivae, oral mucosa
  - jaundice: sclerae, palates, palms
  - hyperpigmentation: increased (Results from variation in melanin deposits or blood flow; palpate for skin temperature and for edema over these areas to assess circulation.)
  - hypopigmentation: decreased vascular/venous patterns, usually symmetric
  - scars and bruises for location, color, length, and width.

Palpation
- Moisture: perspiration

- Edema: extremities, sacrum, eyes
- Tenderness
- Turgor, elasticity
- Texture

Olfaction
- Normal body odor
- Absence of pungent odor
- May indicate presence of bacteria or infection
- Poor hygiene

Observation of hair and nails
- Hair
  - Hirsutism: excessive body hair
  - Alopecia: hair loss
- Nails (can reflect the patient's overall health)
  - Color, shape, contour
  - Clubbing, texture, thickness

Skin alterations
- Previous scars
- Graft sites
- Healed ulcer sites

According to a retrospective study conducted by Malone and colleagues,[8] skin tears occur most commonly in the upper extremities. Almost one-half were found to have occurred without any apparent cause. When the cause is known, approximately one-quarter resulted from wheelchair injuries, and one-quarter were caused by accidentally bumping into objects. Transfers and falls accounted for 18% and 12.4%, respectively.

Whereas nearly 80% of skin tears occur on the arms and hands,[8,10,11] these wounds may occur on other areas of the body as well. Skin tears that occur on the back and buttocks are commonly mistaken for stage II pressure ulcers. Pressure may be a related cause in skin tears, but the etiology of skin tears differs from that of pressure ulcers. (See chapter 13, Pressure ulcers.)

According to a retrospective review by White et al.,[12] the patients most at risk for sustaining skin tears are those who require total care for all activities of daily living. These patients frequently experienced skin tears resulting from routine activities, such as dressing, bathing, posi-

EVIDENCE-BASED PRACTICE

Skin Integrity Risk Assessment Tool

White, et al. (1994) recommend implementing a skin-tear risk prevention care plan for patients who meet any of the criteria in group I below, patients who meet four or more criteria in group II, patients who meet five or more criteria in group III, and patients who meet three criteria in group II and three or more criteria in group III.

Group I
- History of skin tears within last 90 days
- Actual number of skin tears

Group II
- Decision-making skills impaired
- Vision impaired
- Extensive assistance/total dependence for activities of daily living (ADLs)
- Wheelchair assistance needed
- Loss of balance
- Bed or chair confined
- Unsteady gait
- Bruises

Group III
- Physically abusive
- Resists ADL care
- Agitation
- Hearing impaired
- Decreased tactile stimulation
- Wheels self
- Manually or mechanically lifted
- Contracture of arms, legs, shoulders, hands
- Hemiplegia or hemiparesis
- Trunk: partial or total inability to balance or turn body
- Pitting edema of legs
- Open lesions on extremities
- 3 to 4 senile purpura on extremities
- Dry, scaly skin

Reprinted from White, M., et al. "Skin Tears in Frail Elders: A Practical Approach to Prevention," *Geriatric Nursing* 15(2):95-99, March-April 1994, © 1994 Mosby, with permission from Elsevier.

tioning, and transferring. Independent ambulatory residents sustained the second highest number of skin tears, which occurred primarily on the lower extremities. Many of these patients had edema, purpura, or ecchymosis. Slightly impaired residents made up the third highest risk category. These patients sustained injury from hitting stationary equipment or furniture as well as the reasons just described in the dependent and independent ambulatory patients.

Little has been written about the prevention of skin tears. A skin integrity risk assessment tool with three groups of patients at risk for skin tears was developed by White et al. in 1994.[12] (See *Skin Integrity Risk Assessment Tool.*) This tool can be used to identify patients at risk for skin tears.

Common-sense protocols gleaned from the literature could prevent many skin injuries. If the patient is at risk, consider the following:
- Encourage your colleagues and the patient's family members to use proper positioning, turning, lifting, and transferring.
- Promote the use of long sleeves and pants to add a layer of protection.
- Secure padding to bed rails, wheelchair arm and leg supports, and any other equipment that may be used.

EVIDENCE-BASED PRACTICE

Payne-Martin classification system for skin tears

This classification system augments documentation and allows for better tracking of outcomes of care for patients with skin tears.

Category I: Skin tears without tissue loss

A. Linear type—Epidermis and dermis pulled apart as if an incision has been made.
B. Flap type—Epidermal flap completely covers the dermis to within 1 mm of the wound margin.

Category II: Skin tears with partial tissue loss

A. Scant tissue loss type—25% or less of the epidermal flap lost.
B. Moderate to large tissue type—More than 25% of the epidermal flap lost.

Category III: Skin tears with complete tissue loss

Adapted with permission from Payne, R.L., and Martin, M.L. "Defining and Classifying Skin Tears: Need for a Common Language," *Ostomy/Wound Management* 39(5):16-20, 22-24, 26, June 1993.

• Use paper tape or nonadherent dressings on frail skin. Always remove these products gently to prevent skin injury.
• Use stockinettes, gauze wrap, or a similar type of wrap to secure dressings and drains.
• Use pillows and blankets to support dangling arms and legs.
• Move and turn the patient with a lift sheet.
• Minimize the use of soap and alcohol solvents; consider the use of waterless cleansers.
• Avoid scrubbing skin when bathing.
• Pat skin dry rather than rubbing it dry.
• Apply a moisturizing agent to dry skin.
• Provide a well-lit environment to prevent falls.
• Educate staff on the importance of gentle care.

The initial classification system for skin tears evolved in the late 1980s, thanks to the work of Regina Payne and Marie Martin.[11] This pilot research study led to the development of the Payne-Martin Classification for Skin Tears.[11] This system provides health care professionals with a method to enhance documentation and track outcomes of care. Several researchers have used this new taxonomy in their studies as tool validation continues. The Payne-Martin system is a useful tool for addressing the needs for assessment, prevention, and treatment of skin tears.

According to the revised 1993 Payne-Martin Skin Tear Classification System, "a skin tear is a traumatic wound occurring principally on the extremities of older adults, as a result of friction alone or shearing and friction forces which separate the epidermis from the dermis (partial thickness wound) or which separate both the epidermis and the dermis from underlying structures (full thickness wound)."[13] The system is divided into three categories based on whether tissue is lost in the skin tear.[13] (See *Payne-Martin classification system for skin tears.*)

The management or treatment of skin tears varies according to institution. Many types of skin and wound care products are used to promote a healing environment. Little has been published regarding preferred treatments for skin tears. A review of the literature reveals that the following are used to treat skin tears: petrolatum ointment and nonadherent dressings;[14-18] hydrogels, Telfa, and collagen dressings;[14-16,18] foams and transparent films;[14-16,19] and hydrocolloids and adhesive strips.[11,16,18,20]

Skin tears are common in elderly patients. It's reported that 1.5 million skin tears occur each year in institutionalized adults.[19] Alterations in skin integrity may cause undue pain and suffering to patients. Health care professionals should have up-to-date information about prevention techniques, the appropriate use of dressings and tapes and, most important, the prevention of skin integrity injuries. Skin tears need to be documented as separate occurrences and not grouped into pressure ulcer categories. As so eloquently stated by White et al., "The problem of skin tears in the frail elderly population is, perhaps, a hidden phenomena that deserves more attention."[12]

Summary

The skin is the largest organ of the body and commonly the most forgotten. Skin is exposed daily to environmental irritants and chemicals as well as physical and mechanical injury, any of which may lead to impaired skin integrity. One such impairment is a skin tear. This chapter presented an overview of skin structure, presented criteria for doing a skin assessment versus a wound assessment, and identified and classified skin tears, including risk factors and prevention opportunities.

Show what you know

1. While bathing a patient, you notice some flakes of skin on the washcloth. Which layer of the skin is this?

- **A.** Stratum granulosum
- **B.** Stratum spinosum
- **C.** Stratum lucidum
- **D.** Stratum corneum

ANSWER: D. The cells of the stratum corneum can shed and look like flakes during routine cleaning activities such as bathing.

2. Which one of the following is a normal function of the skin?

- **A.** Synthesis of vitamin K
- **B.** Elimination of carbon dioxide
- **C.** Regulation of glucose levels by the Langerhans cells
- **D.** Thermal regulation by skin blood flow dilation or constriction

ANSWER: D. Upon stimulus from the hypothalamus, skin blood vessels will either vasoconstrict (heat needs to be conserved to elevate temperature) or vasodilate (heat needs to be eliminated to lower temperature) depending upon specific needs. Skin can synthesize vitamin D, not K. Carbon dioxide is eliminated via the lungs. Glucose regulation is from the islets of Langerhans in the pancreas, not the Langerhans cells in the skin.

3. Which one of the following changes in aging skin best explains why an elderly person is at increased risk for skin tear injury?

- **A.** Increased epidermal migration
- **B.** Increased secretion of sebum
- **C.** Decreased size of rete ridges
- **D.** Decreased dermal thickness over bony prominences

ANSWER: C. The decrease in size of the rete ridges from the epidermis results in less attachment of the epidermis to the dermis, therefore making accidental skin tear injury more likely to occur. Aging decreases epidermal migration. Sebum secretion is decreased. While aging does decrease dermal thickness over bony prominences, D isn't the best answer as this patient is more at risk for pressures ulcers.

4. Which one of the following is NOT considered part of a routine skin assessment?

A. Color
B. Turgor
C. Temperature
D. Ankle-brachial index (ABI)

ANSWER: D. ABI is a test used for peripheral vascular disease; it doesn't tell you skin assessment. A, B, and C should all be part of a skin assessment.

5. Which one of the following patients is most at risk for skin tear injury?

A. A 22-year-old male postoperative for an inguinal hernia repair
B. A 37-year-old male with a fractured humerus
C. A 64-year-old female 3 days post-cataract extraction
D. A 72-year-old female with rheumatoid arthritis on steroid therapy

ANSWER: D. This person is oldest, least mobile, and receiving steroids, which are known to further cause thinning of the skin, so her skin is at highest risk.

6. A partial thickness skin tear with less than 25% of the epidermal flap loss using the Payne-Martin method would be classified as:

A. category I.
B. category II.
C. category III.
D. category IV.

ANSWER: B. A and C are incorrect, and the Payne-Martin classification system contains no category IV.

7. Which of the following interventions for a resident in a long-term care facility with a skin tear on the lower right leg should you question?

A. Clean the patient daily using detergent.
B. Pad the wheelchair arm and leg supports.
C. Apply a nonadherent dressing to the skin tear.
D. Encourage the patient to wear soft, fleece-lined pants.

ANSWER: A. Nonemollient soaps should be used instead of detergent, which dries the skin. The literature suggests that routine every other day bathing for elderly people is adequate (unless the skin is soiled) and can reduce skin tear injury.

References

1. Wysocki, A. "A Review of the Skin and Its Appendages," *Advances in Wound Care* 8(2 part 1):53-54, 56-62, 64 passim., March-April 1995.
2. Smeltzer, S.C., and Bare, B.G. Brunner and Suddarth's *Textbook of Medical-Surgical Nursing*. Philadelphia: Lippincott Williams & Wilkins, 2000.
3. Hughes, E., and Van Onselen, J. *Dermatology Nursing: A Practical Guide*. London: Churchill Livingstone, Inc., 2001.
4. Guyton, A.C., and Hall, J.E. *Human Physiology and Mechanisms of Disease*, 6th ed. Philadelphia: W.B. Saunders Co., 1997.
5. Kaminer, M., and Gilchrest, B. "Aging of the Skin," in *Principles of Geriatric Medicine and Gerontology*, edited by Hazzard, W. New York: McGraw-Hill Book Co., 1994.
6. Mason, S. "Type of Soap and the Incidence of Skin Tears among Residents of a Long-term Care Facility," *Ostomy/Wound Management* 43(8):26-30, September 1997.
7. Frantz, R., and Gardner, S. "Clinical Concerns: Management of Dry Skin,"

Journal of Gerontological Nursing 20(9):15-18, 45, September 1994.

8. Malone, M.L., et al. "The Epidemiology of Skin Tears in the Institutionalized Elderly," *Journal of the American Geriatric Society* 39(6):591-95, June 1991.

9. Baranoski, S. "Skin: The Forgotten Organ." 16th Annual Clinical Symposium of *Advances in Skin & Wound Care.* Lake Buena Vista, Florida, September 2001.

10. McGough-Csarny, J., and Kopac, C.A. "Skin Tears in Institutionalized Elderly: An Epidemiological Study," *Ostomy/ Wound Management* 44(3A suppl):14S-24S, March 1998.

11. Payne, R.L., and Martin, M.L. "The Epidemiology and Management of Skin Tears in Older Adults," *Ostomy/Wound Management* 26(1):26-37, January-February 1990.

12. White, M., et al. "Skin Tears in Frail Elders: A Practical Approach to Prevention," *Geriatric Nursing* 15(2):95-99, March-April 1994.

13. Payne, R.L., and Martin, M.L. "Defining and Classifying Skin Tears: Need for a Common Language," *Ostomy/Wound Management* 39(5):16-20, 22-24, 26, June 1993.

14. Baranoski, S. "Skin Tears: The Enemy of Frail Skin," *Advances in Skin & Wound Care* 13(3 part 1):123-26, May-June 2000.

15. Baranoski, S. "Skin Tears: Guard Against this Enemy of Frail Skin," *Nursing Management* 32(8):25-31, August 2001.

16. Thomas-Hess, C. "Fundamental Strategies for Skin Care," in *Chronic Wound Care: A Clinical Source Book for Healthcare Professionals,* edited by Krasner, D., and Kane, D. Wayne, Pa.: Health Management Publications, 1997.

17. Krasner, D. "An Approach to Treating Skin Tears," *Ostomy/Wound Management* 32(1):56-58, January-February 1991.

18. O'Regan, A. "Skin Tears: A Review of the Literature," *WCET Journal* 22(2):26-31, April-June 2002.

19. Thomas, D., et al. "A Comparison of an Opaque Foam Dressing Versus a Transparent Film Dressing in the Management of Skin Tears in Institutionalized Subjects," *Ostomy/Wound Management* 45(6):22-24, 27-28, June 1999.

20. Camp-Sorrell, D. "Skin Tears: What Can You Do?" *Oncology Nursing Forum* 18(1):135, January-February 1991.

CHAPTER 5

Acute and chronic wound healing

Vanessa Jones, MSc, RN, NDN, RCNT, PGCE
Sue Bale, BA, PG Dip, RGN, NDN, RHV, Dip N
Keith Harding, MB, ChB, MRCGP, FRCS

OBJECTIVES

After completing this chapter, you'll be able to:

- describe the physiology of wound healing

- compare acute and chronic wound healing

- discuss the cascade of wound healing events

- compare tools to measure healing.

Wound healing events

When a patient experiences tissue injury it's essential that hemostasis is rapidly achieved and tissues are repaired to prevent invasion by pathogens and restore tissue function. The process of wound healing is a complex sequence of events that starts when the injury occurs and ends with complete wound closure and successful, functional scar tissue organization. Although tissue repair is commonly described as a series of stages, in reality it's a continuous process during which cells undergo a number of complicated biological changes to facilitate hemostasis, combat infection, migrate into the wound space, deposit a matrix,

form new blood vessels, and contract to close the defect.

However, wound closure isn't a marker of healing completion; the wound continues to change, in a process called remodeling, for up to 18 months postclosure. During this prolonged phase of remodeling and maturation, the closed wound is still quite vulnerable.

The process of healing is usually divided into four phases — hemostasis, inflammatory, proliferation, and maturation — each of which overlaps the others while remaining distinct in terms of time after injury. (See *Phases of wound healing*, page 62.)

Phases of wound healing

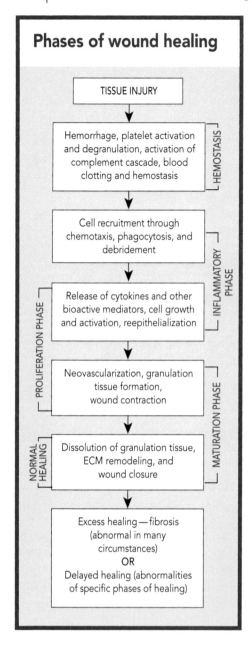

TISSUE INJURY

Hemorrhage, platelet activation and degranulation, activation of complement cascade, blood clotting and hemostasis

— HEMOSTASIS

Cell recruitment through chemotaxis, phagocytosis, and debridement

Release of cytokines and other bioactive mediators, cell growth and activation, reepithelialization

— INFLAMMATORY PHASE

Neovascularization, granulation tissue formation, wound contraction

PROLIFERATION PHASE

Dissolution of granulation tissue, ECM remodeling, and wound closure

— MATURATION PHASE

NORMAL HEALING

Excess healing — fibrosis (abnormal in many circumstances)
OR
Delayed healing (abnormalities of specific phases of healing)

Hemostasis

The disruption of tissues following injury causes hemorrhage, which initially fills the wound and exposes the blood to various components of the extracellular matrix (ECM).[1] Platelets aggregate and degranulate, which activates factor XII (Hageman factor), resulting in clot formation and hemostasis. Hemostasis is the arrest of hemorrhage at the site of blood vessel damage. This is essential as it preserves the integrity of the closed and high-pressure circulatory system to limit blood loss. A fibrinous clot forms during coagulation, acting as a preliminary matrix within the wound space into which cells can migrate.

After the fibrin clot forms, another mechanism is activated as part of the body's defense mechanism — fibrinolysis, in which the fibrin clot starts to break down. This process prevents clot extension and dissolves the fibrin clot to allow ease of further cell migration into the wound space,[2] allowing the next stage of healing to proceed.

Inflammatory phase

As the fibrin clot is degraded, the capillaries dilate and become permeable, allowing fluid into the injury site and activating the complement system. The complement system is composed of a series of interacting, soluble proteins found in serum and extracellular fluid that induce lysis and the destruction of target cells. C3b, a complement molecule, helps bind (opsonize) neutrophils to bacteria, facilitating phagocytosis and subsequent bacterial destruction.

Cytokines and some proteolytic fragments that are hemoattractive are also found in the wound space.[2] Their abundance and accumulation at the site of injury initiate a massive influx of other cells. The two main inflammatory cells — neutrophils and macrophages — are attracted to the wound space to mount an acute inflammatory response.[3] Neutrophils appear in a wound shortly after injury and reach their peak number within 24 to 48 hours. Their main function is to destroy bacteria by the process of phagocytosis. Neutrophils have a very short life span and their numbers reduce rapidly after 3 days in the absence of infection.

Tissue macrophages are derived from blood monocytes and arrive approximately 2 to 3 days after injury, followed by lymphocytes. Like neutrophils, macrophages also destroy bacteria and debris through phagocytosis; however, macrophages are also a rich source of biological regulators, including cytokines and growth factors, bioactive lipid products, and proteolytic enzymes, which are also essential for the normal healing process.[2,4]

Cytokines, growth factors, and chemotaxis

Cytokine is a broad term that includes such molecules as growth factors, interleukins, tumor necrosis factors, and interferons. These molecules act on a variety of cells by exerting a wide range of biological functions by means of their specific receptors on target cells or proteins. Pathogens, endotoxins, tissue degradation products, and hypoxia are all factors that stimulate cells to produce cytokines following injury. The main cellular sources for these cytokines are platelets, fibroblasts, monocytes and macrophages, and endothelial cells. These cells are involved in physiological as well as pathological conditions (for example, tumors), though in wound healing they play an important role as mediators. Cytokines regulate cell proliferation, migration, matrix synthesis, deposition and degradation, and inflammatory responses in the repair process.

Immediately after injury, platelet degranulation releases numerous cytokines, including platelet-derived growth factor (PDGF), transforming growth factor β (TGFβ), and epidermal growth factor (EGF). These cytokines, together with other chemotactic agents, such as tissue debris and pathogenic materials, attract neutrophils and, later, macrophages. In time these cells contribute to a larger number and variety of cytokines, which participate in the healing process.[4]

Cytokines have diverse effects on the healing process, interacting in additive, synergistic, or inhibitory ways. (See *Effects of growth factors on wound healing,* page 64.) For example, keratinocyte growth factor enhances the stimulation of collagenase synthesis exerted by insulin-like growth factor. TGFβ is inhibitory to fibroblast growth in the presence of EGF but stimulates cell division when PDGF is present.

PRACTICE POINT

Keep in mind that the induration, heat, discomfort, redness, and swelling experienced during the inflammatory phase are part of the normal wound healing processes and aren't, at this stage, likely to be due to wound infection. Remember to share this information with your patients.

Proliferation phase

The proliferation phase usually begins 3 days after an injury and lasts for a few weeks. This phase is characterized by the formation of granulation tissue in the wound space. The new tissue consists of a matrix of fibrin, fibronectin, collagens, proteoglycans, glycosaminoglycans (GAGs), and other glycoproteins.[5] Fibroblasts move into the wound space and proliferate. Because the type III collagen in the wound has decreased tensile strength, the patient is at risk for wound dehiscence. Abnormalities at this stage can result in serious medical problems, including wound dehiscence or opening of wound edges in a previously closed wound that healed by primary intention. If organs are protruding from the now opened wound, this is called evisceration. Wound evisceration is a medical emergency, requiring im-

Effects of growth factors on wound healing

The chart below shows which cells the different growth factors target, as well as their effects on wound healing.

Growth factor	Target cells in the wound	Effect on wound healing
Platelet derived growth factor	Keratinocytes Fibroblasts	• Collagen and protein synthesis • Granulation tissue
Transforming growth factor α	Epithelial cells Macrophages Platelets Endothelial cells	• Chemotaxis • Epithelialization
Transforming growth factor β	Epithelial cells Macrophages Platelets Neutrophils	• Collagen • Fibroblasts • Angiogenesis
Basic fibroblast growth factor	Macrophages Fibroblasts Endothelial cells Keratinocytes	• Angiogenesis
Epidermal growth factor	Keratinocytes Fibroblasts	• Neovascularization • Collagen • Fibroblasts • Macrophages

mediate surgery. Cover the organ with saline soaked gauze and prepare the patient for immediate surgery.

PRACTICE POINT

The first 3 weeks after surgery, the patient is at high risk for wound dehiscence and evisceration.

Role of fibroblasts

Fibroblasts play a key role during the proliferation phase, appearing in large numbers within 3 days of injury and reaching peak levels on the 7th day. During this period they undergo intense proliferative and synthetic activity. Fibroblasts synthesize and deposit extracellular proteins during wound healing, producing growth factors and angiogenic factors that regulate cell proliferation and angiogenesis.[6]

Granulation tissue is comprised of many mesenchymal and non-mesenchymal cells with distinct phenotypes, inflammatory cells and new capillaries embedded in a loose ECM composed of collagens, fibronectin, and proteoglycans.

Role of ECM proteins

ECM consists of proteins and polysaccharides and their complexes produced by cells in the wound space. The two main classes of matrix proteins are fibrous (collagens and elastin) and adhesive proteins (fibronectin and laminin). In addition, the ECM contains polysaccharides called proteoglycans and GAGs. Collagen is the most abundant protein in animal tissue and accounts for 70% to 80% of the dry weight of the dermis.[7] The collagen molecule consists of three identical polypeptide chains bound together in a triple helix. Mainly made by fibroblasts, at least 19 genetically distinct collagens have been identified. Collagen synthesis and degradation is finely balanced.[4]

Elastin is a protein that provides elasticity and resilience.[7] Elastin fibers form coils that enable it to stretch and return to its former shape, much like metallic coils. Because of these properties, elastin helps maintain tissue shape. Elastin represents only 2% to 4% of the human skin's dry weight, and it's also found in other organs, including the lungs and blood vessels, as well as the skin. It's secreted into the extracellular space as a soluble precursor, tropoelastin, which binds with a microfibrillar protein to form an elastic fiber network.

Laminin and fibronectin are two fiber-forming molecules. Their function is to provide structural and metabolic support to other cells. Fibronectin is found in plasma and contains specific binding sites on its molecular wall for cells, collagens, fibrinogens, and proteoglycans. It plays a central role in tissue remodeling, acting as a mediator for physical interactions between cells and collagens involved in ECM deposition, thereby providing a preliminary matrix.

Proteoglycans consist of a central core protein combined with a number of GAG chains that may be one or several types. GAGs consist of long, unbranched chains of disaccharide units that can vary in number from 10 to 20,000.[8] Proteoglycans are a highly complex group of molecules, which is demonstrated by their many diverse structural and organizational functions in tissue. Forming a highly hydrated gel-like "ground substance," they can contain up to 95% (w/w) carbohydrates. Originally, they were thought to contribute to tissue resilience due to their capacity to fill much of the extracellular space.

Angiogenesis

Angiogenesis, or formation of new vessels in the wound space, is an integral and essential part of wound healing.[9] The major cell involved in angiogenesis is the vascular endothelial cell, which arises from the damaged end of vessels and capillaries. New vessels originate as capillaries, which sprout from existing small vessels at the wound edge. The endothelial cells from these vessels are detached from the vascular wall, degrade and penetrate (invade) the provisional matrix in the wound, and form a knob-like or cone-shape vascular bud or sprout. These sprouts extend in length until they encounter another capillary, to which they connect to form vascular loops and networks allowing blood to circulate. This pattern of vascular growth is similar in skin, muscle, and intestinal wounds.

Epithelialization

Reepithelialization, which begins a few hours after injury, is another important feature of healing. Marginal basal cells, which are normally firmly attached to the underlying dermis, change their cell adhesion property and start to lose their firm adhesion, migrating in a leapfrog or train fashion across the provisional matrix. Horizontal movement is stopped when cells meet. This is known as contact inhibition.

Wound contraction

The final feature of the proliferation phase is wound contraction, which normally starts 5 days after injury. Wound contraction appears to be a dynamic process in which cells organize their surrounding connective tissue matrix, acting to reduce the healing time by reducing the amount of ECM that needs to be produced. The contractile activity of fibroblasts and myofibroblasts provides the force for this contraction. These cells may use integrins and other adhesion mechanisms to bind to the collagen network and alter its motility, bringing the fibrils and, subsequently, wound edges closer. Such contraction may not be important in a sharply incised, small, and noninfected wound; however, it's critical for wounds with large tissue loss.[10]

Although several theories exist to explain the wound contraction process, its exact mechanism remains unclear. In particular, the type and origin of fibroblasts that appear in the wound haven't yet been determined.[1,3,11-13]

The myofibroblast theory suggests that the contraction force occurs when the movement of microfilament (actin) bundles (also termed stress fibers) contracts the myofibroblast in a musclelike fashion. Because the myofibroblast displays many cell:cell and cell:matrix (fibronexus) contacts, the cellular contraction pulls collagen fibrils toward the body of the myofibroblast and holds them until they're stabilized into position. This gathering of collagen fibers toward the myofibroblast cell "body" leads to the shrinkage of granulation tissue. The ECM of the wound is continuous with the undamaged wound margin, enabling the granulation tissue shrinkage to pull on the wound margin, leading to wound contraction. The myofibroblast theory further proposes that the coordinated contraction (cellular shortening) of many myofibroblasts, synchronized with the help of gap junctions, generates the force necessary for wound contraction.[13]

The traction theory proposes that fibroblasts bring about a closer approximation of matrix fibrils by exerting "traction forces" (analogous to the traction of wheels on tarmac) on extracellular matrix fibers to which they're attached. This theory proposes that fibroblasts neither shorten in length nor do they act in a coordinated multicellular manner (as proposed by the myofibroblast theory); rather, a composite force, made up of traction forces of many individual fibroblasts, is responsible for matrix contraction. Such traction forces act as shearing forces tangential to the cell surface generated during cell elongation and spreading. According to the traction theory, the composite effect of many fibroblasts gathering collagen fibrils within the wound is thought to bring about wound contraction.[14]

Maturation phase

The maturation phase normally starts 7 days after injury and may last for 1 year or more. The initial component in the deposited ECM is fibronectin and this forms a provisional fiber network. Other components include hyaluronic acid and proteoglycans. The network has two main roles: as a substratum for the migration and growth of cells, and as a template for subsequent collagen deposition. Collagen deposition becomes the predominant constituent of the matrix and soon forms fibrillar bundles and provides stiffness and tensile strength to the wound.

Collagen deposition and remodeling contribute to the increased tensile strength of skin wounds. Within 3 weeks of injury, the tensile strength is restored to approximately 20% of normal, uninjured skin. As healing continues, the skin gradually reaches a maximum of 70% to

Summary of wound healing

The following is a summary of the events that occur during the phases of wound healing.

HEMOSTASIS

Platelets ⟶ Release cytokines (PDGF, TGFβ, EGF)

INFLAMMATORY PHASE

Tissue debris and pathogens ⟶ Attract macrophages and neutrophils, which are responsible for:
- phagocytosis
- producing biological regulators, bioactive lipids, and proteolytic enzymes.

PROLIFERATIVE PHASE

Fibroblasts ⟶ Responsible for:
- synthesizing and depositing extracellular proteins
- producing growth factors
- producing angiogenic factors.

Extracellular matrix (ECM) and granulation tissue ⟶ ECM comprised of:
- collagens and elastin
- adhesive proteins
- fibronectin and lamina
- polysaccharides
- proteoglycans
- glycosaminoglycans.

Angiogenesis ⟶ Capillary growth into ECM

ECM

Capillaries

Reepithelialization ⟶ Migration of marginal basal cells across the provisional matrix

Wound contraction ⟶ Contraction of fibroblasts and myofibroblasts to bring wound edges closer

(continued)

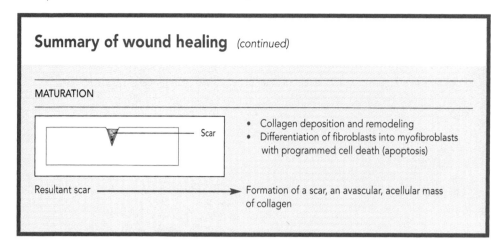

Summary of wound healing (*continued*)

MATURATION

- Collagen deposition and remodeling
- Differentiation of fibroblasts into myofibroblasts with programmed cell death (apoptosis)

Scar

Resultant scar ⟶ Formation of a scar, an avascular, acellular mass of collagen

80% tensile strength. Different organs regain tensile strengths to differing degrees. The remodeling process involves the balance between the synthesis and degradation of collagen. A range of collagenases regulates the latter. This process is also characterized by a gradual reduction in cellularity and vascularity. Differentiation of fibroblasts into myofibroblasts with resultant apoptosis (programmed cell death) are also features of tissue remodeling.[13]

PRACTICE POINT

A patient history should always include information about prior wounds. Healed wounds never achieve the same tensile strength as uninjured skin, thereby increasing the potential for reinjury.

The scar is the final product of wound healing and is a relatively avascular and acellular mass of collagen, which serves to restore tissue continuity and some degree of tensile strength and function. However, the strength of the scar remains less than that of normal tissue, even many years following injury, and it's never fully restored. (See *Summary of wound healing*, page 67.)

Healing in acute and chronic wounds

There would appear to be little consensus regarding the definition of acute and chronic wound etiologies. Chronicity implies a prolonged or lengthy healing process, whereas acute implies uncomplicated, orderly or organized, or rapid healing. Bates-Jensen and Wethe[15] define an acute wound as "a disruption in the integrity of the skin and underlying tissues that progress through the healing process in a timely and uncomplicated manner." Typically, surgical and traumatic wounds, which heal by primary intention, are classified as acute. (See *Wound healing by primary intention*.)

On the other hand, Sussman[16] defines a chronic wound as "one that deviates from expected sequence of repair in terms of time, appearance, and response to aggressive and appropriate treatment." The Wound Healing Society uses the definition of chronic wound as proposed in 1992 by Lazarus and colleagues: Chronic wounds "fail to progress through a normal, orderly, and timely sequence of repair or wounds that pass through the repair process without restoring anatomic and functional results."[17] Such wounds usually heal by

Wound healing by primary intention

The illustrations below depict wound healing by primary intention. This involves little tissue loss; the wound edges can be brought together without tension and glued or sutured.

In primary closure, epithelial migration is short-lived and may be completed within 72 hours.[38] Within 24 to 48 hours, epithelial cells migrate from the wound edges in a linear movement along the cut margins of the dermis. In partial-thickness wounds, such as superficial burns and traumatic injuries, epithelial cells also migrate from sweat and sebaceous glands and hair follicles, forming islands of epithelial tissue and producing more rapid closure.

1. TISSUE INJURY IS PRESENT WITHOUT TISSUE LOSS.

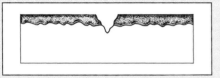

2. SKIN EDGES ARE BROUGHT TOGETHER AND GLUED.

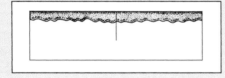

3. SKIN EDGES ARE BROUGHT TOGETHER AND SUTURED.

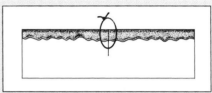

4. HEALING OCCURS WITH MINIMAL SCARRING.

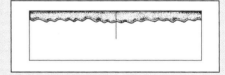

secondary intention and are associated with pathology; for example, diabetes, ischemic disease, pressure damage, and inflammatory diseases. (See *Wound healing by secondary intention,* page 70.)

The physiological differences between wounds that heal slowly and those that heal rapidly have been studied in a variety of ways. (See *Biochemical differences in healing wounds,* page 71.) One experiment explored the effect of chronic wound fluid on cell function.[18] Researchers cultured fibroblasts from human neonatal foreskin to use as a laboratory model of acute wounds. They then exposed the model to either chronic wound fluid or a control, and found that chronic wound fluid dramatically inhibited the growth of the fibroblasts. According to Phillips et al.,[18] these re-

sults indicate that the microenvironment of chronic wounds impairs wound healing.

Nonresolving inflammation has also been associated with chronic wounds by other researchers.[5,19] Prolonged inflammation is believed to be the most significant factor in delayed healing, as these wounds contain abnormally high levels of proteinases and proinflammatory cytokines. In acute wounds the chemical signals that control inflammation aren't active after the first few days following injury, and the healing process proceeds to the next stage. Hart[5] suggests several factors that may induce chronicity, including recurrent physical trauma; ischemic reperfusion injury; subclinical bacterial contamination, and foreign bodies. In particular, Hart[5] proposes

Wound healing by secondary intention

1. In a surgical excision with tissue loss, skin edges can't be brought together.

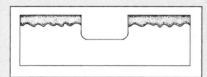

2. In a chronic wound such as a pressure ulcer, the ulcer undermines the skin edges.

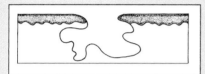

3. A layer of granulation tissue gradually covers the wound.

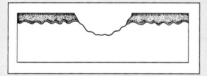

4. Wound contraction brings the wound edges together.

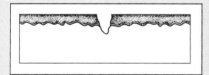

5. Wound closure is complete with scar.

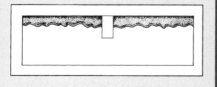

that the prolonged inflammatory phase is due to the presence of inflammatory leukocytes, typically neutrophils and their production of proinflammatory cytokines that perpetuate inflammation. He argues that a further process delays healing — the release of tissue-damaging proteinases, which degrade newly formed tissues — delaying or preventing the normal wound healing processes to proceed.

Chronic wounds are typically characterized by full-thickness tissue loss. Reepithelialization will take longer in full-thickness wounds due to the loss of appendages.[3] Normally, epithelial cells require the smooth, moist surface of the basement membrane to move across the wound. In wounds healing by secondary intention, epithelial cells latch on to and pull themselves across the scaffolding of macromolecules of the provisional matrix such as laminin and fibronectin.

PRACTICE POINT

The width of the resultant scar of a wound healing by secondary intention will be about 10% of the original defect. This is due to the process of wound contraction, working in conjunction with proliferation.

Wound measurement tools and techniques

Evaluating and measuring wound healing over time provides clinicians, patients, and reimbursement agencies with an indication of the success of treatment. In the United States, proper documentation of the wound healing status also becomes paramount in litigation cases.[20] A number of methods for measuring healing

Biochemical differences in healing wounds

Acute wounds	Chronic wounds
BIOCHEMICAL ANALYSIS OF WOUND FLUIDS	
• High cell mitosis	• Low cell mitosis
• Low inflammatory cytokines	• High inflammatory cytokines
• Low proteases (MMP)	• High proteases (MMP)
BIOCHEMICAL RESPONSE OF CELLS	
• Increased levels of growth factors	• Decreased response to growth factors
• Cells capable of rapid response	• Senescent cells

Adapted with permission of HMP Communications from "Biochemical Differences in the Molecular Environments of Healing and Chronic Wounds." In: Schultz, G., and Mast, B. "Molecular Analysis of the Environment of Healing and Chronic Wounds: Cytokines, Proteases, and Growth Factors," *Wounds* 10:(6 Suppl F) 1F9F, 1998.

have been developed. (See *Techniques for measuring wound area and volume,* page 72.) Elements of measurement include area and volume, and these measurements may be obtained in a variety of ways. Some methods are better-suited for use in clinical practice, whereas others are more suited for research. Some measurement tools are specific for certain types of wounds. For example, the Pressure Sore Status Tool and the Pressure Ulcer Scale for Healing were created to measure healing over time in pressure ulcers. (See chapter 13, Pressure ulcers.)

Measuring wound area

For wounds that have superficial tissue loss, are shallow, and don't extend under the skin edge, regular measurement of wound area provides an indication of progress toward complete healing. The techniques described below will enable you to calculate a numerical value and chart the patient's progress over time.

Surface tracing

The surface area of a wound can be calculated in a number of ways. In acetate tracing, for example, a sheet of clear acetate film is placed directly onto the surface of a wound, and the wound perimeter is traced using an indelible ink pen. (See *Acetate tracing,* page 73.) In addition, acetate sheets with printed squares may be used, and the squares counted. Acetate tracing requires no special equipment, but the technique is time-consuming and if the wound extends over several half or quarter squares, its size can be difficult to estimate. Sussman[21] suggests that in addition to calculating area, acetate sheets can also be used to record different wound bed conditions, such as area of necrosis and erythema.

Computerized systems, which have been demonstrated to be accurate in calculating wound area,[22,23] can be used in conjunction with acetate tracings. The outline of the wound is retraced using a

Techniques for measuring wound area and volume

Techniques used to measure wound area include:

- surface tracing
- photography (including Polaroid photography, stereophotogrammetry, and digital photography)
- digital imaging (tracing on a computer model instead of directly on the patient's skin)
- structured light.

Techniques used to measure wound volume include:

- linear measurement (measuring length, depth, and width using a ruler, Kundin gauge, Wound Stick Tunneler, or Wound Stick Wand)
- stereophotogrammetry
- molding or liquid displacement
- structured light.

computer mouse or pen, and the area is calculated using a software package. This system is much easier to use than acetate tracings alone; however, its accuracy may be limited due to the subjectivity inherent in determining the edge of a wound. Interobservers may perceive the wound edge differently, thereby further affecting the accuracy of the technique.[24]

Photography

If taken from the same distance and angle, a photograph can provide a clear and permanent image of the progress of a wound over time. Compared with assessments undertaken at the bedside, the use of photographs for assessing wounds has shown good interobserver and intra-observer reliability.[25] Several types of photography, varying in sophistication, can be used.

Polaroid photography

Polaroid film is available with and without grids imprinted on the film. The grid film can be used to calculate wound area, and the non-grid film used to record the condition of the wound bed. The camera has a toggled string attached to it to help the user keep the camera at the same distance from the wound when taking photographs on subsequent occasions. The greatest advantage of this system is that it allows the user to see the photograph develop immediately after it's taken. In addition, Polaroid photographs are inexpensive, can be stored in the patient's notes, and allow both clinicians and patients to see the progress the wound has made. One disadvantage of Polaroid photographs is that the quality isn't as good as more modern techniques such as digital photographs.

Stereophotogrammetry

In stereophotogrammetry, a video camera is used to take an image of the wound, which is then downloaded into a computer and a software package is used to calculate the area. Langemo et al.[24] report that this system is an accurate, unbiased method of calculating wound area. Stereophotogrammetry provides a printed image of the wound that can be stored in the patient's record, while also storing the information on computer and monitoring progress over time. However, this technology is expensive and not readily available to many clinicians. It's reported to require specialized training, and can take up to 20 minutes per patient to capture the wound image.[26]

Digital photography

Small and easily portable, digital cameras are becoming increasingly popular and are an inexpensive method of capturing and storing wound images. These images can be transferred onto a computer and stored as a record of the patient's progress over time. It's likely that this method will become more widespread in the future.

PRACTICE POINT

Consider your working environment. What's the most useful and practical type of photography that you could employ?

Digital imagery and mouse

A digital camera can be used to record an image of a wound while avoiding direct contact with the patient's skin. The recorded image is brought up on the computer screen and the mouse is used to trace around the wound perimeter, after which the specially designed software calculates the wound area. Taylor[27,28] and Richard et al.[29] report this method to be both reproducible and accurate in calculating wound area. Other researchers report that measuring leg ulcer areas using a computer-aided tracing of digital camera images is more accurate and quicker than using acetate tracings.[30] They recommend that care be taken when capturing the image, as the system requires digital images of good quality. Samad et al.[30] also suggest that digital cameras have much potential in the future. The increasing use of telemedicine has been beneficial in the management of patients with pressure ulcers.[31] However, some researchers have argued that because computerized images may be modified by saving, processing, and resolution, the color quality

Acetate tracing

The photo below shows how to use an ink marker and acetate sheet to trace the perimeter of a wound. Acetate sheets are available as two-layer systems. The inner layer, which comes into contact with the wound, is discarded, and the outer layer remains clean and is retained as a permanent record.

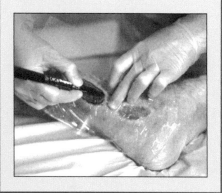

may not accurately reflect the real-life wound situation.[32]

Structured light

Parallel rays of light are shone at an angle over the wound and a camera connected to a computer records the image at a right angle to the surface of the wound.[33] The perimeter of the wound is traced using the mouse and the software is used to calculate wound area.

Measuring wound volume

For wounds that are deep and extend under the skin edge, calculating volume provides an indication of progress toward closure. As with calculating area, the following techniques describe a numerical value to be determined and used to chart progress over time.

Kundin gauge

The Kundin gauge is a disposable paper measurement device comprised of three rulers at right angles to each other. The device is placed into a cavity wound to measure its length, width, and depth.

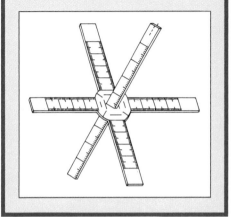

Linear measurements

Dealey[26] describes using a ruler to measure wound length, depth, and width as one of the simplest ways of estimating wound volume. However, she highlights the inaccuracy associated with using this technique, especially when it's used over time and by different clinicians.

Cooper[34] suggests marking the length, width, and depth of a wound using an ink marker, either on a cotton-tipped applicator or on a gloved finger. Sussman[21] describes the use of commercially available devices—the Wound Stick Tunneler and Wound Stick Wand. These devices are sterile, long, thin rulers, one made of metal and the other of plastic, which are gently inserted into the wound cavity until they touch the wound edge. Kundin[35] described the development of the Kundin gauge as a method for measuring wounds with an irregular shape, or those that un-

dermined the skin edges. Three flexible paper rulers are placed at right angles into the wound, where the length, width, and depth can be read. (See *Kundin gauge.*) Cooper[34] reviewed the research related to the use of the Kundin gauge and reported problems associated with reliability when this device is used by different clinicians. She cites one study in particular[36] in which the correlation between acetate tracings and photographs was higher (r = 0.99) than between the Kundin gauge, photographs, and tracings.

> **PRACTICE POINT**
>
> Consider how the wound documentation system currently used in your facility supports the wound measurement techniques described here. Could you easily document the measurement values provided?

Stereophotogrammetry

Previously described for measuring wound area, stereophotogrammetry can also be used to calculate wound volume. When estimating volume, a three-dimensional image is obtained by taking two photographs simultaneously from different angles.[26]

Molding or liquid displacement

Wound volume can be estimated by filling a wound with a solid material (typically an alginate dental impression material) and using the mold to displace water and calculate volume. Alternatively, the wound can be filled with a known volume of water, estimating volume in a similar way. These methods have been described since 1966 and are frequently reported to be impractical, time-consuming, and messy.[34,37] Techniques that use molding and fluid displacement would appear to have limited application in modern wound management.

Structured light

Parallel beams of structured light can also be used to calculate wound volume. When measuring volume, the computer calculates where the surface of the wound should be and where it is from the deflection of the rays. The software uses the angles of deflection to produce a three-dimensional representation of the wound, and from these measurements calculates volume. This device can't measure what it can't see, and is only of benefit in measuring wounds of even contour rather than wounds that are deep or undermine the skin edge.

PRACTICE POINT

Ask your patient what he'd like to know about wound measurements. Try to ascertain his level of knowledge regarding measurements.

Summary

Understanding the processes by which wounds heal and incorporating this knowledge into practice is a key responsibility for clinicians who treat patients with wounds. The ability to recognize the normal wound healing process also enables the clinician to recognize what's abnormal when wounds are failing to heal.

Link the physiology of wound healing to your practical management of patients. Review wound documentation practices used in your facility — do they facilitate the application of theory to practice?

By identifying wound healing problems early, clinicians are in a position to facilitate referral to colleagues. For example, a patient's surgical wound that remains in the inflammatory phase for too long may require further investigation and possibly more surgery.

Measuring the wound as it proceeds from injury toward complete closure is a vital component of evaluating the success or progress of treatment. Regular and ongoing wound measurements provide documentation of the care given to patients for the purposes of communicating with colleagues. This also provides a way of auditing patient outcomes. The wound measurement technique employed and the wound measurement tool selected will depend upon the needs of the patient, the availability of the technology, and the skills of the clinician. For example, a community-based nurse might elect to use acetate tracings or digital photographs, which are downloaded onto a computer upon returning to the office. On the other hand, a researcher may elect to use stereophotogrammetry in carrying out a study investigating the effectiveness of leg ulcer treatments.

As we care for patients in a rapidly changing world, new knowledge about the biochemical processes in wound healing and their application to clinicians is imperative. Technology has improved communication, as clinicians and researchers can access research and information from all around the world. By seeking the answers to the complex questions of the biochemical processes and differences of how acute and chronic wounds heal, we'll continue to enhance our understanding of wound healing and incorporate new theories into practice.

Show what you know

1. Immediately following tissue injury, the priority is:

  A. to modify the immature scar tissue.
  B. to achieve rapid hemostasis.
  C. to rapidly fill the wounded area with granulation tissue.
  D. to destroy bacteria.

ANSWER: B. Rapid hemostasis is essential as it preserves the integrity of the closed and high-pressure circulatory system to limit blood loss.

2. The main mechanism by which chronic wounds fail to heal is believed to be:

  A. too rapid progress from hemostasis to maturation.
  B. a failure of fibroblasts and myofibroblasts to facilitate wound contraction.
  C. a dysfunction of collagen remodeling.
  D. a prolonged inflammatory phase.

ANSWER: D. Because chronic wounds contain abnormally high levels of proteinases and proinflammatory cytokines, prolonged inflammation is believed to be the most significant factor in delayed healing.

3. During the proliferative phase, the framework that new tissue grows into is commonly called:

  A. the extracellular matrix.
  B. the complement system.
  C. chemotaxis.
  D. apoptosis.

ANSWER: A. New tissue, or granulation tissue, grows into the extracellular matrix, which is composed of neovascular tissue, collagens, fibronectin, and proteoglycans.

4. In everyday clinical practice, the most straightforward method of measuring the area of a leg ulcer is likely to be:

  A. to use a Kundin gauge.
  B. to take an acetate tracing.
  C. to use structured light.
  D. to use a Wound Stick Tunneler.

ANSWER: B. Because no special equipment is required, acetate tracing is a straightforward method for measuring the area of a wound.

References

1. Witte, M., and Barbul, A. "General Principles of Wound Healing," *Surgical Clinics of North America* 77:509, June 1997.
2. Steed, D. "The Role of Growth Factors in Wound Healing," *Surgical Clinics of North America* 77:575, June 1997.
3. Martin, P. "Wound Healing: Aiming for Perfect Skin Regeneration," *Science* 276:75, April 1997.
4. Slavin, J. "Wound Healing: Pathophysiology," *Surgery* 17(4):I-V, April 1999.
5. Hart, J. "Inflammation 2: Its Role in the Healing of Chronic Wounds," *Journal of Wound Care* 11:245-49, July 2002.
6. Stephens, P., and Thomas, D.W. "The Cellular Proliferative Phase of the Wound Repair Process," *Journal of Wound Care* 11:253-61, July 2002.
7. Wysocki, A.B. "Anatomy and Physiology of Skin and Soft Tissue," *Acute and Chronic Wounds: Nursing Management.* Edited by Bryant, R.A. St. Louis: Mosby–Year Book, Inc., 2000.
8. Clark, R.A.F. *The Molecular and Cellular Biology of Wound Repair,* 2nd ed. New York: Plenum Publishing Corp., 1996.
9. Neal, M. "Angiogenesis: Is It the Key to Controlling the Healing Process?" *Journal of Wound Care* 10(7):281-87, July 2001.
10. Calvin, M. "Cutaneous Wound Repair," *Wounds* 10(1):12, January 1998.
11. Rohovsky, S., and D'Amore, P. "Growth Factors and Angiogenesis in Wound Healing," in Ziegler, T., et al., eds. *Growth Factors and Wound Healing: Basic Science and Potential Clinical Applications.* New York: Springer-Verlag New York, Inc., 1997.

12. Berry, D.P., et al. "Human Wound Contraction: Collagen Organisation, Fibroblasts and Myofibroblasts," *Plastic and Reconstructive Surgery* 102(1):124-31, July 1998.

13. Tejero-Trujeque, R. "Understanding the Final Stages of Wound Contraction," *Journal of Wound Care* 10(7):259-63, July 2001.

14. Ehrlich, P. "The Physiology of Wound Healing: A Summary of the Normal and Abnormal Wound Healing Processes," *Advanced Wound Care* 11(7):326, November-December 1998.

15. Bates-Jensen, B.M., and Wethe, J. "Acute Surgical Wound Management," in Sussman, C., and Bates-Jensen, B.M., eds. *Wound Care: A Collaborative Practice Manual for Physical Therapists and Nurses.* Gaithersburg, Md.: Aspen Pubs., Inc, 1998.

16. Sussman, C. "Wound Healing Biology and Chronic Wound Healing," in Sussman, C., and Bates-Jensen, B.M., eds., *Wound Care: A Collaborative Practice Manual for Physical Therapists and Nurses.* Gaithersburg, Md.: Aspen Pubs., Inc, 1998.

17. Lazarus, G.S., et al. "Definitions and Guidelines for Assessment for Wounds and Evaluation of Healing," *Archives of Dermatology* 130(4):489-93, April 1994.

18. Phillips, T.J., et al. "Effect of Chronic Wound Fluid on Fibroblasts," *Journal of Wound Care* 7(10):527-32, November 1998.

19. Yager, D.R., and Nwomeh, B.C. "The Proteolytic Environment of Chronic Wounds," *Wound Repair and Regeneration* 7(6):433-41, November-December 1999.

20. Goldman, R.J., and Salcido, R. "More than One Way to Measure a Wound: An Overview of Tools and Techniques," *Advances in Skin & Wound Care* 15(5):236-45, September-October 2002.

21. Sussman, C. "Wound Measurement," in Sussman, C., and Bates-Jensen, B.M., eds., *Wound Care: A Collaborative Practice Manual for Physical Therapists and Nurses.* Gaithersburg, Md.: Aspen Pubs., Inc., 1998.

22. Charles, H. "Wound Assessment: Measuring the Area of a Leg Ulcer," *British Journal of Nursing* 7(13):765-68, July 1998.

23. Oien, R.F., et al. "Measuring the Size of Ulcers by Planimetry: A Useful Method in the Clinical Setting," *Journal of Wound Care* 11(5):165-68, May 2002.

24. Langemo D K, et al. "Two-dimensional Wound Measurement: Comparison of Four Techniques," *Advances in Wound Care* 11(7):337-43, November-December 1998.

25. Houghton, P.E., et al. "Photographic Assessment of the Appearance of Chronic Pressure and Leg Ulcers," *Ostomy/Wound Management* 46(4):20-30, April 2000.

26. Dealey, C. "General Principles of Wound Management," in *The Care of Wounds: A Guide for Nurses.* Oxford: Blackwell Science, 1999.

27. Taylor, R.J. "Mouseyes: An Aid to Wound Measurement Using a Computer," *Journal of Wound Care* 6(3):123-26, March 1997.

28. Taylor, R.J. "Mouseyes Revisited: Upgrading a Computer Program that Aids Wound Measurement," *Journal of Wound Care* 11(6):213-16, June 2002.

29. Richard, J.L., et al. "Of Mice and Wounds: Reproducibility and Accuracy of a Novel Planimetry Program for Measuring Wound Area," *Wounds* 12(6):148-54, November 2000.

30. Samad, A., et al. "Digital Imaging Versus Conventional Contact Tracing for the Objective Measurement of Venous Leg Ulcers," *Journal of Wound Care* 11(4):137-40, April 2002.

31. Vesmarovich, S., et al. "Use of Telerehabilitation to Manage Pressure Ulcers in Persons with Spinal Cord Injuries," *Advances in Wound Care* 12(5):264-69, June 1999.

32. Berriss, W.P., and Sangwine, S.J. "Automatic Quantitative Analysis of Healing Skin Wounds Using Colour Digital Image Processing, 1997" [Online]. Available: *www.smtl.co.uk/World-Wide-Wounds/2002/* [2002 October].

33. Plassman, P., and Jones, T.D. "MAVIS – A Non-invasive Instrument to Measure the Area and Volume of Wounds," *Medical Engineering and Physics* 20(5):325-31, July 1998.

34. Cooper, D. "Assessment, Measurement, and Evaluation: Their Pivotal Role in Wound Healing," in Bryant, R.A., ed. *Acute and Chronic Wounds: Nursing Management.* St. Louis: Mosby–Year Book, Inc., 2000.

35. Kundin, J.I. "Designing and Developing a New Measurement Instrument," *Perioperative Nursing Quarterly* 1(4):40, December 1985.

36. Thomas, A.C., and Wysocki, A.B. "The Healing Wound: A Comparison of Three Clinically Useful Methods of Measurement," *Decubitus* 3(1):18, February 1990.

37. Bale, S., and Jones, V. *Wound Care Nursing: A Patient-centred Approach.* London: Baelliere Tindall, 1997.

38. Waldrop, J., and Doughty, D. "Wound-healing Physiology," in Edited by Bryant, R.A. *Acute and Chronic Wounds: Nursing Management.* St. Louis: Mosby–Year Book, Inc., 2000.

CHAPTER 6

Wound assessment

Sharon Baranoski, MSN, RN, CWOCN, APN, FAAN
Elizabeth A. Ayello, PHD, RN, APRN,BC, CWOCN, FAAN

OBJECTIVES

After completing this chapter, you'll be able to:

- state the reasons for doing a wound assessment

- differentiate between partial- and full-thickness injury

- list the parameters of a complete wound assessment.

The wound

The management of acute and chronic wounds has evolved into a highly specialized area of practice. An accurate and detailed wound assessment is vital to the care of patients with wounds. Care plans, treatment interventions, and ongoing management are based on initial and subsequent wound assessments. Assessment provides the key elements about the current status of a wound and is essential to the developments of all health care discipline interventions. The total patient assessment, inclusive of any comorbid conditions and lifestyle, must be a part of any comprehensive wound assessment. This chapter addresses the key assessment parameters of a patient with a wound admitted to any health care setting. The chapter content includes an explanation for the importance of a history and a physical examination, how to assess a wound, essential practice points, and documentation.

A wound is a disruption of normal anatomic structure and function.[1] Wounds are classified as acute or chronic. Acute wounds can be the result of trauma or surgery. According to Larazus,[1] acute wounds proceed through an orderly and timely healing process with the eventual return of anatomic and functional integrity. Chronic wounds, on the other hand, fail to proceed through this orderly and timely process and lose the cascade effect

The nine Cs of wound assessment

Wound assessment is needed for the nine reasons below:
- **C**ause of the wound
- **C**lear picture of what the wound looks like
- **C**omprehensive picture of the patient
- **C**ontributing factors
- **C**ommunication to other health care providers
- **C**ontinuity of care
- **C**entralized location for wound care information
- **C**omponents of the wound care plan
- **C**omplications from the wound.

of wound healing and sustained anatomic and functional integrity. "Simply stated, wounds may be classified as those that repair themselves or can be repaired in an orderly and timely process (acute wounds) and those that don't (chronic wounds)."[1]

The pathology or cause of the wound must be determined before appropriate interventions can be implemented. Wounds may have a surgical, traumatic, neuropathic, vascular, or pressure related etiology. For example, an acute wound caused by a bite (animal, insect, spider, or human) needs a different care plan than a burn wound. A patient who has an animal bite may require additional testing to rule out damage to nerves, tendons, ligaments, or bone, as well as determination of rabies or rabies vaccination status of the animal and the need for tetanus immunization.[2] The pathologic etiology will provide the basis for additional testing and evaluation to start the assessment process. (See *The nine Cs of wound assessment*.)

tient is taking, and a family history of conditions that can have an impact on the etiology of the wound. In addition, the patient history may reveal information that explains poor healing. A thorough patient history helps focus your questioning on issues that could direct your initial interventions, such as vascular studies, glucose testing, and oxygen perfusion testing.[3] Therapies received as part of a prior health condition, such as radiation at the site of the wound, are also important factors that can contribute to impaired healing and delay appropriate management strategies.[1]

Family support and functional abilities should be evaluated as well. Can the patient care for himself? Is there anyone at home to assist with care after discharge? Can the patient change his own dressings? Who will put on compression stockings? Can the patient afford to purchase the necessary items? These questions are essential elements of a comprehensive assessment of the patient with a wound.

Initial assessment

Obtain a thorough history and a complete physical examination on every patient admitted to your care. Obtaining a patient history provides information on disease processes, medications the pa-

Physical examination

A head-to-toe physical examination should be done to evaluate all skin areas, pressure points, old scars, indications of any prior surgeries, and the presence of vascular or pressure ulcers. The appearance of the skin, nails, and hair on the extremities should be noted. Evaluation of skin color, temperature, capillary refill, pulses, and edema are essential elements of a good physical examination.[3]

Different types of wounds require many different considerations. Dehisced surgical wounds may have opened due to an infection, or may heal poorly due to underlying disease processes or current medications (such as steroids). Hemosiderin staining due to the chronic leakage of red blood cells into the soft tissue of the lower leg is a classic sign of venous insufficiency. If not managed with compression, this leakage often leads to venous ulcers. Hemosiderin deposits (reddish-brown color) are often seen in patients with venous ulcers. Arterial ulcers often present with the classic signs of hair loss, weak or absent pulse, and very thin, shiny, taut skin. Neuropathic ulcers require intense evaluation of the extent of the neuropathy.[4] Patients with diabetes are prone to callus formations and off-loading tension pressure points, both of which are easily noted on an examination. Examination of the total patient will reveal areas of concern and areas that can relate to why the patient has a wound and, if it isn't healing, why healing isn't taking place. Developing a realistic goal and care plan, performing regular follow-up, and ensuring patient compliance are the markers for successful outcomes.

Wound assessment

Wound assessment—a written record or picture of the progress of the wound—is a cumulative process of observation, data collection, and evaluation. As such, it's an important component of patient care. A wound assessment includes a record of your initial assessment, ongoing changes, and treatment interventions.

>
>
> PRACTICE POINT ▬
>
> ### When to reassess a wound
>
> Assessment provides indicators of successful treatment interventions and attainment of achievable outcomes, and guides decisions about product changes. Reassess the patient's wound:
> - after the patient returns from surgery
> - if the wound noticeably deteriorates
> - if the wound becomes odorous or has new purulent exudate
> - upon observing any other significant change in the condition of the wound
> - after the patient has returned from another facility.

Frequency of wound assessment is often determined by the patient's health care setting. Acute-care patients receive wound assessments daily or with each dressing change. Long-term care facilities may assess on admission and weekly. Home-care assessments are usually based on the frequency of the home visits. Regardless of setting, the frequency of reassessment should be determined by the wound characteristics observed at the previous dressing change, or on the physician's or other practitioner's orders. The effectiveness of interventions can't be ascertained unless baseline assessment data are compared to follow-up data.[5] (See *When to reassess a wound*.)

No written standard exists outlining the type and amount of information to include in a wound assessment; likewise, no single documentation chart or tool has been designated as the most effective. Several studies[6,7] found that wound assessments were documented significantly more frequently when an assessment chart is used (and that using a chart improves the nurses' assessment skills). Numerous documentation methods are available.[1,3-4,8] The most successful assessment form in any facility is the one completed and used by the facility's staff. If the staff finds a form too long or difficult to use, it won't be utilized. Forms that can be completed easily and quickly will be used.

A minimal wound assessment should include the following: a thorough look at the whole patient, etiology or type of wound, and wound characteristics such as location, size, depth, exudate, tissue type. (See chapter 4, Skin: An essential organ.) Wounds can be classified using several different approaches. The partial- versus full-thickness model is used primarily by physicians and clinicians for wounds other than pressure ulcers. Damage to the epidermis and part of the dermis constitutes a partial-thickness wound. Abrasions, skin tears, blisters, and skin-graft donor sites are common examples of partial-thickness wounds. Full-thickness wounds extend through the epidermis and dermis and may extend into the subcutaneous tissue, fascia, and muscle.[3] Partial-thickness wounds heal by resurfacing or reepithelialization. Full-thickness wounds heal by secondary intention through the formation of granulation tissue, contraction and, finally, reepithelialization.

Pressure ulcers and neuropathic ulcers have their own staging and classification systems to indicate the depth of injury and healing methods. (See chapter 13, Pressure ulcers, and chapter 15, Diabetic foot ulcers.) Assessing the severity of a burn is a two-part process. Burn injuries are described by the extent of the body burned using one of several methods for estimating burn size, such as the Rule of Nines or Lund and Browder Chart. The depth of a burn injury is described by clinical observation of the anatomic layer of the skin involved (superficial, partial-thickness, full-thickness, or subdermal burns).[9]

Many parameters should be considered when you're performing a compre-hensive wound assessment. Whether using a stage, grade, or partial- and full-thickness terminology, the one constant is clinical assessment. Assessment data gives the health care provider a mechanism to communicate, improve continuity among disciplines, and establish appropriate treatment modalities.

Elements of a wound assessment

In 1992, Ayello[8] developed a mnemonic for pressure ulcer assessment and documentation. (See *Pressure ulcer ASSESSMENT chart*.) The mnemonic has been adapted for use with any type of wound to provide a thorough look at the parameters that complete and enhance an assessment. It provides a support structure, in chart format, for clinical decision-making regarding ongoing assessment and reassessment. The mnemonic can be used in any practice setting and according to the guidelines set up by your facility. You may choose to use this assessment chart daily, weekly, or monthly. It's simple, fast, and can be further adapted to fit individual use. (See *Wound ASSESSMENTS chart*, page 84.)

Location and age of wound

Wound location should be documented using the correct anatomical terms—for example, right great trochanter rather than right hip. How long has the patient had the wound? Are you dealing with a new, acute wound or a wound that has failed to heal for several weeks or months. Include a drawing of the human body with the wound's location noted on the drawing in your assessment record to provide complete admission documentation.

Size and stage

Measurement of a wound is an important part of the initial assessment. Wound measurements are also an invaluable tool for documenting the progres-

Pressure ulcer ASSESSMENT chart[8]

PATIENT'S NAME: _____ AGE: _____ ❑ M ❑ F

DATE: _____ TIME: _____ NUMBER OF PRESSURE ULCERS _____

A ANATOMIC LOCATION OF WOUND
❑ Sacrum ❑ Elbow ❑ R ❑ L
❑ Trochanter ❑ R ❑ L ❑ Incisional
❑ Ischium ❑ R ❑ L ❑ Other
❑ Heel ❑ R ❑ L
❑ Lateral malleolus ❑ R ❑ L
AGE OF WOUND
____days or ____months patient has had the pressure ulcer

S SIZE
____cm length ____cm width ____cm depth
SHAPE
❑ Oval ❑ Round
❑ Other _____
STAGE
Pressure ulcer stage:
❑ Stage I ❑ Stage II ❑ Stage III ❑ Stage IV
❑ Unable to determine stage; ulcer is necrotic
Wagner ulcer grade for neurotrophic ulcers:
❑ 0 ❑ 1 ❑ 2 ❑ 3 ❑ 4 ❑ 5

S SINUS TRACT, TUNNELING,
UNDERMINING, FISTULAS
❑ Sinus tract, tunneling (narrow tracts under the skin) at ____ o'clock
❑ Undermining (bigger area [than tunneling] of tissue destruction — area is more like a cave than a tract)

E EXUDATE
Color
❑ Serous ❑ Serosanguineous ❑ Sanguineous
Amount
❑ Scant ❑ Moderate ❑ Large
Consistency
❑ Clear ❑ Purulent

S SEPSIS
❑ Local ❑ Systemic ❑ None

S SURROUNDING SKIN
❑ Dark ❑ Discolored ❑ Erythematous
❑ Intact ❑ Swollen
❑ Other _____

M MARGINS
❑ Attached (edges are connected to the sides of the wound)
❑ Not attached (edges aren't connected to the sides of the wound)
❑ Rolled (edges appear rounded or rolled over)
MACERATION
❑ Present ❑ Not present

E ERYTHEMA
❑ Present ❑ Not present
EPITHELIALIZATION
❑ Present ❑ Not present
ESCHAR (NECROTIC TISSUE)
❑ Yellow slough ❑ Black ❑ Soft ❑ Hard
❑ Stringy
Area around eschar is:
❑ Dry ❑ Moist ❑ Reddened

N NECROTIC TISSUE
❑ Present ❑ Not present
NOSE
❑ Odor present ❑ Odor not present
NEOVASCULARIZATION
(BLOOD VESSELS ARE VISIBLE)
❑ Present ❑ Not present

T TISSUE BED
❑ Granulation tissue present ❑ Not present
TENDERNESS TO TOUCH
❑ No pain
❑ Pain present:
❑ On touch
❑ Anytime
❑ Only when performing ulcer care
Patient getting pain medication:
❑ Yes ❑ No
TENSION
❑ Tautness, hardness present ❑ Not present
TEMPERATURE
❑ Skin warm to touch ❑ Skin cool to touch
❑ Normal

Wound ASSESSMENTS chart

PATIENT'S NAME: _____ AGE: _____

ASSESSMENT DATE: _____ REASSESSMENT DUE DATE: _____

Wound etiology:
❑ Surgical ❑ Arterial ❑ Venous ❑ Pressure ulcer
❑ Diabetic or neurotrophic ulcer ❑ Other

A **ANATOMIC LOCATION OF WOUND**
❑ Upper/lower chest ❑ Abdomen ❑ Back
❑ Sacrum ❑ Foot ❑ R ❑ L ❑ Other ❑ R ❑ L
❑ Trochanter ❑ R ❑ L ❑ Ischium ❑ R ❑ L
❑ Elbow ❑ R ❑ L ❑ Arm ❑ R ❑ L
❑ Leg ❑ R ❑ L ❑ Heel ❑ R ❑ L
❑ Lateral malleolus ❑ R ❑ L
❑ Medial malleolus ❑ R ❑ L
AGE OF WOUND
❑ Acute: post op < 7 days ❑ Acute: post op > 7days
❑ Chronic: < 1 month
❑ Chronic: > 1 month _____ Days/months

S **SIZE, SHAPE, STAGE**
_____cm width_____cm length_____cm diameter
SHAPE
❑ Oval ❑ Round ❑ Irregular ❑ Other _____
STAGE
Stage of pressure ulcer
❑ I ❑ II ❑ III ❑ IV ❑ Unable to stage; ulcer necrotic
Wagner ulcer grade for neurotrophic ulcers
❑ 0 ❑ 1 ❑ 2 ❑ 3 ❑ 4 ❑ 5

S **SINUS TRACT, TUNNELING, UNDERMINING,**
FISTULAS
❑ None ❑ Present: located _____ at
_____ o'clock, _____ cm depth

E **EXUDATE**
Amount
❑ None ❑ Scant ❑ Moderate ❑ Large
Color ❑ Serous ❑ Serosanguineous ❑ Sanguineous
Consistency: ❑ Thick ❑ Purulent ❑ Milky

S **SEPSIS**
❑ Systemic ❑ Local ❑ Both ❑ None
❑ Odor present

S **SURROUNDING SKIN**
❑ Intact ❑ Erythematous ❑ Edematous
❑ Induration ❑ Warm ❑ Cool
❑ Discolored ❑ Dry ❑ Other

M **MACERATION**
❑ Not present
❑ Present: _____cm, location_____

E **EDGES, EPITHELIALIZATION**
❑ Edge attached ❑ Edge not attached
❑ Edges rolled
❑ Surgical incision approximated
❑ Surgical incision open ❑ Sutures/staples intact
❑ Epithelialization present: _____ cm
❑ Epithelialization not present

N **NECROTIC TISSUE**
❑ Not Present ❑ Present
Type
❑ Yellow slough ❑ Black ❑ Soft ❑ Hard ❑ Stringy
Percentage of wound (check closest percentage):
❑ 100% of wound ❑ 75% of wound
❑ 50% of wound ❑ 25% of wound
❑ Other: _____ %

T **TISSUE BED**
❑ Granulation tissue not present
❑ Granulation tissue present _____ amount%
❑ Moist ❑ Dry
Tenderness or pain
(0 being no pain, 10 being intense pain)
Pain scale score
0   1   2   3   4   5   6   7   8   9   10
Circle appropriate number
Pain present:
❑ on touch ❑ anytime
❑ only when performing wound care
❑ other (specify) _____
Pain management: Specify method _____
❑ Not effective ❑ Effective

S **STATUS**
Wound status: Initial assessment date _____
❑ Improved: date _____ ❑ Unchanged: date _____
❑ Healing: date _____ ❑ Deteriorating:* date _____
*Notify physician
❑ Supportive therapy
    ❑ compression ❑ off-loading
    ❑ pressure relieving mattress ❑ other _____
❑ Patient's perception on quality of life _____
❑ Referrals Specify to whom _____
Initial assessment:
Signature _____ Title _____ Date _____
Reassessment (per policy):
Signature _____ Title _____ Date _____

© Baranoski, S., and Ayello, E.A.

sion — or lack — of healing. Consistency in how the wound is measured is important for accuracy in determining wound improvement. Numerous centimeter (cm) measurement devices are available for use. Wounds shouldn't be measured using inches or an object, but by "cm" measurement, which is the preferred dimension of most clinicians. Linear measurements (length and width) are the most common recorded sizing dimensions in clinical practice. Linear measurements should be taken *at the greatest length and width perpendicular to each other*. (See *Wound measurement*.)

Wounds can also be measured by multiplying the length, width, and the greatest depth of the wound to determine the surface measurement. More experienced wound clinicians use this method to monitor healing — a decrease in surface measurement indicates progression of wound healing. Surgical incisions can be measured using length (for example, "Incision line is 8 cm long"). If the incision edges aren't closed by sutures, a width may also be obtained. If the wound is open, depth should also be assessed.

Wound area is calculated by multiplying the wound's perpendicular linear dimensions; the resulting number is recorded in cubic centimeters (cm^2). Although linear measurements may not be the most accurate because many wounds aren't rectangular in shape, they are still the most frequently used method in clinical settings. Other wound measurement methods include digital images, molds, planimetry, wound tracings, and computerized mapping programs. (See chapter 5, Acute and chronic wound healing.) More detailed measurements are often needed in research studies.

Wound depth is often excluded during assessment. Depth can be measured by using a cotton swab applicator or centimeter measuring device. (See *Determining wound depth*, page 86.) The NPUAP stag-

Wound measurement

Linear measurements of a wound should be taken at the greatest length and width perpendicular to each other, as shown below.

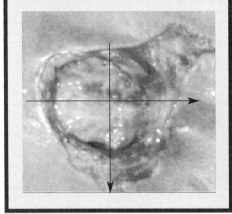

ing system is only intended to be used for pressure ulcers. (See chapter 13, Pressure ulcers.) The staging system addresses the depth of insult in stages I through IV. A pressure ulcer covered with eschar or necrotic tissue is unstageable as far as depth, but its length and width should still be measured to document the outer, visible wound size. (See *Necrotic, unstageable pressure ulcer*, page 87.)

Sinus tracts, undermining, and fistulas

A sinus tract (or tunnel) is a channel that extends from any part of the wound and may pass through subcutaneous tissue and muscle. The channel or pathway involves an area larger than the visible surface of the wound and may result in dead space and abscess formation, further complicating the healing process. Documenting sinus tracts is an important element in assessment because it enables the clinician to evaluate potential treatment interventions. Sinus tracts are

Determining wound depth

The depth of a wound can be measured by using a cotton swab applicator, as shown in the photographs below, or centimeter measuring device.

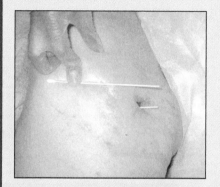

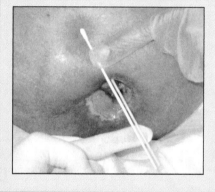

88.) Pressure ulcers that have been subjected to a shearing force often present with undermining in the area of the greatest shear. Undermining is also seen when the opening of the wound is smaller than the affected tissue of the wound below the dermis. Documentation of the location and amount of undermining is important. Clinicians can document using the clock figure, using the head as the 12 o'clock position (for example, "Undermining from 2 to 6 o'clock, measures 3 cm") or using percentages (for example, "75% of the wound has undermining measuring 2 cm"). Undermining may be more extensive in one part of a wound than another; that is, one part may exhibit extensive undermining whereas another part may not have any undermining. This, too, should be documented appropriately. Interventions include loosely packing or tucking all undermined areas to prevent buildup of debris and dead tissue, and applying an appropriate dressing, such as hydrogel, gauze, or alginate dressing.

Fistulas can develop in surgical wounds and in deep, severe pressure ulcers. Fistulas are named by using the point of origin, such as the rectum, and the point of exit, such as the vagina, which would be designated a rectovaginal fistula. A fistula connects viscous organs together (for example, rectovaginal fistula), or to the skin (for example, enterocutaneous fistula).[3] Management of patients with fistulas is complex and intense, and demands critical thinking skills as well as technical skills.[10] Fistulas can take weeks or months to heal. In addition, the patient with a fistula is often malnourished and may require weeks of intense nutrition therapy to improve.

Sinus tracts, undermining, and fistula formation delay the healing cascade and require added interventions and treatment costs. Intervening early with the appropriate medical, surgical, and nurs-

common in dehisced surgical wounds and may also be present in neuropathic and arterial wounds. Treatment interventions involve packing the dead space with an appropriate dressing to stimulate granulation and the contraction process. The tract is closed first, while the outside of the wound is allowed to remain open.

Undermining is tissue destruction that occurs around the wound perimeter underlying intact skin; in these wounds, the edges have pulled away from the wound's base. (See *Undermining,* page

ing actions is paramount to healing these complicated wounds.

Exudate

Exudate is the accumulation of fluids in the wound. The fluid may contain serum, cellular debris, bacteria, and leukocytes. It can appear as dry, dehydrated, dead, or nonviable tissue (nondraining) or be moist and draining. Exudate assessment includes the amount (scant, moderate, large), color, and consistency.

Exudate may be serous (clear or pale yellow), serosanguineous (serous or blood tinged), or sanguinous (bloody). The consistency of the exudate is also important (thick, milky, or purulent).

Sepsis

Sepsis is caused by anaerobes and gram-negative bacteria and can occur in any susceptible wound. To determine the presence of sepsis an assessment should include consideration of erythema, warmth, edema, purulent or increased drainage, induration, and increased tenderness or pain. If sepsis is present, it's important to determine whether the infection is local or systemic. Interventions are based on accurate assessment and laboratory support.

The best method to culture a wound to determine the presence of sepsis remains controversial. Tissue biopsy is the gold standard, followed by fluid aspiration. These options, however, may not be available in all settings and many clinicians lack the skill necessary to perform them. Many settings continue to use the swab method, in which the wound must be cleaned and thoroughly dried prior to swabbing for a culture.

Malodorous wounds should also be documented. However, make sure the odor is from the wound — not the dressing change, which is a common mistake. Not all odor indicates infection; certain dressings develop a distinct odor when exudate interacts with them. Odor can

---

Necrotic, unstageable pressure ulcer

Shown here is a pressure ulcer that is unstageable because it is covered with necrotic tissue.

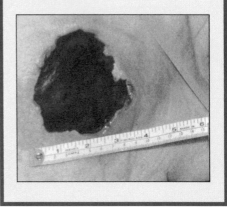

---

indicate the need to change the dressing more often. Certain organisms — such as pseudomonas — have a very distinct odor that's easily recognized by the trained clinician. (See chapter 7, Wound bioburden, for more detailed information on infection and culturing.)

 PRACTICE POINT

Remember that odor doesn't always indicate infection; it may signal the need for a dressing change.

Surrounding skin

The skin surrounding a wound also provides valuable information to the assessing clinician. Erythema and warmth may indicate an infection. Interruptions in periwound skin integrity (denudation, erosion, papules, or pustules) may indicate allergic reactions to tape or dressing adhesive. Maceration or desiccation may be a sign that the dressing isn't appropriate for the amount or type of exudate.

Undermining

Undermining, shown in the photographs below, is tissue destruction that occurs around the wound perimeter underlying intact skin.

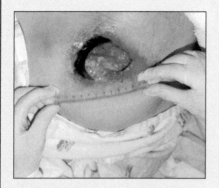

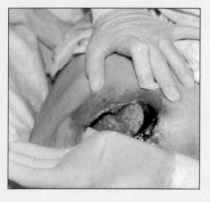

Palpation should be done with the fingertips around a wound surface. This may reveal induration or fluctuance, an abnormal fluid accumulation indicative of further tissue damage or abscess. Assessment of surrounding skin, while not the actual wound, provides useful information for the ongoing evaluation and future wound-care interventions.

Maceration

Maceration is a softening of the skin surrounding a wound due to excess drainage or pooling of fluid on intact skin. It appears as a white, waterlogged area. It may be due to inadequate management of exudate or an increase in exudate due to changes in the wound tissue. Maceration may be prevented by using an appropriate barrier cream around the wound, changing the dressing more often, or by selecting a more absorbent dressing.

Edges and epithelialization

Epithelialization is the regeneration of the epidermis across a wound surface.[10] The epithelial wound edge is continuous and often difficult to see. As wound migration occurs from the edges, the portion covered with epithelium is pearly or silver and shiny. It's also thin and fragile, and thereby easily insulted. The edge of a wound may be attached to the wound bed, unattached (undermining occurring), or rolled inward. Wound edges should be assessed as part of a thorough evaluation of the wound.

Examining the wound edges may reveal whether the wound is acute or chronic, and can often provide clues to the wound's etiology. For example, a wound with inflamed edges or violaceous with undermined borders may indicate pyoderma gangrenosum. A wound with edges rolled inward may be too dry, causing the wound edges to seek more moisture from the wound bed. A wound covered in necrotic tissue, desiccated, or deprived of oxygenation will exhibit poorly defined wound margins.[10]

Epithelialization can also occur in the middle of a wound bed if hair follicles or new cell growth are present. The appearance of new tissue at the wound edge can be measured in centimeters or by percentage of wound coverage (for example,

"0.3 cm of epithelial tissue surrounds the wound," or "wound is 25% epithelialized"). The degree of epithelialization is often overlooked.

PRACTICE POINT

Be sure to assess and record the wound's epithelialization.

Necrotic tissue

Necrotic tissue is dead, devitalized avascular tissue that provides an ideal medium for bacterial proliferation and may inhibit the microenvironment for healing. It's a well-known theory that wound healing is optimized when all necrotic tissue is removed from the wound bed. Necrotic tissue may present as yellow, gray, brown, or black. As it becomes dry, it presents as thick, hard, leathery black eschar.[10,11] Yellow, stringy necrosed tissue is referred to as slough.[10] Document necrotic tissue by quantifying the percentage of tissue at the wound bed. For example, the wound bed may be 100% necrotic or 25% granular with 75% necrotic tissue.

Tissue bed

The wound bed tissue reveals the phase and progress of wound healing through observation of its tissue color, degree of wetness, and amount of epithelialization.[12] The wound bed may be pale pink, pink, red, yellow, or black. Clean, granular wounds are typically described as red and wounds with devitalized slough are described as yellow. Brown and black wounds are typically those with necrotic tissue or eschar or desiccated tissue.[10]

Is the wound bed moist or dry? The presence of moisture or dry tissue will guide you in selecting the right dressing to create an environment that supports healing. Do you see new tissue growth — ep-ithelialization at the wound edges or within the wound bed? Is granulation tissue present — that is, beefy red tissue with a granular or gritty appearance?

Assessment and documentation should be based on your observations. Is the wound 100% granular tissue, or is it 25% filled with slough (yellow tissue) or necrotic (dead) tissue? All three tissue types can be found in the same wound, and assessing the amount of each type of tissue will help you document the outcome of care based on improvement or deterioration of characteristics seen in the wound tissue. Outcomes can then be tracked by percentage of improvement toward a clean granular wound bed (for example, "the wound progressed from 75% necrotic tissue to 100% granular tissue").

Tenderness to touch or the amount of pain the patient reports — both in the wound itself and in the surrounding tissue — are also essential parts of your assessment. Wound pain is one of the secondary signs of infection. It's important to differentiate between constant and episodic pain (such as pain that occurs only with dressing changes). Use a pain assessment scale accepted by your facility. (See chapter 7, Wound bioburden, and chapter 12, Pain management and wounds.)

Summary

Wound assessment — an appraisal of a patient's condition based on clinical signs and symptoms, laboratory data, and medical history — is an integral part of wound management. Assessment has become a highly specialized area of care, requiring well-developed observational skills and current knowledge. The use of current terminology is imperative to accurate assessment and communication.

Use of the newly created Wound AS-SESSMENTS chart can provide a fast, ongoing, and accurate assessment for patients with wounds. Assessment of wound parameters provides clinicians with the information needed to make decisions affecting the outcome of care. These decisions will guide the wound care team to suitable interventions, management, and care strategies.

Show what you know

1. Wound assessment involves all of the following except:

A. observation.
B. data collection.
C. evaluation.
D. dressing change.

ANSWER: D. Wound assessment involves observation, data collection and ongoing evaluation process. Dressing change is an intervention for the management of wound care.

2. A wound that has tissue damage through the epidermis and partially into the dermis would be classified as:

A. superficial.
B. partial-thickness.
C. full-thickness.
D. subdermal.

ANSWER: B. A superficial wound involves only the epidermis and the dermis is still intact. A full-thickness wound extends through the dermis. A subdermal wound extends into underlying structures below the skin such as bone, muscle, or tendon.

3. In assessing a wound, you find an area of tissue destruction under the edge of the patient's wound. This is best described as:

A. a sinus tract.
B. maceration.

C. fistula.
D. undermining.

ANSWER: D. A sinus tract is a channel that involves an area larger than the visible surface of the wound. Maceration is the softening of the surrounding skin usually from exposure to or excess wound drainage. A fistula is an opening between two organs or an organ and the skin.

References

1. Larazus, G.S., et al. "Definitions and Guidelines for Assessment of Wounds and Evaluation of Healing," *Archives of Dermatology* 130(4):489-93, April 1994.
2. Bower, M.G. "Evaluating and Managing Bite Wounds," *Advances in Skin & Wound Care* 15(2): 88-90, March-April 2002.
3. Stotts, N.A., and Cavanaugh, C.C. "Assessing the Patient with a Wound," in *Home Health Care Nurse*. Philadelphia: Lippincott Williams & Wilkins, 1999.
4. Bates-Jensen, B. "The Pressure Sore Status Tool a Few Thousand Assessments Later," *Advances in Wound Care* 10(5):65-73, 1997.
5. van Rijswijk, L. "The Fundamentals of Wound Assessment," *Ostomy/Wound Management* 42(7):40-46, August 1996.
6. Banfield, K.R., and Shuttleworth, E. "A Systematic Approach with Lasting Benefits: Designing and Implementing a Wound Assessment Chart," *Professional Nurse* 8(4):234-38, January 1993.
7. Morison, M.J. "Wound Assessment," *Professional Nurse* 2(10):315-17, July 1987.
8. Ayello, E. "Teaching the Assessment of Patients with Pressure Ulcers," *Decubitus* 5(7):53-54, July 1992.
9. Richards, R. "Assessment and Diagnosis of Burn Wounds," *Advances in Wound Care* 12(9): 468-71, November-December 1999.
10. Bryant, R.A. *Acute and Chronic Wounds, Nursing Management.* St. Louis: Mosby–Year Book, Inc., 1992.
11. Maklebust, J., and Sieggreen, M. *Pressure Ulcers: Guidelines for Prevention and Management,* 3rd ed. Springhouse, Pa.: Springhouse Corp., 2000.
12. *www.ruralfamilymedicine.org*

CHAPTER 7

Wound bioburden

Sue E. Gardner, PhD, RN, CWCN
Rita A. Frantz, PhD, RN, FAAN

OBJECTIVES

After completing this chapter, you'll be able to:

- distinguish between colonization and infection in a chronic wound
- identify the most valid method of determining a wound infection
- explain the effects of antiseptics on chronic wound tissue
- identify conditions when antimicrobial therapy is indicated for treatment of a chronic wound.

Bioburden in wounds

The human body is in constant contact with multiple microorganisms originating from both endogenous and exogenous sources.[1] Usually, these microorganisms are present without any evidence of infection because a balance exists between host resistance and microbial growth. Infection occurs when this equilibrium is upset, either because of lowered host defenses or increased microorganism quantity or virulence. Infection is directly related to the number of organisms and to the virulence of the organisms, and is inversely related to host resistance.[2]

The skin provides a physical and chemical barrier to microorganisms. Many microorganisms are able to survive on the skin and are known as skin colonizers, or normal flora. Normal flora may actually inhibit the growth of more virulent microorganisms and, therefore, serve a protective function. This mutually beneficial relationship between host and microorganism is referred to as a commensal relationship. Some normal flora are transient colonizers; they merely survive, don't multiply, and can easily be removed. Resident flora, on the other hand, multiply and are permanent.

Breaks in the skin, including wounds, allow microorganisms access to deeper tissue and structures where they can more readily adhere and multiply.[2] Host response to microorganisms in the wound is multifaceted. Nonspecific host responses occur regardless of microbial species; specific host responses are triggered by specific microorganisms and involve the immune system. Nonspecific and specific responses are essential for preventing invasion of wound microorganisms into vital tissues and organs.

Nonspecific responses include phagocytosis by polymorphonuclear leukocytes (PMNs) and macrophages and inflammation. Although the mechanisms of inflammation evolved to protect humans from microorganisms,[3] these responses can be elicited from any type of tissue injury. Thus, the first phase of wound healing is referred to as the inflammatory phase (see chapter 5, Acute and chronic wound healing); the cascade of events that occur during this phase are essential to activating the healing process.

Inflammation

Inflammation is integral to microbial resistance. It's triggered by both endogenous (host sources) and exogenous (microbial) mediators. Endogenous mediators, such as cytokines and growth factors, arise from mast cells, PMNs, macrophages, the complement system, and immune cells. These cells release mediators in response to contact with microorganisms or microbial products. Endogenous mediators are also released in response to tissue injury unrelated to microorganisms such as injury caused by surgical procedures or trauma.

Exogenous mediators of inflammation are produced by microorganisms. Most notable is endotoxin, which is produced by gram-negative bacteria. If released into the blood, endotoxin activates all inflammatory mechanisms at once, resulting in septic shock. Exotoxins are inflammatory mediators released by bacteria. Many bacterial exotoxins are extremely chemotactic; that is, they attract leukocytes. However, many bacterial toxins don't elicit inflammation directly. They indirectly elicit inflammation by activating mast cells and macrophages or by evoking an adaptive immune response, which then produce inflammatory mediators.[3,4]

The release of inflammatory mediators results in localized vasodilation and increased blood flow to the area of injury. The accompanying increase in vascular permeability promotes a rapid influx of phagocytic cells, complement, and antibody to the wound site. Collectively, these events remove microorganisms and debris as well as bacterial toxins and enzymes. These physiological responses to injury are expressed by the signs of inflammation including erythema, heat, edema, and pain.[3,5,6]

PRACTICE POINT

Signs and symptoms of inflammation include erythema, heat, edema, and pain.

Inflammation is characterized as being either acute or chronic.[3,7] Acute inflammation is the initial response to tissue invasion or injury and includes pronounced vascular changes and the predominance of PMNs at the site of injury.[7] Again, this type of inflammation can result from microorganisms or any type of tissue injury. Chronic inflammation occurs if the invasion or injury of tissue isn't resolved and persists over a long period. The vascular response becomes less pronounced during chronic inflammation and the predominant leukocyte at the site of injury shifts to macrophages.[3,7] Chronic inflammation is also characterized by the proliferation of fibroblasts and scar tissue.[7]

Infection

When host resistance fails to control the growth of microorganisms, localized wound infection results. Uncontrolled localized infection of a wound can lead to deep, more severe infections such as extensive cellulitis, osteomyelitis, bacteremia, and sepsis. More subtly, localized wound infection impairs healing and is thought to be an important cause of wound chronicity.[8]

The persistent presence of microorganisms leads to the influx of phagocytes, which release proteolytic enzymes, inflammatory mediators, and free radicals. The cumulative effect of these substances in the wound is additional tissue injury and wound deterioration.[9] Moreover, inflammatory mediators produce localized thrombosis and vasoconstriction resulting in a hypoxic wound environment. This hypoxic environment promotes further bacterial proliferation establishing a destructive, prolonged inflammatory cycle.[10] The immune response (that is, specific host responses) may be down-regulated in an attempt to limit self-destruction.

The proliferative phase of wound healing is also affected by wound infection. Bacteria and bacterial toxins stimulate macrophages to produce an excessive angiogenic response. The resultant granulation tissue is edematous, somewhat hemorrhagic, and more fragile.[11] Although the collagen content of infected wounds is higher than the collagen content of noninfected wounds, collagenolytic activity is also higher, resulting in wound breakdown.[12,13] Migration of epithelial tissue is inhibited by bacteria and bacterial toxins, and new epithelium is prone to lysis and desiccation by neutrophil proteases.[14,15] Finally, wound contraction is inhibited in the presence of large numbers of bacteria.[16]

PRACTICE POINT

Wound infection prolongs the inflammatory phase and disrupts the proliferative phase of wound healing.

Defining infection

Wound infection has been defined as the invasion and multiplication of microorganisms in wound tissue resulting in pathophysiologic effects or tissue injury.[22] The most important element in this definition is that invasion and multiplication of microorganisms occurs in the wound tissue. (See *Key elements of wound infection,* page 94.) Thus, wound infection can be contrasted from wound contamination and colonization. As previously noted, humans, and therefore human wounds, are in constant contact with microorganisms. As with human skin, some organisms in the wound are transient colonizers and don't multiply. Wound contamination is the presence of bacteria on wound surfaces with no multiplication of bacteria.[23-25]

Other organisms are permanent colonizers and replicate, or multiply, on the wound surface. Wound colonization is characterized by the replication of microorganisms on the wound surface without invasion of wound tissue and no host immune response.[2] Some of these colonizers may be involved in a mutually beneficial relationship with the host preventing the adherence of more virulent organisms in the wound bed. These organisms include Corynebacteria species, coagulase negative staphylococci, and viridans streptococci.[10]

The mere presence or multiplication of microorganisms on the wound surface

Key elements of wound infection

- Wound infection occurs in wound tissue, not on the surface of the wound bed.
- Wound infection occurs in viable wound tissue; it isn't a phenomenon of necrotic tissue, eschar, or other debris contained in the wound bed.
- Wound infection is caused by invasion and multiplication of microbes in the wound.
- Wound infection is manifested by a host reaction or tissue injury.

doesn't necessarily constitute wound infection. Contamination and colonization with wound microorganisms is a condition common to all wounds healing by secondary intention and in fact is a prerequisite to the formation of granulation tissue.[1,2,26] In contrast, wound infection is the invasion and multiplication of microorganisms in the wound tissue beneath the wound surface. Thus, for an infection to be present, the microorganisms must be present in viable tissue.

PRACTICE POINT

Contamination and colonization of a wound with microorganisms doesn't constitute infection.

The presence of microorganisms in wound pus, necrotic tissue, or slough isn't evidence of tissue invasion. These nonviable substances are known to support bacterial growth[27] and debridement of this tissue is essential to prevent infection. However, the presence of microorganisms in necrotic tissue, without invasion of viable tissue, doesn't constitute

wound infection. Microorganisms must be present in viable tissue for infection to occur is an essential element in the definition of wound infection.

Multiplication of microorganisms is another key element of the definition of infection; that is, microorganisms must replicate and produce large enough numbers to cause injury or impair healing.

Another key element in the definition of wound infection is that the invading organisms must produce host responses or tissue injury. The concepts of host response and pathophysiologic tissue injury are related in that both present clinical signs and symptoms. As previously described, host response produces the signs and symptoms associated with inflammation. Tissue injury produces other signs and symptoms.

Identifying infection

Despite the known deleterious effect of infection on healing,[17,18] the identification and diagnosis of localized wound infection is wrought with uncertainty in clinical practice. This is especially true for chronic wounds, which heal by secondary intention. (See chapter 5, Acute and chronic wound healing.)

Conversely, the identification and diagnosis of localized infection of acute wounds — such as surgical incisions — is less equivocal because most of these wounds will display a clinically apparent, robust inflammatory response. The normal time frame for inflammation associated with the wounding event (for example, a surgical procedure) is 3 to 5 days. Inflammation that persists past 3 to 5 days is considered indicative of wound infection.[19]

Like acute wound infections, the identification of deep, more severe infections is often easier to identify due to the development of overt systemic signs and symptoms. For example, extensive erythema, elevated body temperature, elevated white count, and elevated blood sugar in people with diabetes are readily evident. Similarly, osteomyelitis should always be considered if a wound can be probed to bone because exposed bone is usually indicative of osteomyelitis, especially in diabetic foot ulcers.[20]

EVIDENCE-BASED PRACTICE

A wound that has exposed bone or that can be probed to the bone with a sterile instrument should be evaluated for osteomyelitis.

However, identifying milder, localized infection in chronic wounds is much more problematic for a variety of reasons. First, chronic wounds by definition are slow to heal or don't heal at all. Although many factors may account for impaired healing, wound bioburden has always been suspected as a major deterrent to healing and an important cause of wound chronicity. Second, the manifestation of inflammation may be altered in chronic wounds because of population-specific factors. The inflammatory response to bacteria may be influenced by age,[21] diabetes, tissue perfusion and oxygenation, and other aspects of immunocompetence and anti-inflammatory drug use. These factors are of particular relevance in chronic wounds because chronic wounds predominantly occur in the aged who have decreased immune capacity and high prevalence of diabetes, peripheral vascular disease, and autoimmune disorders. On the other hand, the persistence of mechanisms that caused the chronic wound may elicit inflammatory responses that are unrelated to multiplying microorganisms in wound tissue.

Finally, considerable disagreement exists regarding what constitutes wound infection in the chronic wound. In addition to this lack of consensus, the value of different types of wound cultures in identifying infection is a source of confusion for clinicians and a source of debate among experts. Despite the factors that contribute to the confusion surrounding identification of localized chronic wound infection, an operative definition of wound infection can provide a foundation from which clinicians can approach identification and diagnosis in a rational, consistent manner.

Methods to identify wound infection

In practice, wound infection is identified and diagnosed based on clinical signs and symptoms of infection or on the findings from wound cultures. The advantages and disadvantages of using these methods can be evaluated in light of the key elements contained in the definition of wound infection.

Clinical signs and symptoms

The most common and clinically practical method for identifying wound infection is to monitor for clinical signs and symptoms of infection. Clinical signs and symptoms of wound infection reflect host response to invasion or tissue injury. They can be detected by direct observation of the wound and periwound area or self-reported by the patient. The clinical signs and symptoms of wound infection can be divided into those that comprise the classic signs of infection and those that are specific to secondary wounds (that is, tissue injury).

The classic signs and symptoms of infection have been recognized since antiquity. These signs and symptoms are erythema, heat, edema, pain, and purulent exudate.[3,5,6] As indicators of infection, they're a reflection of the host's response to invading organisms. The first four of these signs — pain, erythema, edema,

CDC criteria for surgical site infection

The Centers for Disease Control and Prevention (CDC) has established the following criteria to define surgical site infection (SSI).

Superficial incisional SSI	Deep incisional SSI	Organ/space SSI
Involves only skin or subcutaneous tissue of the incision and at least one of the following: • purulent drainage from the superficial incision • organisms isolated from aseptically obtained culture of fluid or tissue from the incision • at least one of the following, unless negative culture: – pain or tenderness – localized swelling – redness or heat – incision opened by surgeon • diagnosis of SSI by the surgeon or attending physician.	Involves deep soft tissues (such as fascia and muscle layers) of the incision and at least one of the following: • purulent drainage from the deep incision but not organ/space • deep incision spontaneously dehisces or is deliberately opened by surgeon with one of the following symptoms, unless negative culture: – fever greater than 100.4° F (38° C) – localized pain • an abscess • diagnosis of deep SSI by surgeon or attending physician.	Involves any part of the anatomy (other than the incision) opened or manipulated during operation and at least one of the following: • purulent drainage from a drain placed in organ/space • organisms isolated from aseptically obtained culture of fluid or tissue in organ/space • an abscess or other evidence of infection • diagnosis of an organ/space SSI by a surgeon or attending physician.

and heat — are also known as the signs of inflammation, which can be elicited by tissue damage unrelated to infection.[3] Purulent exudate is the result of bacterial exotoxins recruiting white cells to the wound. However, it's the host reaction, expressed by the classic signs and symptoms of infection, that distinguishes an infected wound from one that's merely colonized or contaminated according to some authors.[2,26]

PRACTICE POINT

The classic signs of infection are erythema, heat, edema, pain, and purulent exudate.

The classic signs and symptoms of infection are believed to be reliable indicators of infection in acute wounds such as surgical incisions. In surgical wounds, in-

flammation occurs after wounding, but should subside within 5 days.[28] The Centers for Disease Control and Prevention's (CDC) definition of a surgical site infection (SSI) reflects the confidence placed in clinical signs and symptoms to identify SSIs.[29] (See *CDC criteria for surgical site infection*.) SSIs are defined as occurring within 30 days of the operative procedure and are categorized as superficial incisional, deep incisional, or organ/space. The presence of purulent drainage is sufficient criteria as are signs of inflammation accompanied by a positive culture.

Unlike acute wounds, the classic signs and symptoms don't always present in the chronic wounds with high wound bioburden.[30] This may be due to diminished systemic or local inflammatory responses among populations with high prevalence of chronic wounds, such as elderly people or those with diabetes, peripheral vascular disease, or autoimmune disorders. Similarly, immunosuppressed patients with acute wounds may not express classic signs of infection despite high wound bioburden. The only exception is the symptom of pain,[31] which may occur in people with compromised immune function and be the only apparent symptom of infection.[32]

EVIDENCE-BASED PRACTICE

The classic signs and symptoms of infection may not be present in chronic wounds or in patients who are immunosuppressed.

EVIDENCE-BASED PRACTICE

Pain may be the only classic sign of wound infection present in immune compromised patients.

Additional signs and symptoms specific to secondary wounds have been proposed as indicators of infection.[33] These signs and symptoms include:
• serous drainage with concurrent inflammation
• delayed healing
• discoloration of granulation tissue
• friable granulation tissue
• pocketing at the base of the wound
• foul odor
• wound breakdown.

All of these signs and symptoms, with the exception of pocketing, were found to be valid indicators of localized infection in chronic wounds.[31] In fact, delayed healing may be the only sign apparent. Delayed healing is the lack of progress toward wound closure with no decrease in the size of the wound. The filling of the tissue defect with granulation tissue causes the wound volume to de-

crease, while migration of epithelial tissue and wound contraction cause the wound surface area to decrease. According to the clinical practice guideline published by the Agency for Healthcare Research and Quality, "a clean pressure ulcer should show some evidence of healing within 2 to 4 weeks."[34] Although many factors have been associated with delayed healing, wound infection may be a primary contributor.[8] When it's the only sign readily apparent, delayed healing should stimulate further assessment of wound bioburden by clinicians.[34]

PRACTICE POINT

Signs of infection specific to secondary wounds include serous drainage with concurrent inflammation, delayed healing, discoloration of granulation tissue, friable granulation tissue, pocketing of the base of the wound, foul odor, and wound breakdown. Many of these signs represent disruption of the proliferative phase of wound healing.

PRACTICE POINT

Delayed healing may be the only sign of infection in some wounds.

Although using clinical signs and symptoms of infection to monitor wounds for infection is congruent with the definition of infection, the assessment of these parameters is quite subjective.[35] The Clinical Signs and Symptoms Checklist (CSSC) was developed to assess the presence of the clinical signs and symptoms of wound infection in chronic wounds. (See *Clinical signs and symptoms checklist*, pages 98 and 99.) The CSSC provides a precise description for each of the clinical signs and symptoms. It was developed in an effort to standardize and more objectively measure

Clinical signs and symptoms checklist

SIGNS AND SYMPTOMS   CHECK (+) IF PRESENT

Increasing pain in the ulcer area
The patient reports increased level of peri-ulcer pain since the ulcer developed. Ask him to select the most appropriate statement for current level of ulcer pain from the following choices:
1. I can't detect pain in ulcer area.
2. I have less ulcer pain now than I had in the past.
3. The intensity of the ulcer pain has remained the same since the ulcer developed.
4. I have more ulcer pain now than I had in the past.
If the patient selects number 4, his pain is increasing. Write n/a if the patient can't respond to
the question.

Erythema
The presence of bright or dark red skin or darkening of normal ethnic skin color immediately
adjacent to the ulcer opening indicates erythema.

Edema
The presence of shiny, taut skin or pitting impressions in the skin adjacent to the ulcer but within 4 cm from the ulcer margin indicates edema. Assess pitting edema by firmly pressing the
skin within 4 cm of ulcer margin with a finger, release and waiting 5 seconds to observe indentation.

Heat
A detectable increase in temperature of the skin adjacent to the ulcer but within 4 cm of the ulcer margin as compared to the skin 10 cm proximal to the wound indicates heat. Assess differences in skin temperature using the back of your hand or your wrist.

Purulent exudate
Tan, creamy, yellow, or green, thick fluid that's present on a dry gauze dressing removed from
the ulcer 1 hour after the wound was cleaned and dressed indicates purulent exudate.

Sanguinous exudate
Bloody fluid that's present on a dry gauze dressing removed from the ulcer 1 hour after the
wound was cleaned and dressed indicates sanguinous exudate.

Serous exudate
Thin, watery fluid that's present on a dry gauze dressing removed from the ulcer 1 hour after
the wound was cleaned and dressed indicates serous exudate.

Delayed healing of the ulcer
The patient reporting no change, or an increase in the volume or surface area of the ulcer, over
the preceding 4 weeks indicates delayed healing. Ask the patient if the ulcer has filled with tissue or is smaller around than it was 4 weeks ago.

Discoloration of granulation tissue
Granulation tissue that is pale, dusky, or dull in color compared to surrounding, healthy tissue.
Note variations of normal, beefy-red appearance of granulation tissue.

Friable granulation tissue
Bleeding of granulation tissue when gently manipulated with a sterile cotton-tipped applicator
indicates friable tissue.

Clinical signs and symptoms checklist *(continued)*

SIGNS AND SYMPTOMS	CHECK (+) IF PRESENT
Pocketing at base of wound The presence of smooth, nongranulating pockets of ulcer tissue surrounded by beefy red granulation tissue indicates pocketing.	☐
Foul odor The ulcer may have a putrid or distinctively unpleasant smell.	☐
Wound breakdown Small open areas in newly formed epithelial tissue not caused by reinjury or trauma indicate wound breakdown.	☐

Adapted with permission of HMP Communications from Gardner, S.E., et al. "A Tool to Assess Clinical Signs and Symptoms of Localized Chronic Wound Infection: Development and Reliability," *Ostomy/Wound Management* 47(1):40-47, January 2001.

clinical signs and symptoms. Although more research regarding the validity and reliability of the tool is needed, preliminary findings indicate that the interrater reliability of the items on the CSSC are acceptable.[31] Moreover, the CSSC provides clinicians with information on assessing the less well-known signs and symptoms specific to secondary wounds.

Compounding the subjective limitations of using signs and symptoms to identify wound infection is the lack of clear guidelines regarding the number of signs and symptoms that need to be present to constitute infection. Increasing pain and wound breakdown were found to be sufficient signs of infection in a small study (n = 36) of chronic wounds, but none were necessary.[30] It's unclear how assessment of clinical signs and symptoms leads to decisions regarding wound infection status.[35] In practice, the presence of frankly obvious signs and symptoms of infection triggers treatment or wound cultures to guide selection of antimicrobials. However, when infection is only suspected but not blatantly obvious, wound cultures are often ordered to confirm the diagnosis of infection.

EVIDENCE-BASED PRACTICE

Increasing pain and wound breakdown are sufficient signs of wound infection.

PRACTICE POINT

Wound cultures are used to diagnose wound infection when it isn't clinically obvious.

Wound cultures and specimens

Like clinical signs and symptoms, the identification of wound infection based on culture findings can be inconclusive. This problem has led many clinicians to abandon wound cultures altogether, especially with respect to chronic wounds. Nonetheless, numerous methods are available for clinical and research purposes. The methods presented here are limited to those most commonly used in practice.

Wound cultures can be conceptualized as consisting of two steps. The first step is the acquisition of a specimen from the wound. The second step includes the laboratory procedures used to grow, identify, and quantify the microorganisms. Clinicians are directly responsible for the first part and must be aware of laboratory processes included in the second to acquire an appropriate wound specimen and effectively transport the specimen to the microbiology laboratory. This requires close communication with the microbiologist and the microbiology laboratory.

The three most common types of wound specimens are:
- wound tissue
- needle-aspirated wound fluid
- swabs.

The tissue biopsy method consists of aseptically removing a piece of viable wound tissue with a scalpel or punch biopsy instrument. Wound tissue specimens are the most congruent with the first two elements that define wound infection if the specimens are samples from viable tissue rather than necrotic tissue. Among a sample of 41 wounds of mixed etiology, the quantitative tissue biopsy method had a sensitivity of 100%, a specificity of 93.5%, and an accuracy of 95.1% in predicting the success of delayed closure.[36] Based on this and other data, the tissue biopsy became the gold standard specimen for wound cultures.[37] Unfortunately, tissue biopsy cultures are invasive, skill-intensive (both from clinician and laboratory perspectives), and unavailable in many settings. Therefore, they aren't commonly used in practice but are often used in research of wound microbiology.

PRACTICE POINT

Wound tissue is considered the best specimen for culture from which to identify wound infection.

Needle-aspiration technique obtains fluid through multiple insertions of a 22G needle into the tissue surrounding the wound. The needle is attached to a 10-cc syringe.[38] Although studies have compared needle aspiration technique with both quantitative tissue biopsy and swab cultures, the sensitivity, specificity, and accuracy of quantitative needle-aspiration remains unclear due to methodological limitations.[37-39] However, this may be the best technique for specimen collection when focal collections of tissue fluid or abscess formations exist close to the wound.[40]

The most practical and widely available method for obtaining wound specimens is the swab culture. The usefulness of this method is extremely contentious. Since this method samples only wound surface organisms (as opposed to organisms within the tissue), many believe it's ineffectual as a measure of infection[34] because it can't distinguish between infection and contamination. In addition, it may be difficult to recover anaerobic organisms from swab specimens.[19] However, others defend the role of swab cultures in monitoring infection, emphasizing its entrenchment in clinical practice.[41]

Although the accuracy of swab cultures as compared to biopsy cultures has been studied, the findings from these studies provide little information from which to base clinical practice. [39,42-46] Perhaps the most serious methodological problem presented by these studies is that the specific swabbing techniques employed were not described. Swabbing techniques vary greatly according to wound preparation, area of the wound sampled, duration of sampling, and even the type of swab employed (for example, alginate).[37] Given this variation, the specific technique employed may be an unrecognized, though significant, confounding factor on the findings of studies aimed at examining their diagnostic validity. Despite the lack of evidence-based recommendations, the utility of swab cultures in practice can be enhanced if specimens are collected recognizing the key elements contained in a clear definition of wound infection.

The swab techniques most commonly used or advocated in the literature are swabs of wound exudate, swabs taken using a broad Z-stroke over the entire wound bed, and swabs using the technique described by Levine and colleagues.[19,40,43,47-51] Swabs of wound exudate are self-descriptive and are usually taken prior to wound cleaning. Specimens obtained is this manner sample microorganisms on the surface and aren't congruent with the first or second key elements of infection, which establish that infection occurs in viable wound tissue.

Wound cleaning is advocated prior to obtaining swabs using either Z-stroke or Levine's technique in order for the culture to isolate wound tissue microorganisms as opposed to microorganisms associated with wound exudate, topical therapies, or nonviable tissue.[19,50] Moistening the swab with normal saline or transport medium is also recommended prior to specimen collection.[39,50] Moistening the swab is believed to provide more precise data than a dry swab.[52] Swabs using the broad Z-stroke entail rotating the swab between the fingers as the wound is swabbed from margin to margin in a 10-point zigzag fashion.[40] Because a large portion of the wound surface is sampled, the specimen collected may reflect surface contamination rather than tissue bioburden.[19]

The Levine technique consists of rotating a swab over a 1-cm square area with sufficient pressure to express fluid from within the wound tissue.[43] This technique is believed to be more reflective of "tissue" bioburden than swabs of exudate or swabs taken with a Z-stroke.[19] Theoretically, the Levine technique is the best technique of wound swabbing provided the wound is cleaned first and the

area sampled is over viable tissue, not necrotic tissue or eschar.[19]

PRACTICE POINT

The swab technique most consistent with the key elements of wound infection is Levine's technique because this technique attempts to sample microorganisms from within the wound tissue, not just from the wound surface.

Analyzing cultures and specimens
Laboratory procedures for the bacteriological analysis of wound specimens include isolation and identification of the microorganisms alone or in combination with quantification of the microorganisms isolated. When done alone, isolation and identification is referred to as qualitative culture, and when done in conjunction with quantification, it's referred to as quantitative culture. Quantitative cultures provide information regarding the type of organisms present in addition to the number of organisms present, which is usually expressed as number per gram of tissue, milliliter of fluid, or swab. The number of organisms present provides information regarding the rate of microorganism multiplication; therefore, quantitative cultures reflect the third key element of wound infection more completely than qualitative cultures.

Qualitative cultures
The recovery, isolation, and identification of microorganisms gained importance in identifying wound infection following the post-World War I (WWI) development of organism-specific antimicrobials.[53] According to the CDC, one sufficient criteria of surgical site infection is an "organism isolated from an aseptically obtained culture of fluid or tissue."[29] By this definition, an organism

present in the tissues of the wound indicates infection. It's important to note that this CDC criterion implies that isolation of organisms must be from within the tissue or tissue fluid, not isolation of organisms from the wound surface. The CDC defines pressure ulcer infection as the presence of two of the following clinical findings: redness, tenderness, or swelling of wound edges and organisms are isolated from a needle aspiration, tissue biopsy, or blood culture.[54] Clinical signs and symptoms of infection must be present along with isolation of an organism known to cause disease.

Acute wounds often contain skin flora, such as staphylococci and diphtheroids.[2] Chronic wounds, with their distinctive environment, often contain larger numbers and types of microorganisms than acute wounds. These wounds have large amounts of exudate, necrotic tissue and eschar, large surface areas, and deep cracks and crevices suitable for a variety of microbial species. Chronic wounds have been associated with anaerobes and multiple types of organisms.[55-57] Common organisms isolated from chronic wounds are *Proteus mirabilis, Escherichia coli,* and *Streptococcus, Staphylococcus, Pseudomonas, Corynebacteria,* and *Bacteroides* species.[55,56,58-60] Limited data indicate that the presence of *Proteus mirabilis, Pseudomonas aeruginosa,* and *Bacteroides,* an anaerobe, deter chronic wound healing.[61,62] Nonhealing chronic wounds were also associated with the presence of *E. coli,* group D *Streptococci,* and other anaerobic cocci.[44] Although the presence of methicillin-resistant *Staphylococcus aureus* (MRSA) in chronic wounds presents a problem for infection control in health care settings, the association between colonization with MRSA and subsequent infection or bacteremia is unclear.[63] Only the presence of β-hemolytic *Streptococcus* is considered to be a notable threat in the chronic wound at lev-

els less than 10^5 organisms per gram of tissue.[40,53,64] Nonetheless, qualitative cultures have a role in the monitoring of wounds and in guiding antibiotic selection for infected wounds. Qualitative cultures are accomplished by plating wound specimens on solid media, identifying isolates using standard microbiological procedures, and testing for antibiotic sensitivity.

PRACTICE POINT

β-hemolytic *Streptococcus* is considered a notable threat in wounds regardless of the number of these microorganisms present.

Quantitative cultures

Although Pasteur suggested that the invasion of microorganisms in the body was related to quantity of inoculation, French WWI surgeons were the first to base wound management on the number of organisms present.[65-67] The relationship between bacterial quantity, wound infection, and sepsis was given attention in the 1960s. Krizek and Davis[68] found that fatal sepsis was associated with visceral or blood cultures greater than 10^6 or 10^7 organisms per gram of tissue or milliliter of blood. These researchers also demonstrated that fatal wound sepsis was related to the number of bacteria in the wound.[69] In addition, Noyes and colleagues[70] found that wound exudates with greater than 10^6 bacteria per milliliter were associated with invasive infection. The U.S. Army Surgical Research Unit provided a series of studies that found burn wound sepsis was associated with bacterial levels exceeding 10^5 organisms per gram of tissue.[71-73] Quantity of bacteria was also inversely linked to chronic wound healing.[17,36,61,62] These studies, along with earlier findings that clean wounds harbor microorganisms, provided the foundation from which quantitative culturing was added as a method of diagnosing infection.[36] The Agency for Healthcare Research and Quality (AHRQ) clinical practice guideline, *Treatment of Pressure Ulcers*, embraced quantitative cultures as the gold standard method to diagnose pressure ulcer infection.[34,74] Greater than 10^5 organisms per gram of tissue, milliliter of fluid, or swab has been adopted by many as the critical value for diagnosing wound infection.[17,21,26,34,53,75] Although references to greater than 10^5 have been interpreted as 100,000[1] or 1,000,000[76] organisms per gram of tissue, greater than 1,000,000 organisms per gram of tissue is the preferred critical value.[77]

Most wound specimens can be quantitatively processed in the microbiology laboratory. Wound tissue specimens must be of sufficient weight to ensure validity of findings, around 0.25 g of tissue.[76] In the microbiology laboratory, the tissue is weighed, ground, serially diluted, plated, and incubated in both aerobic and anaerobic conditions. Plates are read for type as well as number of colony forming units and expressed as number of organisms per gram of tissue. Similarly, wound aspirate is diluted, plated, and incubated. Quantification is expressed as the number of organisms per ml of fluid.[38]

Swab specimens can be quantitatively or semi-quantitatively processed. Quantitative swab cultures are placed in 1 ml of dilutant and vortexed to release microorganisms from the swab. This fluid is then serially diluted, plated, and incubated, usually in aerobic conditions only. Plates are read for type and quantity of organisms and quantification is expressed as number or organisms per swab. Semi-quantitative swabs are inoculated onto solid media and streaked on four quadrants. Number of colony form-

ing units is counted in each quadrant and results are reported from 1 to 4+. Dow and colleagues[40] suggest 4+ should be used as cut-off for diagnosing infection.

PRACTICE POINT

Wounds with greater than 1,000,000 organisms per gram of tissue, milliliter of fluid, or swab are considered to be infected.

PRACTICE POINT

Semi-quantitative swab cultures may be a good alternative to quantitative cultures if quantitation is unavailable. Culture results of 4+ are considered positive for infection.

In summary, the identification of wound infection remains ambiguous and uncertain. Monitoring wounds for the clinical signs and symptoms of infection is an important component of wound assessment. Indicators of inflammation are especially important markers in acute wounds, such as SSIs. However, the signs and symptoms associated with inflammation may not be present in some patients with acute wounds or in patients with chronic wounds. The signs specific to secondary wounds may be useful in these cases and should be incorporated into clinical assessment. Wounds suspected of infection, especially those with delayed healing, are often cultured to confirm the diagnosis. While qualitative cultures provide useful information in wounds that are demonstrating obvious clinical signs of infection, they may not be as useful in diagnosing infection in the absence of signs and symptoms unless certain pathogens are isolated. In the absence of clinical signs and symptoms, quantitative cultures are the gold standard method for diagnosing localized wound infection.

Managing wound bioburden

Controlling wound bioburden requires a multifaceted approach consisting of one or more of the following:
• correction of the host factors that contributed to the infection.
• removal of devitalized tissue and foreign debris.
• initiation of antimicrobial therapy.

While not all of these interventions will be indicated in every case of wound infection, they each have a role to play in either reducing the number of microorganisms or enhancing host resistance.

The presence of host factors that reduce resistance to infection are often overlooked in management of wound bioburden. Judicious attention to restoration of adequate blood supply, provision of nutritional support, maintenance of glycemic control, reduction of edema, and protection from mechanical forces on the wounded tissue will aid in restoring the balance between host resistance and microorganisms. Failure to address these host factors may contribute to continued proliferation of microorganisms despite initiation of other treatment modalities.

PRACTICE POINT

In managing wound bioburden, attention should be given to supporting or restoring host defenses to microorganism invasion, such as adequate blood supply, nutrition, management of blood sugar, and control of edema.

Removal of devitalized tissue and debris is an essential step in treating wound infection, since necrotic tissue provides an excellent media for growth of microorganisms. When devitalized tissue is adherent to the wound bed, wound debridement is indicated. Methods of wound debridement are addressed in chapter 8.

Wound cleaning

The presence of foreign debris and contaminants on the surface of the wound can harbor microorganisms or provide nutrients for their growth. Wound cleaning is a process that removes these less adherent inflammatory contaminants from the wound surface and renders the wound less conducive to microbial growth. However, the process of wound cleaning can create tissue trauma. Effective wound cleaning requires selection of methods that minimize chemical and mechanical trauma to wound tissue while removing surface debris and contaminants. Although definitive research is lacking to guide selection of wound cleaning methods, the available practice evidence suggests using a nontoxic cleaning solution in combination with a delivery device that will create sufficient mechanical forces to remove the surface debris while limiting tissue injury.

Cleaning agents

The usefulness of specific agents depends on a balance between their antibacterial properties and their cytotoxicity to wound healing cells, such as white blood cells (WBCs) and fibroblasts.[78] For the majority of wounds, isotonic saline is adequate to clean the wound surface. Water, although not isotonic, is a suitable alternative, as long as it's free of any potential contaminants. Since the fluid has only brief contact with the wound surface, it isn't crucial that the solution be isotonic (0.9% sodium chloride). An inexpensive saline solution can

PATIENT TEACHING
Preparing saline solution at home

To prepare saline solution at home, tell the patient to bring 1 quart of water to a boil and allow it to boil for 5 minutes. He should then add 2 teaspoons of noniodized salt and stir until the salt is completely dissolved. Warn him to allow the solution to cool completely before using. The solution can be stored for up to 1 week, at room temperature, in a tightly covered glass or plastic container.

be prepared by combining two teaspoons of noniodized salt in one liter of boiling water. (See *Preparing saline solution at home.*)

If the wound surface is heavily laden with surface debris, a commercial wound cleaner may be used. These agents contain surface-active agents or surfactants that by the nature of their chemical polarity break the bonds that attach wound contaminants. The intensity of their chemical reactivity is directly related to their cleaning capacity and cytotoxicity. Thus, selection of a wound cleaner needs to weigh cleaning capacity against potential toxicity to cells in the wound.

Evidence regarding the safety of wound cleaners is difficult to interpret due to the lack of standardized methods for testing these agents. At present, the preponderance of available evidence comes from in-vitro studies comparing wound cleaners under experimentally controlled conditions. The earliest such study evaluated the relative toxicity of various commercial wound and skin cleaners according to their effect on the viability of PMNs.[79] PMNs were exposed to increasing 1:10 dilutions of test cleaners for 30 minutes and analyzed for viability and phagocytic function. The toxicity index was defined as the amount of dilution required to achieve PMN viability and phagocytic function compara-

ble to that obtained by cells exposed to a balanced salt solution. Toxicity indices ranged from a low of 10 to a high of 10,000 for the agents tested. Generally, the toxicity levels of wound cleaners were 10 to 1,000 while skin cleaners were 10,000. A second study of wound cleaner cytotoxicity evaluated the effects of five wound cleaning products on the viability of human fibroblasts, red blood cells, and white blood cells in culture.[80] The range of performance was found to be similar, although the findings related to specific agents varied somewhat from those reported by Foresman et al.[79] One cleaner was found to be considerably more toxic in this study, a result of the sample tested failing to meet the manufacturer's specification for pH.

Collectively, these studies confirm that skin cleaners, which are formulated to break the chemical bonds that bind fecal matter to the skin, are stronger and more toxic than wound cleaners. For this reason, skin cleaners should never be used for wound cleaning.

EVIDENCE-BASED PRACTICE

Skin cleaners should never be used for wound cleaning.

Antiseptic agents have historically been used to control bacterial levels in chronic wounds. This practice was based on the well-documented finding that bacteria suspended in a test tube of fluid medium are rapidly killed when exposed to an antiseptic. However, in order for an agent to be effective in the environment of a chronic wound, an agent must be able to penetrate into contaminated tissue in an active form and in sufficient concentration to achieve bactericidal activity. Since antiseptics bind chemically to multiple organic substrates that are normally present in chronic wounds, they may fail to reach bacteria in the wound tissue when used in standard clinical concentrations.[81-83] Thus, they're unable to create an effective antibacterial effect. Furthermore, antiseptics are toxic to all cells with which they come in contact, including white cells and fibroblasts. The cytotoxic properties of antiseptics have been well documented in vitro and in vivo.[78,84-91] Furthermore, the addition of an antiseptic to wound cleaners has been shown to increase the toxicity index of the agent to 10,000 on average.[92] Although multiple clinical studies are cited to support the benefits of using antiseptic agents in healing chronic wounds, they fail to distinguish the antimicrobial effect of the antiseptic from other bacteria-reducing treatments that are being simultaneously administered, such as debridement or absorption of wound exudate, including bacteria and their toxins.[93-96] To date, no scientifically valid clinical studies have documented the antibacterial benefits of using antiseptic agents in chronic wounds.

PRACTICE POINT

Antiseptics shouldn't be used as a cleaning agent for wounds.

Cleaning devices

The effectiveness of wound cleaning is influenced by the type of cleaning device used to deliver the solution to the wound surface. It's essential that the method used provide sufficient force to remove surface contaminants and debris while minimizing trauma to the wound. A variety of scrubbing cloths, sponges, and brushes are available for wound cleaning. Although evidence related to their efficacy is limited, it has been demonstrated that wounds cleaned with coarse sponges were significantly more susceptible to infection than those scrubbed with a smoother sponge.[97] Furthermore, when compared to saline, wound cleaners containing surfactant were found to decrease the coefficient of friction between the scrubbing device and wound tissue.

Wound irrigation promotes wound cleaning by creating hydraulic forces generated by the fluid stream. In order for the irrigation to be effective in cleaning the wound, the force of the irrigation stream must be greater than the adhesion forces that hold the debris to the surface of the wound. Multiple studies have substantiated that increasing pressure of a fluid stream improves removal of bacteria and debris from the wound.[98,99] Wound irrigation pressures of 10 lb per square inch (psi) and 15 psi are more effective than 1 psi and 5 psi in removing debris and bacteria from the wound surface. While 15 psi is more effective than 10 psi in removing bacteria, increasing the irrigation pressure to 20 psi or greater doesn't significantly improve the efficacy of cleaning.

When irrigation is delivered with a mechanical irrigation device, such as those used for dental hygiene, greater pressures are attainable than with other methods. Although clinical studies of mechanical irrigation devices used on crushing trauma wounds have confirmed that cleaning with 70 psi produces significantly more effective removal of bacteria and debris than 25 psi or 50 psi,[100-102] lower pressures are generally desirable in chronic wounds. With pressures as low as 10 psi, bacteria and debris removal with mechanical irrigation devices was significantly more effective than results obtained from irrigation with a bulb syringe.

Although high pressure optimizes wound cleaning, the risk of dispersing fluid into adjacent wound tissue or along tissue planes is increased when higher pressures are used for irrigation.[103-105] The magnitude of this dispersion is related to the amount of fluid stream pressure. Research on the animal model established that irrigation at 70 psi produced greater dispersion of fluid into the tissues than irrigation with a 35-ml syringe and a 19G needle (8 psi).[105] Moreover, when a single orifice tip was used to irrigate experimental wounds, extensive fluid penetration occurred at pressures greater than 30 psi.[104] This dispersion of fluid did not occur when a multi-jet tip was used to deliver the irrigation stream. Collectively, this evidence supports avoiding irrigation pressures of greater than 15 psi for wound cleaning.

While high pressures should be avoided in performing wound irrigation, it's also necessary to create sufficient hydraulic forces with the fluid stream to overcome the adhesion forces holding debris to the wound surface. Research on experimental wounds in the animal model has found that irrigation pressures of 1 psi and 5 psi produced significantly less removal of wound debris than results achieved with 10 psi and 15 psi.[99] The use of a needle and syringe to deliver fluid to wound tissue is generally regarded as a convenient method of providing effective irrigation pressure. A 35-cc syringe and a 19G needle or angiocatheter has been shown to deliver an irrigation stream at 8 psi.[106] This study also demonstrated that irrigation with a 19G needle and a 35-cc syringe was significantly more effective than a bulb syringe in removing wound bacteria and preventing the development of infection in experimental wounds.[106] Additional evidence of the effectiveness of a needle and syringe method of irrigation over the bulb syringe was established in a clinical experimental study of trauma wounds treated within 24 hours of injury with either a standard bulb syringe (0.05 psi) or a 12-cc syringe and 22G needle (13 psi).[107] A significant decrease was observed in both wound inflammation and wound infection in those wounds cleaned with the syringe and needle compared with the bulb syringe. The collective evidence regarding the effect of fluid stream pressure on removal of wound debris and bacteria supports using an irrigation pressure of 5 psi to 15 psi for wound cleaning.

A variety of needle and syringe combinations can be used to achieve the desired range of irrigation pressure. The size of the syringe and the needle gauge determine the amount of pressure of the fluid stream. Since the force depressing the plunger is distributed over a larger surface area, the larger the syringe, the less the force. With a 19G needle, 6-cc, 12-cc, and 35-cc syringes will produce pressures of 30, 20, and 8 psi, respectively. The opposite effect occurs by increasing the size of the needle. Since the larger the lumen of the needle, the greater will be the flow of fluid, needles of 25-, 21-, and 19G will create pressures of 4, 6, and 8 psi, respectively, when used with a 35-cc syringe.

A number of pressurized canisters capable of delivering saline under pressure are now available commercially. Although the claim is made that these devices produce a 19G stream at 8 psi, no evidence exists to support this assertion. In a preliminary report of the pressure dynamics of one of these devices, measurement of pressure was limited to the pressure within the pressurized canister system, not the actual force of the fluid stream against the wound surface.[108]

PRACTICE POINT

Wound irrigation can be accomplished with a variety of medical tools and specially made devices.

EVIDENCE-BASED PRACTICE

Research indicates that the optimum pressure for wound cleaning is between 5 and 15 psi.

In addition to varying the amount of pressure used for wound irrigation, the fluid steam can be delivered in either a pulsatile or continuous flow pattern. The benefit of delivering wound irrigation with a pulsatile as compared to a continuous fluid stream hasn't been substantiated in experimental studies.[98,101,102] Although several commercially available battery-powered, disposable irrigation systems (Davol, Inc., Cranston, Rhode Island; Stryker Instruments, Kalamazo, Michigan; Zimmer, Inc., Dover, Ohio) deliver pulsatile fluid streams with different spray patterns and remove the fluid and wound debris with suction, their efficacy in comparison to other irrigation methods remains to be established.[109-112] At the present time, their primary benefit appears to be their portability and capability to serve as an alternative to whirlpool therapy for patients with chronic wounds, which aren't amenable

to whirlpool, or for patients when whirlpool therapy isn't accessible.

PRACTICE POINT

Pulsatile irrigation devices don't appear to be better than nonpulsatile devices, but they may be useful for patients who don't have access to a whirlpool.

An alternate approach to wound irrigation is the whirlpool bath. It cleans the wound by exposing the entire wound bed and surrounding skin to agitating water generated by jets in the sides of the whirlpool tub. Only two studies have investigated the cleaning effectiveness of whirlpool and these are methodologically confounded with wound irrigation, which was provided at the end of the whirlpool therapy.[113,114] The benefit of whirlpool is thought to be derived from the prolonged exposure of the wound to water, which softens wound debris and makes it more amendable to removal. For this reason, the whirlpool is best suited for use with chronic wounds containing thick slough or necrotic tissue. Since it isn't possible to control the amount of pressure being exerted on the wound surface in a whirlpool bath, once the devitalized tissue has been cleared from the wound, the whirlpool should be discontinued to avoid disrupting new granulation tissue forming in the wound. Extreme caution must also be taken to ensure that the wound doesn't come in close contact with the water jets, since the high pressure they generate could cause further tissue injury.

Antimicrobial therapy

When removal of necrotic tissue doesn't reduce bacterial burden to a level compatible with healing, additional interventions that act directly on the bacteria are indicated. The clinical use of antibiotics to control bacterial burden in chronic wounds has been characterized by misconceptions and controversy. As a result, antibiotics have frequently been used too extensively or for too long a time. The lack of valid indicators of chronic wound infection has further complicated the selection and use of antimicrobial therapy. Research evidence has documented that systemic antibiotics are of no value in reducing bacterial counts in chronic, granulating wounds.[115] Furthermore, the presence of purulent exudate, a recognized sign of infection in an acute wound, isn't a sufficient indicator of the need to initiate antibiotic therapy to treat a chronic wound. Given the current state of ambiguity regarding valid clinical signs and symptoms of chronic wound infection, the decision to initiate antimicrobial therapy is best guided by the failure of a wound to make progress toward healing despite the absence of devitalized tissue.

Research studies have suggested the potential utility of topical antibiotics in reducing bacterial burden in chronic wounds. In a randomized controlled trial of 31 pressure ulcers, all ulcers treated with topical gentamicin cream and standard treatment consisting of debridement, cleaning, pressure reduction and nutritional support demonstrated significant improvement, while only three of the nine given standard treatment alone improved.[61] Serial bacteriological and pathological observations made over a 1- to 4-week treatment period showed a rapid reduction in bacterial counts to levels less than 10^6 per ml in all ulcers treated with gentamicin. Furthermore, analysis of quantitative bacterial counts in relation to clinical outcome revealed an absolute correlation between significant clinical improvement and a fall in the bacterial count to less than 10^6 per ml and between no clinical improvement

and the persistence of counts greater than 10^6 per ml.

The efficacy of topical antibiotics in reducing bacterial burden in chronic wounds was substantiated further in a randomized trial of 45 patients with a single infected pressure ulcer that were randomly assigned to receive silver sulfadiazine cream, povidone-iodine solution, or saline gauze dressings.[93] Standard care consisting of debridement, pressure reduction, and nutritional support was provided to all subjects. In 100% of the ulcers treated with silver sulfadiazine cream, the bacterial levels were reduced to 10^5 or less per gram of tissue during the 3-week protocol, while only 78.6% of the povidone-iodine solution-treated ulcers and 63.6% of the saline gauze-treated ulcers achieved these reductions in bacterial levels. Overall, ulcers treated with silver sulfadiazine responded more rapidly, with one-third achieving bacterial levels of less than 10^5 within 3 days and half the ulcers reaching this level within 1 week. These data support limiting treatment with topical antibiotics to no more than 2 weeks. If clinical evidence of improvement has not occurred in this time, other host factors that may be contributing to decreased bacterial resistance should be explored.

 EVIDENCE-BASED PRACTICE

Research suggests that topical antibiotic therapy be limited to 2 weeks.

Recent advances in technology have produced dressings that incorporate silver directly into the dressing material, thus eliminating the necessity of applying and removing the silver sulfadiazine cream. While such dressings would appear to possess the same antibacterial benefits as direct application of the cream, this hasn't been substantiated in controlled clinical studies. These types of dressings are designed to provide an antimicrobial barrier and have not been demonstrated to reduce bacterial levels in chronic wounds.

Although clinical studies provide evidence supporting the utility of topical antibiotics in reducing bacterial burden in chronic wounds, these agents can cause adverse reactions in some patients. Reports of permanent hearing loss with topical 1% neomycin solution and acute anaphylactic reactions with topically applied Bacitracin suggest that careful monitoring is indicated when using these agents.[116,117] Additionally, since there's a risk of selecting out resistant strains of bacteria, antibiotics that are used to treat infections systemically shouldn't be used in a topical form on chronic wounds. For this reason, despite the reported effectiveness of gentamicin in reducing bacterial levels in pressure ulcers, alternative topical antibiotics are indicated that won't produce resistant bacterial strains to systemic forms of the antimicrobial agent.

While topical antibiotics have demonstrated effectiveness in reducing bacterial burden when the area of involvement is localized, they're generally regarded as inadequate to control more extensive tissue involvement, such as advancing cellulitis. In these instances, systemic antibiotic therapy is indicated. Since the type of organisms and degree of invasiveness will vary, the choice of antimicrobial therapy will need to be individualized. Unfortunately, little research evidence exists to guide selection of antibiotics to treat chronic wound infections. Generally, chronic wound infections are treated empirically with broad-spectrum antibiotics administered orally. Parenteral therapy may be indicated when the infection involves deeper tissue and is accompanied by systemic signs, such as fever, chills, and elevated WBC count. Regardless of the route, the effectiveness of any systemic antibiotic in reducing bacterial burden will be dependent on the adequacy of the patient's peripheral circulation. In those instances where peripheral vascular disease compromises the blood flow to the infected tissue, systemic antimicrobial therapy may produce no clinical improvement in the wound.

 PRACTICE POINT

The effectiveness of systemic antibiotics is dependent on an adequate blood supply to the wound.

Summary

Most of our understanding of wound infection has been derived from the study of acute wounds. As wound healing science has evolved, it has become clear that chronic wounds are distinctly different environments where host resistance has been overwhelmed by bacterial burden. The classic signs and symptoms of infection are well recognized. However, they're based on assessments made of acute wounds and aren't valid in the chronic wound. While indicators of chronic wound infection remain ambiguous, substantial evidence exists showing that necrotic tissue harbors microorganisms. Therefore, debridement of necrotic tissue in the wound bed is an essential first step to reducing bacterial burden. Regular wound cleaning with a noncytotoxic solution, using sufficient force to remove surface contaminants and debris while minimizing trauma, is an important adjunct to reduce surface contaminants. In those instances where these measures aren't sufficient to restore a balance between host resistance and bacterial burden, antimicrobials that act directly on the bacteria are indicated.

Show what you know

1. Which of the following distinguishes a wound colonized with bacteria from one that's infected?

   A. An infected wound will have purulent exudate; a colonized wound won't.
   B. An infected wound will have organisms present in viable tissue; a colonized wound won't.
   C. An infected wound will always have necrotic tissue; a colonized wound won't.
   D. An infected wound will have a positive swab culture; a colonized wound won't.

ANSWER: B. For a wound to be infected, organisms must be present in viable tissue and not limited to the wound surface. Purulent exudate may be observed in a colonized wound as well as one that's infected. While necrotic tissue does contain organisms, a wound can be infected without the presence of necrotic tissue. Both an infected wound and a colonized wound will produce a positive swab culture. For the wound to be infected, the organisms must be present in the tissue and not limited to the surface of the wound that has contact with the culture swab.

2. Which of the following is the most valid indicator of a wound infection?

   A. A swab culture showing large amounts of *Staphylococcus*
   B. The presence of erythema in the periwound area
   C. Quantitative culture of tissue showing 1,000,000 organisms/g of tissue
   D. Large amounts of serosanguinous exudate on dressings

ANSWER: C. Quantitative cultures provide a count of the actual number of organisms present in a standard gram of tissue taken from beneath the wound surface in the wound tissue. Swab cultures provide information regarding surface bacteria only. They don't assess bacterial level in the tissue. Erythema is one of the classic signs of inflammation and may arise in response to any type of tissue injury, including, but not limited to, infection. Serosanguinous exudate contains serum and a small number of red blood cells, and may be indicative, but not conclusive, of infection.

3. Antiseptics are a deterrent to healing of clean, granulating wounds because they:

   A. interfere with absorption of nutrients.
   B. discolor the wound tissue.
   C. irritate surrounding skin.
   D. are harmful to fibroblasts and other cells.

ANSWER: D. Antiseptics have been documented as toxic to fibroblasts. Topical antiseptics have no effect on nutrient absorption from the bloodstream. Although some antiseptics can bleach out the color of wound tissue, this isn't what causes them to disrupt the repair process. While many antiseptics can cause skin irritation if allowed to come in contact with the periwound surface, this isn't the mechanism that interferes with wound repair.

4. The use of topical antibiotics for treatment of chronic wounds should be:

   A. used routinely to reduce high bacterial levels.
   B. used routinely to prevent infection.
   C. avoided unless necrotic tissue is present.

D. avoided in absence of signs of infection.

ANSWER: D. Treatment with topical antibiotics is indicated only when signs of infection are present. However, it's important to recognize that a chronic wound may not present with the same signs of infection as an acute wound. Treatment with topical antibiotics isn't indicated unless the wound is infected. Routine use of topical antibiotics for prevention of infection is unnecessary and can lead to development of resistant organisms. Using topical antibiotics in the presence of necrotic tissue isn't effective. The necrotic tissue harbors microorganisms and should be removed to decrease bacterial burden.

References

1. Robson, M.C. "Wound Infection: A Failure of Wound Healing Caused by an Imbalance of Bacteria," *Surgical Clinics of North America* 77(3):637-50, June 1997.
2. Mertz, P.M., and Ovington, L.G. "Wound Healing Microbiology," *Dermatology Clinics* 11(4):739-47, October 1993.
3. Majno, G., and Joris, I. *Cells, Tissues, and Disease: Principles of General Pathology.* Cambridge: Blackwell Science, 1996.
4. Abraham, S.N. "Discovering the Benign Traits of the Mast Cell," *Science and Medicine* pp. 46-55, September-October 1997.
5. McGeer, A., et al. "Definitions of Infection for Surveillance in Long-term-care Facilities," *American Journal of Infection Control* 19(1):1-7, February 1991.
6. Thomson, P.D., and Taddonio, T.E. "Wound Infection," in Krasner, D., and Kane, D., eds., *Chronic Wound Care,* 2nd ed. Wayne, Pa.: HMP Communications, 1997.
7. Larocco, M. "Inflammation and Immunity," in Porth, C.M., ed., *Pathophysiology: Concepts of Altered Health States,* 4th ed. Philadelphia: Lippincott Williams & Wilkins, 1994.
8. Tarnuzzer, R.W., and Schultz, G.S. "Biochemical Analysis of Acute and Chronic Wound Environments," *Wound Repair and Regeneration* 4(3):321-26, July-September 1996.
9. Heggers, J.P., and Robson, M.C. "Prostaglandins and Thromboxanes," in Ninneman, J., ed., *Traumatic Injury-infection and Other Immunological Sequelae.* Baltimore: University Park Press, 1983.
10. Dow, G. "Infection in Chronic Wounds," in *Chronic Wound Care: A Clinical Source Book for Healthcare Professionals,* 3rd ed. Wayne, Pa.: HMP Communications, 2001.
11. Hunt, T.K., et al. "A New Model for the Study of Wound Infection," *Journal of Trauma* 7(2):298-306, March 1967.
12. Bucknall, T.E. "The Effect of Local Infection upon Wound Healing: An Experimental Study," *British Journal of Surgery* 67(12):851-55, December 1980.
13. Dunphy, J.E. "The Cut Gut," *American Journal of Surgery* 119(1):1-8, January 1970.
14. Lawrence, J.C. "Bacteriology and Wound Healing," in Fox, J.A., and Fischer, J., eds., *Cadexomer Iodine.* Stuttgart: Schattauer Verlag, 1983.
15. Orgill, D., and Demling, R.H. "Current Concepts and Approaches to Wound Healing," *Critical Care Medicine* 16(9):899-908, September 1988.
16. Stenberg, B.D., et al. "Effect of bFGF on the Inhibition of Contraction Caused by Bacteria," *Journal of Surgical Research* 50(1):47-50, January 1991.
17. Lookingbill, D.P., et al. "Bacteriology of Chronic Leg Ulcers," *Archives of Dermatology* 114(12):1765-68, December 1978.
18. Robson, M.C., et al. "Wound Healing Alterations Caused by Infection," *Clinics in Plastic Surgery* 17(3):485-92, July 1990.
19. Stotts, N.A., and Whitney, J.D. "Identifying and Evaluating Wound Infection," *Home Healthcare Nurse* 17(3):159-65, March 1999.
20. Grayson, M.L., et al. "Probing to Bone in Infected Pedal Ulcers: A Clinical Sign of Underlying Osteomyelitis in Diabetic Patients," *JAMA* 273(9):721-23, March 1995.
21. Gilchrist, B. "Infection and Culturing," in Krasner, D., and Kane, D., eds., *Chronic Wound Care,* 2nd ed. Wayne, Pa.: HMP Communications, 1997.
22. Committee on the Control of Surgical Infections of the Committee on Pre- and Postoperative Care of the American

College of Surgeons. *Manual on Control of Infection in Surgical Patients.* Philadelphia: Lippincott Williams & Wilkins, 1976.

23. Baxter, C., and Mertz, P.M. "Local Factors that Affect Wound Healing," *Nursing RSA Verpleging* 7(2):16-23, February 1992.

24. Gilchrist, B. "Treating Bacterial Wound Infection," *Nursing Times* 90(50):55-58, December 1994.

25. Hutchinson, J.J., and McGuckin, M. "Occlusive Dressings: A Microbiologic and Clinical Review," *American Journal of Infection Control* 18(4):256-68, August 1990.

26. Stotts, N.A., and Hunt, T.K. "Pressure Ulcers. Managing Bacterial Colonization and Infection," *Clinics in Geriatric Medicine* 13(3):565-73, August 1997.

27. Barnett, A., et al. "A Concentration Gradient of Bacteria within Wound Tissue and Scab," *Journal of Surgical Research* 41(3):326-32, September 1986.

28. Stotts, N.A. "Promoting Wound Healing," in Kinney, M.R., et al., eds., *AACN's Clinical Reference for Critical Care Nursing,* 4th ed. St. Louis: Mosby–Year Book, Inc., 1998.

29. Horan, T.C., et al. "CDC Definitions of Nosocomial Surgical Site Infections, 1992: A Modification of CDC Definitions of Surgical Wound Infections," *American Journal of Infection Control* 20(5):271-74, October 1992.

30. Gardner, S.E., et al. "The Validity of the Clinical Signs and Symptoms Used to Identify Localized Chronic Wound Infection," *Wound Repair and Regeneration* 9(3):178-86, May-June 2001.

31. Gardner, S.E., et al. "A Tool to Assess Clinical Signs and Symptoms of Localized Chronic Wound Infection: Development and Reliability," *Ostomy/Wound Management* 47(1):40-47, January 2001.

32. Steed, D.L. "Diabetic Wounds: Assessment, Classification, and Management," in Krasner, D., and Kane, D., eds., *Chronic Wound Care,* 2nd ed. Wayne, Pa.: HMP Communications, 1997.

33. Cutting, K.F., and Harding, K.G. "Criteria for Identifying Wound Infection," *Journal of Wound Care* 3(4):198-201, June 1994.

34. Bergstrom, N., et al. *Treatment of Pressure Ulcers. Clinical Practice Guideline, Number 15. AHCPR Publication No. 95-0652.* Rockville, Md.: Agency for Health Care Policy and Research, Public Health Service, U.S. Department of Health and Human Services, December 1994.

35. Cutting, K.F. "Identification of Infection in Granulating Wounds by Registered Nurses," *Journal of Clinical Nursing* 7(6):539-46, November 1998.

36. Robson, M.C., and Heggers, J.P. "Bacterial Quantification of Open Wounds," *Military Medicine* 134(1):19-24, January 1969.

37. Stotts, N.A. "Determination of Bacterial Burden in Wounds," *Advances in Wound Care* 8(4):46-52, July-August 1995.

38. Lee, P., et al. "Fine-needle Aspiration Biopsy in Diagnosis of Soft Tissue Infections," *Journal of Clinical Microbiology* 22(1):80-83, July 1985.

39. Rudensky, B., et al. "Infected Pressure Sores: Comparison of Methods for Bacterial Identification," *Southern Medical Journal* 85(9):901-903, September 1992.

40. Dow, G., et al. "Infection in Chronic Wounds: Controversies and Treatment," *Ostomy/Wound Management* 45(8): 23-40, August 1999.

41. Donovan, S. "Wound Infection and Wound Swabbing," *Professional Nurse* 13(11): 757-59, August 1998.

42. Bill, T.J., et al. "Quantitative Swab Culture versus Tissue Biopsy: A Comparison in Chronic Wounds," *Ostomy/Wound Management* 47(1):34-37, January 2001.

43. Levine, N.S., et al. "The Quantitative Swab Culture and Smear: A Quick, Simple Method for Determining the Number of Viable Aerobic Bacteria on Open Wounds," *Journal of Trauma* 16(2):89-94, February 1976.

44. Sapico, F.L., et al. "Quantitative Micro-biology of Pressure Sores in Different Stages of Healing," *Diagnostic Micro-biology of Infectious Diseases* 5(1):31-38, May 1986.

45. Basak, S., et al. "Bacteriology of Wound Infection: Evaluation by Surface Swab and Quantitative Full Thickness Wound Biopsy Culture," *Journal of the Indian Medical Association* 90(2):33-34, February 1992.

46. Herruzo-Cabrera, R., et al. "Diagnosis of Local Infection of a Burn by Semi-quantitative Culture of the Eschar Surface," *Journal of Burn Care & Rehabilitation* 13(6):639-641, November-December 1992.

47. Morison, M.J. *A Colour Guide to the Nursing Management of Wounds.* Oxford: Blackwell Scientific, November-December 1992.

48. Pagana, K., and Pagana, T.J. *Mosby's Diagnostic and Laboratory Test Reference.* St. Louis: Mosby–Year Book, Inc., 1992.

49. Alvarez, O., et al. "Moist Environment for Healing: Matching the Dressing to the Wound," *Ostomy/Wound Management* 21:64-83, Winter 1988.

50. Cooper, R., and Lawrence, J.C. "The Isolation and Identification of Bacteria from Wounds," *Journal of Wound Care* 5(7):335-40, July 1996.

51. Cuzzell, J.Z. "The Right Way to Culture a Wound," *AJN* 93(5):48-50, May 1993.

52. Georgiade, N.G., et al. "A Comparison of Methods for the Quantitation of Bacteria in Burn Wounds I: Experimental Evaluation," *American Journal of Clinical Pathology* 53(1):35-39, January 1970.

53. Robson, M.C., and Heggers, J.P. "Quantitative Bacteriology and Inflammatory Mediators in Soft Tissue," in *Biological and Clinical Aspects of Soft and Hard Tissue Repair.* Edited by Hunt, T.K., et al. New York: Praeger Pubs., 1984.

54. Garner, J.S., et al. "CDC Definitions for Nosocomial Infections, 1988," *American Journal of Infection Control* 16(3):128-40, June 1988.

55. Peromet, M., et al. "Anaerobic Bacteria Isolated from Decubitus Ulcers," *Infection* 1(4):205-207, 1973.

56. Chow, A.W., et al. "Clindamycin for Treatment of Sepsis by Decubitus Ulcers," *Journal of Infectious Disease* 135(suppl):S65-S68, March 1977.

57. Vaziri, N.D., et al. "Bacterial Infections in Patients with Chronic Renal Failure: Occurrence with Spinal Cord Injury," *Archives of Internal Medicine* 142(7):1273-76, July 1982.

58. Bryan, C.S., et al. "Bacteremia Associated with Decubitus Ulcers," *Archives of Internal Medicine* 143(11):2093-95, November 1983.

59. Gilchrist, B., and Reed, C. "The Bacteriology of Chronic Venous Ulcers Treated with Occlusive Hydrocolloid Dressings," *British Journal of Dermatology* 121(3):337-44, September 1989.

60. Trengove, N.J., et al. "Qualitative Bacteriology and Leg Ulcer Healing," *Journal of Wound Care* 5(6):277-80, June 1996.

61. Bendy, R.H., et al. "Relationship of Quantitative Wound Bacterial Counts to Healing of Decubiti: Effect of Topical Gentamicin," *Antimicrobial Agents and Chemotherapy* 4:147-55, 1964.

62. Daltrey, D.C., et al. "Investigation into the Microbial Flora of Healing and Non-healing Decubitus Ulcers," *Journal of Clinical Pathology* 34(7):701-705, July 1981.

63. Roghmann, M.C., et al. "MRSA Colonization and the Risk of MRSA Bacteraemia in Hospitalized Patients with Chronic Ulcers," *Journal of Hospital Infection* 47(2):98-103, February 2001.

64. Leaper, D.J. "Defining Infection," *Journal of Wound Care* 7(8):373, September 1998.

65. Absolon, K.B., et al. "From Antisepsis to Asepsis: Louis Pasteur's Publication on "The Germ Theory and its Application to Medicine and Surgery," *Review of Surgery* 27(4):245-58, July-August 1970.

66. Elek, S.D. "Experimental Staphylococcal Infections in the Skin of Man," *Annals of the New York Academy of Science* 65:85, 1956.

67. Hepburn, H.H. "Delayed Primary Suture of Wounds," *British Medical Journal* 1:181-83, 1919.

68. Krizek, T.J., and Davis, J.H. "Endogenous Wound Infection," *Journal of Trauma* 6(2):239-48, March 1966.

69. Krizek, T.J., and Davis, J.H. "Experimental Pseudomonas Burn Sepsis: Evaluation of Topical Therapy," *Journal of Trauma* 7(3):433-42, May 1967.

70. Noyes, H.E., et al. "Delayed Topical Antimicrobials as Adjuncts to Systemic Antibiotic Therapy of War Wounds: Bacteriologic Studies," *Military Medicine* 132(6):461-68, June 1967.

71. Lindberg, R.B., et al. "The Successful Control of Burn Wound Sepsis," *Journal of Trauma* 5(5):601-16, September 1965.

72. Shuck, J.M., and Moncrief, J.A. "The Management of Burns: Part I. General Considerations and the Sulfamylon Method," *Current Problems in Surgery* 3-52, February 1969.

73. Teplitz, C., et al. "Pseudomonas Burn Wound Sepsis. I. Pathogens of Experimental Burn Wound Sepsis," *Journal of Surgical Research* 4:200-16, 1964.

74. Rodeheaver, G.T., and Frantz, R.A. "14. Guideline: Bacterial Control," in *Treating*

Pressure Ulcers. Guideline Technical Report, Number 15, Volume 1. Edited by Bergstrom, N., and Cuddigan, J. Rockville, Md.: U. S. Department of Health and Human Services, Public Health Service, Agency for Health Care Policy and Research, AHCPR Publication No. 96-N014, 1994.

75. Krizek, T.J., and Robson, M.C. "Evolution of Quantitative Bacteriology in Wound Management," *American Journal of Surgery* 130(5):579-84, November 1975.

76. Heggers, J.P. "Variations on a Theme," in *Quantitative Bacteriology: Its Role in the Armamentarium of the Surgeon.* Edited by Heggers, J.P., and Robson, M.C. Boca Raton: CRC Press, 1991.

77. Robson, M.C. Personal communication, May 29, 2002.

78. Lineaweaver, W., et al. "Topical Antimicrobial Toxicity," *Archives of Surgery* 120(3):267-70, March 1985.

79. Foresman, P.A., et al. "A Relative Toxicity Index for Wound Cleansers," *Wounds* 5(5):226-31, September-October 1993.

80. Wright, R.W., and Orr, R. "Fibroblast Cytotoxicity and Blood Cell Integrity Following Exposure to Dermal Wound Cleansers," *Ostomy/Wound Management* 39(7):33-36, 38, 40, September 1993.

81. Zamora, J.L., et al. "Inhibition of Povidone-iodine's Bactericidal Activity by Common Organic Substances: An Experimental Study," *Surgery* 98(1):25-29, July 985.

82. Fleming, A. "The Action of Chemical and Physiological Antiseptics in a Septic Wound," *British Journal of Surgery* 7:99-129, 1919.

83. Lacey, R.W. "Antibacterial Activity of Povidone Towards Non-sporing Bacteria," *The Journal of Applied Bacteriology* 46(3):443-49, June 979.

84. Cooper, M.L., et al. "The Cytotoxic Effects of Commonly Used Topical Antimicrobial Agents on Human Fibroblasts and Keratinocytes," *Journal of Trauma* 31(6):775-84, June 1991.

85. Teepe, R.G., et al. "Cytotoxic Effects of Topical Antimicrobial and Antiseptic Agents on Human Keratinocytes In Vitro," *Journal of Trauma* 35(1):8-19, July1993.

86. Branemark, P.I., and Ekholm, R. "Tissue Injury Caused by Wound Disinfectants," *Journal of Bone and Joint Surgery American* 49(1):48-62, January 1967.

87. Brennan, S.S., et al. "The Effect of Antiseptics on the Healing Wound: A Study Using the Ear Chamber," *British Journal of Surgery* 72(10):780-82, 1985.

88. Cotter, J.L., et al. "Chemical Parameters, Antimicrobial Activities, and Tissue Toxicity of 0.1 and 0.5% Sodium Hypochlorite Solutions," *Antimicrobial Agents Chemotherapeutics* 9(1):118-22, 1985.

89. Brennan, S.S., et al. "Antiseptic Toxicity in Wounds Healing by Secondary Intention," *Journal of Hospital Infection* 8(3):263-67, 1986.

90. Becker, G.D. "Identification and Management of the Patient at High Risk for Wound Infection," *Head and Neck Surgery* 8:205-10, 1986.

91. Viljanto, J. "Disinfection of Surgical Wounds without Inhibition of Normal Wound Healing," *Archives of Surgery* 115:253-56, 1980.

92. Hellewell, T.B., et al. "A Cytotoxicity Evaluation of Antimicrobial and Non-antimicrobial Wound Cleansers," *Wounds* 9(1):15-20, 1997.

93. Kucan, J.O., et al. "Comparison of Silver Sulfadiazine, Povidone-iodine and Physiologic Saline in the Treatment of Chronic Pressure Ulcers," *Journal of the American Geriatric Society* 29(5):232-35, 1981.

94. Carrel, A., and Dehelly, G. *The Treatment of Infected Wounds.* New York: Hoeber, 1917.

95. American Medical Association. *AMA Drug Evaluation,* 10th ed. Chicago: American Medical Association, 1994.

96. Sundberg, J., and Meller, R. "A Retrospective Review of the Use of Cadexomer Iodine in the Treatment of Chronic Wounds," *Wounds* 9(3):68-86, May-June 1997.

97. Rodeheaver, G.T., et al. "Mechanical Cleaning of Contaminated Wounds with a Surfactant," *American Journal of Surgery* 129(3):241-45, 1975.

98. Madden, J., et al. "Application of Principles of Fluid Dynamics to Surgical Wound Irrigation," *Current Topics in Surgical Research* 3:85-93, 1971.

99. Rodeheaver, G.T., et al. "Wound Cleaning by High Pressure Irrigation," *Surgical Gynecology and Obstetrics* 141(3):357-62, September 1975.

100. Grower, M.F., et al. Effect of Water Lavage on Removal of Tissue Fragments from Crush Wounds," *Oral Surgery Oral Medicine Oral Pathology* 33(6):1031-36, June 1972.

101. Green, V.A., et al. "A Comparison of the Efficacy of Pulsed Mechanical Lavage with That of Rubber-bulb Syringe Irrigation in Removal of Debris from Avulsive Wounds," *Oral Surgery Oral Medicine Oral Pathology* 32(1):158-64, July 1971.

102. Stewart, J.L., et al. "The Bacteria-removal Efficiency of Mechanical Lavage and Rubber-bulb Syringe Irrigation in Contaminated Avulsive Wounds," *Oral Surgery Oral Medicine Oral Pathology* 31(6):842-48, June 1971.

103. Bhaskar, S.N., et al. "Effect of Water Lavage on Infected Wounds in the Rat," *Journal of Periodontology* 40(11):671-72, November 1969.

104. Carlson, H.C., et al. "Effect of Pressure and Tip Modification on the Dispersion of Fluid Throughout Cells and Tissues During the Irrigation of Experimental Wounds," *Oral Surgery Oral Medicine Oral Pathology* 32(2):347-55, August 1971.

105. Wheeler, C.B., et al. "Side Effects of High Pressure Irrigation," *Surgical Gynecology and Obstetrics* 143(5):775-78, November 1976.

106. Stevenson, T.R., et al. "Cleansing the Traumatic Wound by High Pressure Syringe Irrigation," *Journal of the American College of Emergency Physicians* 5(1): 17-21, January 1976.

107. Longmire, A.W., et al. "Wound Infection Following High-pressure Syringe and Needle Irrigation" [Letter to the editor], *American Journal of Emergency Medicine* 5(2):179-818, March 1987.

108. Singer, A.J., et al. "Pressure Dynamics of Various Irrigation Techniques Commonly Used in the Emergency Department," *Annals of Emergency Medicine* 24(1): 36-40, July 1994.

109. Loehne, H. "Pulsatile Lavage with Concurrent Suction," In *Wound Care: A Collaborative Practice Manual for Physical Therapists and Nurses,* 1st ed. Edited by C. Sussman, C., and Bates-Jensen, B.M. Gaithersburg, Md.: Aspen Pubs., 1998.

110. Cicione, J. "Making Waves," *Case Review* 26-29, July-August 1998.

111. Ho, C., et al. "Healing with Hydrotherapy," *Advances for Directors in Rehabilitation* 7(5):45-49, 1998.

112. Morgan, D., and Hoelscher, J. "Pulsed Lavage: Promoting Comfort and Healing in Home Care," *Ostomy/Wound Management* 46(4):44-49, April 2000.

113. Bohannon, R.W. "Whirlpool Versus Whirlpool Rinse for Removal of Bacteria from a Venous Stasis Ulcer," *Physical Therapy* 62(3):304-08, March 1982.

114. Neiderhuber, S., et al. "Reduction of Skin Bacterial Load with Use of Therapeutic Whirlpool," *Physical Therapy* 55(5): 482-86, 1975.

115. Robson, M.C., et al. "The Efficacy of Systemic Antibiotics in the Treatment of Granulating Wounds," *Journal of Surgical Research* 16(4):299-306, April 1974.

116. Johnson, C.A. "Hearing Loss Following the Application of Topical Neomycin," *Journal of Burn Care and Rehabilitation* 9(2):162-64, March-April 1988.

117. Schechter, J.F., et al. "Anaphylaxis Following the Use of Bacitracin Ointment. Report of a Case and Review of the Literature," *Archives of Dermatology* 120(7):909-11, July 1984.

CHAPTER 8

Wound debridement

Elizabeth A. Ayello, PhD, RN, APRN,BC, CWOCN, FAAN
Sharon Baranoski, MSN, RN, CWOCN, APN, FAAN
Morris D. Kerstein, MD
Janet Cuddigan, PhD, RN, CWCN

OBJECTIVES

After completing this chapter, you'll be able to:

- state the purpose of debriding a wound

- list criteria for *not* debriding a necrotic wound

- describe four types of debridement: sharp/surgical, mechanical, enzymatic, and autolytic

- list the indications and advantages of four types of debridement

- differentiate when to use a particular method of debridement.

Speeding the healing process

Debridement is the removal of necrotic tissue, exudate, and metabolic waste from a wound to improve or facilitate the healing process. Accumulation of necrotic tissue usually results from poor blood supply at the wound site or from increased interstitial pressure, a common scenario in patients with wounds such as pressure ulcers. In otherwise healthy people, natural debridement keeps pace with accumulation of dying tissue in a wound, but malnourished patients, those who have wounds such as pressure ulcers, or those with comorbidities such

as diabetes, require medical intervention to facilitate wound healing.

The primary purpose of debridement is to reduce the bioburden of the wound to control and prevent wound infection, especially in deteriorating wounds.[1] Debridement allows the practitioner to visualize the wound's walls and base more accurately to determine the presence of viable tissue (without debridement, wounds such as pressure ulcers can't be staged). If necrotic tissue isn't removed, it not only impedes wound healing but results in protein loss, osteomyelitis, generalized infection, and the possibility of septicemia, limb amputation, or death. By removing necrotic tissue, debridement restores circulation and allows adequate oxygen delivery to the wound site.[2]

Wounds must have a microenvironment free from the nonviable tissue that offers a location for bacteria growth.[3] Oxygen is a primary requirement for energy-dependent metabolic processes. The production of free radicals kills bacteria, facilitating the proliferation of fibroblasts and epithelial cells, which are crucial for wound healing. Bacteria present in hypoxic conditions competes with healing tissue for nutrients and produces exotoxins and endotoxins that damage newly generated, mature cells. This setting of hypoxia and bacteria interrupts the process initiated by the migration of fibroblasts into the extracellular matrix, one of the fundamental steps in wound healing. The fibrils of collagen produced by fibroblasts lay the foundation for new cell growth.

The chemicals released from damaged cells initiate inflammatory processes and the chemical and biological cascade that results in recruiting cells necessary to deposit collagen.[3] Leukocytes — primarily polymorphonuclear leukocytes — are the primary cells of the inflammatory process. Leukocytes enter the wound with removal of devitalized tissue and foreign material. Collaboration of local enzymes (proteolytic, fibrinolytic, or collagenolytic) helps dissolve and remove devitalized tissue. Because collagen comprises approximately 75% of the skin's dry weight, the overall endogenous collagenase can be considered one of the regulators of tissue remodeling.

After the cleaning process is initiated, macrophages are recruited; they, in turn, recruit fibroblasts, which are responsible for depositing collagen and filling the wound with scar tissue. A wound with a good blood supply and essential nutrients generally "heals" within 14 days — but this doesn't represent the total healing process. Remodeling — the portion of the healing process in which the wound restructures into its final functional image — typically takes another 4 weeks, making the total healing process take about 6 weeks. Wound sites that appear in areas of rich blood supplies such as the scalp heal faster than areas with a lesser blood supply. Collagen breakdown and collagen buildup occur in equal degrees, resulting in an appropriate-appearing scar. Excess collagen results in formation of a keloid or hypertrophic scar.

Identifying necrotic tissue

Dead or necrotic tissue is identified by its moist, yellow, green, or gray appearance, and may become thick and leathery with a black eschar. Oxygen and nutrients can't penetrate a wound impaired by necrotic tissue. Dead tissue is the breeding ground for bacteria, and the eschar may mask an underlying abscess.[4] Necrotic tissue that's moist, stringy, and yellow is referred to as slough (devitalized connective tissue). If the wound becomes dehydrated, necrotic tissue becomes thick, leathery, and black in color and is described as eschar.

In general, removing necrotic tissue restores circulation to the wound and improves healing. But be careful! Debriding too much tissue can destroy the framework for healing. Some wounds shouldn't be debrided at all. Exercise caution, for example, in dealing with necrotic ulcers on the heels or toes, which may have poor perfusion.

 PRACTICE POINT

Monitor stable necrotic heels for the signs of edema, erythema, fluid wave, or drainage, which signal a need for debridement.

Guidelines from the Agency for Health Care Policy and Research, now the Agency for Health Care Research and Quality,[5] recommend against disturbing a dry, stable eschar ulcer of the heel without signs of edema, erythema, fluctuance (fluid wave), or drainage. In these wounds, eschar acts as a natural barrier to infection. Focus on preventing trauma to the wound. Wrap the foot in a soft dressing material and monitor it for signs of infection and changes in eschar.

Debridement methods

Mechanical, sharp/surgical, enzymatic, and autolytic are the common debridement methods; however, a resurgence in the use of older methods, such as larval therapy, is occurring.

Mechanical debridement

Methods of mechanical debridement include wet-to-dry dressings, hydrotherapy (whirlpool), and wound irrigation (pulsed lavage).[6] Mechanical debridement may be painful, so consider premedicating the patient for pain. Both whirlpool and pulsed lavage require special equipment and skill. These methods are nonselective; that is, they don't always discriminate between viable and nonviable tissue. Therefore, newly formed epithelium and granulation tissue may also be damaged or removed along with the necrotic tissue.

 PRACTICE POINT

Mechanical debridement may be painful, so consider premedicating the patient for pain.

Wet-to-dry dressings

The use of wet-to-dry dressing as a mechanism to debride a wound remains a common treatment in all health care settings. This method involves placing a moist saline gauze dressing on the wound surface and removing it when it's dry. The removal of the dried gauze dressing facilitates removal of devitalized tissue and debris from the wound bed. Unfortunately, newly formed granulation tissue and new cell growth are also removed. To prevent pain and to help remove the dry gauze, clinicians often wet the dressing before removal. This defeats the purpose of aggressively removing dead tissue.

A wet-to-dry dressing should be used when a moderate to large amount of necrotic tissue is present and surgical intervention isn't an immediate option. It shouldn't be used in a clean, granulating wound. Instead, use moist wound therapy dressings. (See chapter 9, Wound treatment options.)

Hydrotherapy

Hydrotherapy or whirlpool debridement may be indicated for patients who need aggressive cleaning or softening of necrotic tissue in large wounds. Hydrotherapy is contraindicated in granulating wounds because it can dry and injure the wound bed. Hydrotherapy should be discontinued after necrotic tissue has been removed from the wound bed.

Hydrotherapy or whirlpool debridement is performed by putting the patient in a whirlpool bath and letting the swirling waters soften and loosen dead tissue. It's usually done in the physical therapy department, with treatment of 10 to 20 minutes once or twice per day. Check the water temperature to prevent burns. The water should be tepid (80° to 92° F [26.7° to 33.3° C]) or neutral (92° to 96° F [33.3° to 35.5° C]).

Hydrotherapy may cause periwound maceration, traumatize the wound bed, and put the patient at risk for waterborne infections such as *Pseudomonas aeruginosa*. The potential for cross-contamination between patients is also a concern. Both patient and health care workers may be exposed to health risks associated with aerolization. To minimize infection risks, the whirlpool tank must be thoroughly cleaned with an appropriate disinfectant after each use.

Pulsed lavage

Pulsed lavage debridement is accomplished by using specialized equipment that combines a pulsating irrigation fluid with suction.[7] With pulsed lavage, you can clean and debride a wound at variable irrigation pressures (measured in pounds per square inch [psi]). The pulsatile action and effective wound bed debridement may improve granulation tissue growth. This treatment takes 15 to 30 minutes and should be done twice daily if more than half of the wound is necrotic tissue. Pulsed lavage debridement is often indicated for patients with large amounts of necrotic tissue and those for whom other debridement methods aren't an option.

Patients may need to be premedicated for comfort before beginning the procedure. Safe and effective ulcer irrigation pressures range from 4 to 15 psi.[5] Controlling the amount of water pressure is critical during this procedure. Because fluid is being forced at the wound directly, the risk of driving organisms down deep into the wound tissue has been expressed as a concern. In addition, inhalation of contaminated water droplets or mist is possible for both the clinician and the patient.

PRACTICE POINT

Always wear personal protective equipment to prevent splash injury, including eye and face protectors as well as an impervious gown. Remember to administer pain medication to the patient before the procedure.

Sharp/surgical debridement

A sharp/surgical debridement includes the use of scalpel, forceps, scissors, or laser to remove dead tissue.[8] Because viable tissue may also be inadvertently removed with this method, excellent judgment must be used when performing sharp debridement. The clinician must be able to differentiate where and what to cut; for example, the clinician must be able to identify a tendon versus slough because both are yellow in color. Sharp debridement is usually done by experienced physicians or surgeons and may require licensing for nurses and therapists in some states.

The use of sharp debridement is based on expert opinion and clinical data. Steed[9] reanalyzed data from the multisite clinical trials testing the use of growth factor rhPDGF in neuropathic diabetic foot ulcers, and found significantly higher healing rates in treatment facilities performing more frequent surgical debridement. Surgical debridement is used for adherent eschar and devitalized tissues. This method can be used in infected wounds and should be the first choice for wounds showing signs of advancing cellulitis or sepsis. Small wounds may be debrided at the bedside, but extensive wounds — for example, a stage IV pressure ulcer — may require debridement in the operating room. Surgical/sharp debridement may not be the best choice for a patient taking anticoagulant medications.

PRACTICE POINT

Exercise caution when performing surgical/sharp debridement on any patient who has been on a prolonged course of anticoagulant therapy.

Enzymatic debridement

Enzymatic debridement is considered safe, effective, and easy to use. Enzymes are effective cleaning agents that accelerate degradation and debridement, resulting in early initiation of anabolic processes and overall enhanced wound healing.[6] They're an ideal option for patients who aren't candidates for surgery, and for patients receiving care in a long-term care facility or at home. Enzymatic debridement is accomplished by applying topical enzymatic agents to devitalized tissue to digest and dissolve necrotic tissue in the wound bed.

If infection has spread beyond the ulcer (as in advancing cellulitis), immediate removal of necrotic tissue is usually recommended. Surgical debridement and then nonenzymatic debridement should be considered. Enzymes often can be used alone to break down the eschar before sharp debridement, or in conjunction with mechanical debridement. Some topical antibiotics are compatible with enzymatic debriding agents and may be used in conjunction with the treatment.

Enzymes that act on necrotic tissue are categorized as proteolytics, fibrinolytics, and collagenases, depending on the tissue component they target. Some enzymes are selective and can be used throughout the treatment phase. Others are nonselective and can harm healthy surrounding tissue; these enzymes should be applied only to the area of eschar or slough. Don't use nonselective enzymes on healthy tissue, such as granulation tissue on exposed tendons. Surrounding tissue can be protected by applying a protective barrier ointment around the wound.

Enzymes are a prescription drug and require a physician or prescriber's order. Some are applied once per day, while others require twice-per-day application. Before reapplying the enzymatic agent, thoroughly clean the wound to remove any residual enzymatic ointment and wound debris.

To use an enzymatic debriding agent, thoroughly clean the wound with normal saline solution to remove debris on the wound bed. Avoid solutions with metal ions such as mercury or silver, which can deactivate the enzymatic activity. The suggested technique is crosshatching or scoring the eschar with a scalpel (if within your scope of practice in your state and permitted by your facility) to let the debriding agent penetrate into the eschar. Apply a thin layer (about the thickness of a nickel) of enzymatic ointment onto the necrotic tissue. Cover the wound with an appropriate dressing to keep it moist and let the debriding agent work. Various types of dressings can be used with enzymatic debriders. (For more information on dressing types, see chapter 9, Wound treatment options.) Follow the manufacturer's directions for the enzyme you're using.

Autolytic debridement

Autolytic debridement uses the body's endogenous enzymes to slowly rid a wound of necrotic tissue. In a moist wound, phagocytic cells and proteolytic enzymatic enzymes can soften and liquefy the necrotic tissue, which is then digested by macrophages. Autolytic debridement may be applied in the superficial wound that contains little necrotic tissue, or a larger, deeper pressure ulcer.[10,11] Underlying these concepts is a requirement of adequate circulation and nutrition.[12] Autolytic debridement may take longer than other methods; however, it represents a less stressful method to the patient and wound than mechanical debridement. This method of debridement is contraindicated in infected wounds.

Autolytic debridement is easy to do and is accomplished through the use of

Dressings for autolytic debridement

Use wound characteristics to help you select the best dressing to use for autolytic debridement.

Appearance of the wound bed
- What type of tissue do you see?
- Is the volume of exudate small, moderate, or large? If you're packing the wound, how many dressings does it soak?

Wound depth
Match the type of dressing to the depth of the wound. For shallow wounds, use a transparent film or hydrocolloid dressing. For deep wounds with cavities, a transparent film dressing shouldn't be used. Instead, a foam or alginate dressing is a better choice. The cavities of deep wounds should be filled with an absorbent product. The secondary or outer dressing must be able to remain in place until the next scheduled dressing change. Transparent films will lift off prematurely with moderate to large amounts of drainage from the wound.

Condition of periwound skin
Is the skin around the wound macerated? Can you use a dressing that has adhesive properties or do you need a dressing that won't stick and damage surrounding skin? If the patient's skin is sensitive to tape or the dressing needs to be changed often, use strips of hydrocolloid dressing to create a "window" around the wound. You'll apply tape to these strips instead of the skin, reducing skin irritation.

semiocclusive or occlusive dressings, such as transparent films, hydrocolloids, and hydrogels. A moisture-retentive topical dressing is applied to the wound. (See *Dressings for autolytic debridement.*) Wound fluid accumulates under the dressing, aiding in the lysis of necrotic tissue. Autolytic debridement is a pain-free process in patients with adequate tissue perfusion.

PATIENT TEACHING

Be sure to tell the patient and his family that fluid accumulating under the dressing is a normal part of the debridement process. Discolored wound fluid may not signal a wound infection.

Monitor the wound for signs of infection, such as odor, inflammation, or increased pain, and discontinue autolytic debridement if these symptoms occur. Immunocompromised patients should be assessed frequently for any indication of infection. Autolytic debridement isn't the treatment of choice in severely infected wounds; in fact, it may lead to more severe infection and is therefore contraindicated in these situations. Surgical consult is warranted with appropriate medical management.

Choosing a debridement method
Answering the following questions can help guide you choose the best method of debridement for your patient.[13] (See *Debridement decision-making algorithm.*)

How much time do you have to debride?
Infected wounds require immediate attention. The patient's clinical condition and the amount of time that you can devote to a treatment may influence your choice.

Debridement decision-making algorithm

The following patient factors drive the debridement decision-making process:

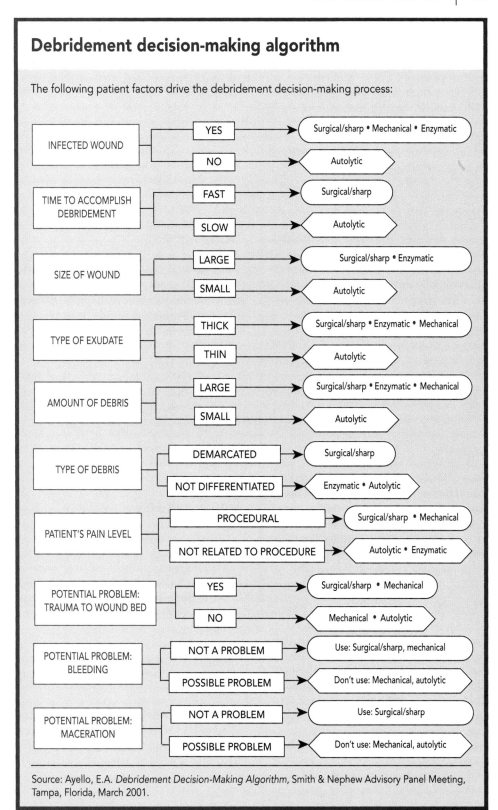

INFECTED WOUND	YES →	Surgical/sharp • Mechanical • Enzymatic
	NO →	Autolytic
TIME TO ACCOMPLISH DEBRIDEMENT	FAST →	Surgical/sharp
	SLOW →	Autolytic
SIZE OF WOUND	LARGE →	Surgical/sharp • Enzymatic
	SMALL →	Autolytic
TYPE OF EXUDATE	THICK →	Surgical/sharp • Enzymatic • Mechanical
	THIN →	Autolytic
AMOUNT OF DEBRIS	LARGE →	Surgical/sharp • Enzymatic • Mechanical
	SMALL →	Autolytic
TYPE OF DEBRIS	DEMARCATED →	Surgical/sharp
	NOT DIFFERENTIATED →	Enzymatic • Autolytic
PATIENT'S PAIN LEVEL	PROCEDURAL →	Surgical/sharp • Mechanical
	NOT RELATED TO PROCEDURE →	Autolytic • Enzymatic
POTENTIAL PROBLEM: TRAUMA TO WOUND BED	YES →	Surgical/sharp • Mechanical
	NO →	Mechanical • Autolytic
POTENTIAL PROBLEM: BLEEDING	NOT A PROBLEM →	Use: Surgical/sharp, mechanical
	POSSIBLE PROBLEM →	Don't use: Mechanical, autolytic
POTENTIAL PROBLEM: MACERATION	NOT A PROBLEM →	Use: Surgical/sharp
	POSSIBLE PROBLEM →	Don't use: Mechanical, autolytic

Source: Ayello, E.A. *Debridement Decision-Making Algorithm*, Smith & Nephew Advisory Panel Meeting, Tampa, Florida, March 2001.

What are the wound characteristics?

Consider the size, depth, location, amount of drainage, presence (and extent) or absence of infection, and etiology of the wound.

How selective a method is needed?

Determine the risk for damage to healthy tissue when necrotic tissue is removed.

What methods are permitted?

Check that the intended debridement method is allowed by your state's practice act and by your facility. For example, using a scalpel to crosshatch eschar requires specialized training and licensure.

What's the care setting?

Some resources available in a hospital aren't practical in the home and may not even be available in a long-term care facility.

How much debridement is enough?

How do you know when you've debrided enough? Assess the tissue in the wound bed: When most of the wound surface is covered with granulation tissue and the necrotic tissue is gone, you've debrided enough. Falanga[14] has proposed that chronic wounds need constant debridement because maintenance debridement is an important part of the wound-bed preparation in these wounds. In the past, debridement was regarded as a singular event based on the visible assessment of the wound. Now, however, it's thought that frequent, limited, maintenance debridement will keep the bioburden low and stimulate growth factors.[15]

PRACTICE POINT

Use of the TIME acronym may be helpful in preparing the wound bed for healing.

Tissue nonviable or deficient
Infection or inflammation
Moisture imbalance
Epidermal margin nonadvancing or undermining[15]

Summary

Debridement is an essential step in the wound management process. Although surgical debridement is the fastest way of removing necrotic tissue from a wound, it may not be appropriate for all patients in all health care settings. The selection of the correct method of debridement should be based on the individual patient and the degree of necrosis present. By knowing the options for debridement, you can help prepare the wound bed and assist your patient on the road to healing.

Show what you know

1. Which one of the following statements about the purpose of debridement is correct? Debridement:

    A. is nonessential for wound healing.
    B. removes debris so cell movement is enhanced.
    C. removes necrotic tissue in order to enhance the wound's biologic burden.
    D. reduces the need for moist wound healing.

ANSWER: B. A is incorrect; most wounds need debridement to heal. C is incorrect because necrotic tissue increases the wound's biologic burden. D is incorrect because wounds need moist healing.

2. *Which one of the following signs in a stable necrotic heel would signal a need for debridement?*

A. Edema
B. Presence of thick, leathery eschar
C. An impending inspection by a regulator
D. Yellow slough

ANSWER: A. Edema is a sign of infection. Other signs are erythema, fluid wave, and drainage.

3. *Which one of the following methods is an example of mechanical debridement?*

A. Collagenases
B. Maggots
C. Film dressings
D. Pulsed lavage

ANSWER: D. Collagenases are enzymes, maggots secrete natural collagenase, and film dressings are a method of autolytic debridement.

4. *A resident in a long-term care facility is on Coumadin and needs debridement for a necrotic ulcer on his forearm. Which of the following methods of debridement would be least indicated?*

A. Surgical
B. Enzymatic
C. Mechanical
D. Autolytic

ANSWER: A. Since this resident is on Coumadin and bleeding can occur, surgical debridement would be least indicated. Also, the appropriate personnel and equipment may not be available in the patient's long-term care facility.

5. *Which method of debridement would be best to use initially for a hospitalized client with an infected large sacral pressure ulcer?*

A. Surgical
B. Enzymatic

C. Mechanical
D. Autolytic

ANSWER: A. Time is of the essence and surgical debridement is the quickest method that can be used with infected wounds. Because the client is hospitalized, the appropriate personnel and equipment to do this method of debridement are available.

References

1. Ramasastry, S.S. "Chronic Problem Wounds," *Clinical Plastic Surgery* 25(3):367-96, July 1998.
2. Ayello, E.A., et al. "Skip the Knife: Debriding Wounds Without Surgery," *Nursing 2002* 32(9): 58-63, September 2002.
3. Wysocki, B. "Wound Fluids and the Pathogenesis of Chronic Wounds," *Journal of Wound, Ostomy, and Continence Nursing* 23(6):283-90, November 1996.
4. Edlich, R.F., et al. "The Biology of Infections: Sutures, Tapes, and Bacteria," in *Wound Healing and Wound Infection: Theory and Surgical Practice*. Edited by Hunt, T.K. New York, NY: Appleton-Century-Crofts, 1980.
5. Treatment of Pressure Ulcer Guideline Panel. *Treatment of Pressure Ulcers, Clinical Practice Guideline*, No. 15. U.S. Department of Health and Human Services, AHCPR Publication No. 95-0652, Rockville, MD, December 1994.
6. Hatz, R.A., et al. *Wound Healing and Wound Management*. Heidelberg, Germany: Springer-Verlag Berlin, 1994.
7. Scott, R., and Loehne, H. "Five Questions and Answers About Pulsed Lavage," *Advances in Skin & Wound Care* 13(3, part I):133-34, May-June 2000.
8. Ashworth, J., and Chivers, M. "Conservative Sharp Debridement: The Professional and Legal Issues," *Professional Nurse* 17(10):585-88, June 2002.
9. Steed, D.L., et al. "Effect of Extensive Debridement and Treatment on the Healing of Diabetic Foot Ulcers. Diabetic Ulcer Study Group," *Journal of the American College of Surgeons* 183(1): 61-64, July 1996.

10. Rodeheaver, G., et al. "Wound Healing and Wound Management: Focus on Debridement. An Interdisciplinary Round Table, September 18, 1992, Jackson Hole, WY," *Advances in Wound Care* 7(1):22-39, January 1992.

11. Jones, G., and Nahai, F. , "Management of Complex Wounds," *Current Problems in Surgery* 35(3):179-270, March 1998.

12. Bale, S. "A Guide to Wound Debridement," *Journal of Wound Care* 6(4):179-82, April 1997.

13. Mosher, B.A., et al. "Outcomes of Four Methods of Debridement Using a Decision Analysis Methodology," *Advances in Wound Care* 12(2):81-88, March 1999.

14. Falanga, V. "Wound Bed Preparation and the Role of Enzymes: A Case for Multiple Actions of Therapeutic Agents," *Wounds* 14(2): 47-57, March 2002.

15. Schultz, G.S., et al. "Wound Bed Preparation: A Systematic Approach to Wound Management," *Wound Repair and Regeneration* 11(Suppl 1):S1-S28, March 2003.

CHAPTER 9

Wound treatment options

Sharon Baranoski, MSN, RN, CWOCN, APN, FAAN
Elizabeth A. Ayello, PhD, RN, APRN,BC, CWOCN, FAAN

OBJECTIVES

After completing this chapter, you'll be able to:

- explain moist wound therapy
- select dressings based on assessment of wound characteristics
- list indications for use of dressings by categories
- state the advantages and disadvantages for each dressing category
- use the principles of care in dressing selection
- discuss the use of dermal skin substitutes
- list three alternate wound care therapies.

A challenge for clinicians

Providing quality care for your wound care patients should start with understanding wound products, cost-effective treatment modalities, and the principles of optimal wound interventions. Wound dressings can present a challenging decision for clinicians. As clinicians try to heal wounds faster, the marketplace continues to provide many more treatment choices. Keeping abreast of wound dressing choices and various application techniques as well as which product to use and when, is an ambitious task for all clinicians. Essential dressing competency recommendations have been suggested. (See *Clinician competencies for dressing selection*, page 128.) Clinicians can benefit from a working knowledge of wound management including dressing options, cost, frequency of product changes, and how they correlate with visit frequency.

Moist wound healing

Health and wound care have certainly changed! During the past 2 decades, wound care has made more advances than over the past 2,000 years. The wound care revolution has occurred due in part to the discovery by Dr. Winter in the 1960s of the importance of moist wound healing in experimental animals.[1] Hinman and Maibach[2] paralleled these

Clinician competencies for dressing selection

- Conduct a thorough wound assessment to identify wound characteristics and treatment options.
- Know the principles of wound care.
- Be able to differentiate among the different types of dressings.
- Know the characteristics of an ideal dressing.
- Consider the patient's health care coverage, financial abilities, and access to appropriate products, and factor in cost as well as clinical benefit when selecting products.
- Take advantage of conferences, seminars, and self-study opportunities to keep abreast of the latest treatment techniques and products.

Adapted with permission from Baranoski, S. "Wound Dressings: Challenging Decisions," *Home Healthcare Nurse* 17(1):19-25, January 1999.

findings of faster resurfacing in partial thickness wounds in humans. This new concept of moist wound healing, coupled with advancement in wound dressing materials, has changed the practice of wound management.

EVIDENCE-BASED PRACTICE

Partial-thickness wounds in pigs covered with a plastic material had two times faster epithelialization than identical wounds left open to air.[1]

We now understand that wound healing must take place in a moist environment. Epithelial cells require this to migrate from the wound edges to reepithelialize or close the wound. This process is likened to "leap-frogging" of the cells. In a dry wound, these cells have to burrow down underneath the wound bed to find a moist area upon which to move to "march" or move forward. (See *Epithelial cell migration in an open wound*.)

This new understanding of the importance of moist wound healing based on wound physiology required that new dressing materials be developed and used. Wound dressings or coverings have evolved from "natural" coverings such as feathers and leafs, to gauze, to more sophisticated dressings based on current research.[3] Since the essential function of a wound dressing is to provide an optimal healing environment, the main objective of moist wound treatment is to imitate the condition of an intact blister. This "humid environment" has a stimulatory effect on cell proliferation and migration of epithelial cells.[3]

Formerly, wound dressings were primarily used to protect the wound from secondary infection by forming a barrier against bacteria and absorbing wound fluid. The greatest advantage of contemporary dressings is the maintenance of moist wound conditions in contrast to the "classical gauze techniques" that lead to the formation of a dry, firmly adhering scab.[4] Today's dressings promote rapid healing, act as a barrier, decrease or eliminate pain, require fewer changes, provide autolytic debridement, and can be cost-effective if used appropriately.[5]

Ovington[6] states "despite the benefits of newer dressing products, gauze is still the most widely used dressing and may be erroneously considered a standard of care." This is based on a study by Pieper and colleagues[7] of 1,638 wounds in the home care setting. The most commonly used dressing for all types of wounds (n = 406) was dry gauze. No dressing (that is, an uncovered wound) was the second most

Epithelial cell migration in an open wound

In a moist environment, epithelial cells can migrate on the wound bed surface to close the wound, as shown below.

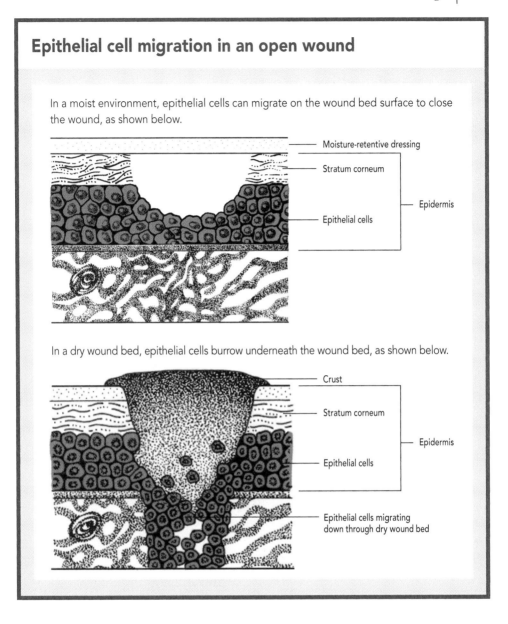

In a dry wound bed, epithelial cells burrow underneath the wound bed, as shown below.

common (n = 252), and saline-moistened gauze (n = 145) was third.[7] Advanced moisture-retentive dressings were less than 25% of all dressings used.

Ovington[6] cautions clinicians about using gauze dressings. (See *The case against gauze dressings*, page 130.) Although intended for wet-to-moist use, gauze dressings are often allowed to dry out before removal. Research by Kim et al.[8] suggests that a saline gauze dressing acts as an osmotic dressing.

As water evaporates from the saline dressing, it becomes hypertonic. Because the body wants to maintain homeostasis by reestablishing isotonicity, wound tissue fluid is drawn into the dressing. In addition to water, wound fluid includes blood and proteins. These substances form an impermeable layer on the dress-

The case against gauze dressings

- A gauze dressing can impair wound healing because it lowers the wound temperature and impedes fluid evaporation.
- Wet-to-dry gauze dressings are a non-selective mechanical debridement method. Removal of healthy tissue causes injury to the wound and pain.
- Clinical studies have shown higher infection rates in wounds for which gauze dressings were used compared to wounds dressed with transparent films or hydrocolloids.
- Changing a dressing more than once per day isn't always effective for patient outcomes and may not be reimbursable.
- Research has shown that bacteria are released into the air when gauze dressings (wet or dry) are removed from the wound.
- Semiocclusive dressings are more financially feasible from a total cost perspective.

Adapted with permission from Ovington, L.G. "Hanging Wet-to-Dry Dressings Out to Dry," *Advances in Skin & Wound Care* 15(2):79-84, March-April 2002.

is that nerve endings in the wound aren't exposed and don't become dehydrated.

Local tissue cools as a gauze dressing becomes dry. As water evaporates from the wound surface, wound temperature decreases. Reduced tissue temperatures (up to 10° below normal) have been found in wounds left open and uncovered (69.8° F [21° C]) as well as those where gauze dressings are used (77° to 80.6° F [25° to 27° C]).[11] Reduced wound temperature results in physiologic effects (effects of local vasoconstriction, hypoxia, impaired leukocyte mobility, phagocytic efficiency, and increased affinity of hemoglobin for oxygen), all which contribute to impaired wound healing.[6] Higher temperatures of 91.4° to 95° F (33° to 35° C) are found in wounds covered with transparent films or foam dressings. Semiocclusive dressings impede moisture loss from the wound, thus preventing local cooling and its associated negative healing effects.[6]

Gauze dressings don't present a barrier to bacteria. An in vitro study by Lawrence[12] demonstrated that bacteria can pass through up to 64 layers of dry gauze. Once the gauze is moistened, it's even less effective as a barrier to bacteria.[6] Infection rates are higher in wounds where gauze is used as compared to wounds covered with transparent films or hydrocolloids.[13,14] Gauze dressings are also labor intensive as they require several changes per day.[6] (See *Why are gauze dressings still used?*)

Film dressings and hydrocolloid dressings were among the first of the dressing materials that could maintain a moist wound-healing environment. New application techniques had to be learned and, more importantly, the clinical significance of wound fluid findings. The accumulation of light greenish-yellow fluid seen collecting under film dressings has caused us to relearn what is a normal expectation in a healing wound. Even the

ing that prevents wound fluid from "wetting" the dressing; the net result is the dressing dries out. Ovington[6] states that "removal of a wet-to-moist dressing that has dried may then cause reinjury of the wound, resulting in pain and delayed wound healing." Decreased pain, including at time of dressing change, has been found when semiocclusive dressings rather than gauze dressings are used.[9,10] The mechanism for this reduction in pain

different nuance of wound odors has been cause for new learning. For example, different odors occur as wound fluid interacts with different dressing materials. A wound being treated with alginate dressings, which are made from seaweed, may smell like "low tide."

Treatment decisions

The myriad products available for wound care have enhanced the overall management of patients, but have also created confusion about selecting the appropriate product. Optimal wound interventions should be dependent on the basic principles of wound care, attentive wound assessment, and expected outcomes. A complete wound assessment should be the driving element in all treatment decisions. (See chapter 6, Wound assessment.) Wound assessment should be based on the principles of wound care. (See *Principles of care: The MEASURES acronym,* page 132.)

Wound treatment decisions start with a thorough assessment of the wound itself and a comprehensive collection of data about the patient's overall status. Wound assessment parameters can assist with treatment choices and decisions for appropriate dressing selection. (See *Wound care decision algorithm,* page 133.)

Once a thorough wound assessment is complete, choosing dressings and treatments becomes a clinical decision based on data collected during the assessment and the overall expected outcome.

PRACTICE POINT

Dressing choices = Wound assessment + Principles of wound care

Treatment goals may be to achieve a clean wound, heal the wound, maintain a clean wound bed, or place the patient in

Why are gauze dressings still used?

Ovington[6] suggests reasons for the continued use of gauze dressings.

- Gauze dressings have a long tradition in wound care—gauze and saline are familiar and readily available.
- Gauze is perceived as being inexpensive; advanced dressings may be incorrectly perceived as being expensive. Frequency of dressing change and caregiver costs must be considered in addition to the cost of the dressing itself when calculating the total cost of dressing changes.
- Most advanced dressings are of discrete dimensions and can't always be adjusted for wounds of different sizes, requiring health care facilities to stock multiple sizes. Gauze, on the other hand, is easily tailored to fit the wound.
- Many practitioners are unaware of the broad array of alternative dressing products available and the way they work. The variations in appearance and performance of new types of dressings may initially confuse the health care provider.
- Advanced dressings may be perceived as more expensive than gauze due to individual rather than bulk purchase pricing.

Adapted with permission from Ovington, L.G. "Hanging Wet-to-Dry Dressings Out to Dry," *Advances in Skin & Wound Care* 15(2):79-84, March-April 2002.

another setting to continue care.[15] Clinicians need to match the wound assessment characteristics with the dressing characteristics from the various dressings available. The goal of care then becomes *using the right product on the right wound at the right time.* For example, a

Principles of care: The MEASURES acronym

Minimize trauma to wound bed

Eliminate dead space (tunnels, tracts, undermining)

Assess and manage the amount of exudate

Support the body's tissue defense system

Use non-toxic wound cleansers

Remove infection, debris, and necrotic tissue

Environment maintenance, including thermal insulation and a moist wound bed

Surrounding tissue, protect from injury and bacterial invasion

Adapted with permission from Baranoski, S. "Wound Dressings: Challenging Decisions," *Home Healthcare Nurse* 17(1):19-25, January 1999.

granular, nondraining moist or wet wound needs to maintain a moisture balance conducive to healing. The primary dressing choice would be a product that maintains a moist environment but doesn't cause maceration or desiccation of the wound bed. In another example, the goal of dressing selection for a necrotic draining wound is to loosen the eschar for surgical debridement or to autolytically debride the wound (see chapter 8, Wound debridement), absorb the excess exudate, and prevent trauma to surrounding tissue.

PRACTICE POINT

If the wound is dry, add moisture. If the wound has drainage, absorb it. If the wound has necrotic tissue, debride it.

Clinicians need to constantly reassess the wound status so that appropriate treatment interventions can be given. It's important to understand that once the characteristics of the wound assessment change, so may the dressing choice. All wound products come with product information and instructions to guide the user in appropriate use of that product. The most appropriate dressing should be selected, considering the patient, the wound, and the site. (See *Characteristics of an ideal dressing*, page 134 and *Wound care products*, pages 136 to 145.)

PRACTICE POINT

Wound dressings should be changed to meet the characteristics of the wound bed.

PRACTICE POINT

Read and understand the information in the package insert before using a wound care product.

Dressings that come in contact with the wound bed are considered primary dressings. Secondary dressings are those dressings that cover a primary dressing or secure a dressing in place. Clinicians should know which dressings are safe to be put into the actual wound and those that are used as securement products.

Wound care decision algorithm

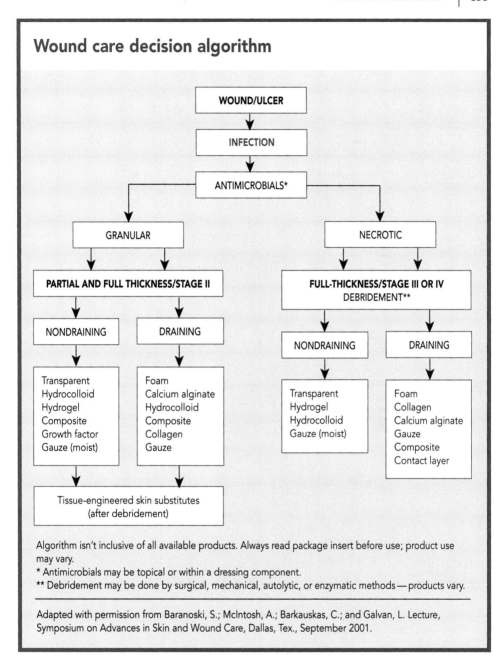

Algorithm isn't inclusive of all available products. Always read package insert before use; product use may vary.
* Antimicrobials may be topical or within a dressing component.
** Debridement may be done by surgical, mechanical, autolytic, or enzymatic methods—products vary.

Adapted with permission from Baranoski, S.; McIntosh, A.; Barkauskas, C.; and Galvan, L. Lecture, Symposium on Advances in Skin and Wound Care, Dallas, Tex., September 2001.

Several dressings on the market act as primary and secondary dressings. Again, what are the wound characteristics that you are addressing?

Dressing selections should also include an assessment of the patient outcome for treatment. High-priced, inappropriate dressings are often utilized when a more cost-effective management would apply. Outcome is commonly driven by institutional setting. Acute care patients with length of stays of 4 to 5 days usually won't achieve healing as their outcome, but will achieve a moist, clean wound

Characteristics of an ideal dressing

Use the following characteristics to determine the ideal dressing for your patient. The ideal dressing should:

- maintain a moist environment
- facilitate autolytic debridement
- be conformable for the range of use needed (such as to fill tunneling, undermining, or sinus tracts to eliminate dead space)
- come in numerous shapes and sizes
- be absorbent
- provide thermal insulation
- act as a bacterial barrier
- reduce or eliminate pain at the wound site and not cause pain on dressing removal
- be cost effective.

The following considerations can be used to evaluate the dressing:

- number of days the dressing can remain in place
- reason for change or removal of dressing
- appearance of dressing (soiled or intact?)
- ease of dressing application
- ease of dressing removal
- ease of dressing maintenance
- ease of teaching about dressing to caregiver.

Adapted with permission from Seaman, S. "Dressing Selection in Chronic Wound Management," *Journal of the American Podiatric Medical Association* 92(1):24-33, January 2002.

of the patient. Wound outcomes need to be patient-focused and realistic to the length of time a patient is in our care.

The old practice of using the same dressing material for the entire wound healing time is no longer valid. All wounds under the care of clinicians should be assessed weekly and more often if notable changes occur. (See chapter 6, Wound assessment.)

Wound assessment is the cumulative process of observation of the actual wound as well as observing the patient, data collection, and evaluation. Weekly reassessment will provide the indices of a successful treatment and guide decisions that suggest product changes. As the wound characteristics change, so too should the choice of the wound dressings. Several different types of products may be needed as the wound progresses through the stages of healing. It's much more likely that dressing choices will change as the wound evolves.

Dressings should be carefully matched to the wound, the patient, and the setting. For example, a deep wound with a large amount of drainage will require a highly absorbent dressing such as an alginate or foam. As the depth and amount of drainage decreases, a dressing such as a hydrogel, hydrocolloid, or film might be used.

PRACTICE POINT

Don't use film dressings with higher moisture vapor rates developed for use over intravenous line sites on open wounds.

Over the course of healing, the treatment plan will change as the wound is filled with granulation tissue and epithelialization occurs. Economic factors should also be considered when selecting dressings. (See *Economic considerations for nurses,* page 146.)

bed that supports the healing environment. Home care and long-term care settings may have a goal of healing or just maintaining the current status of the wound based on the overall health status

The notion that all wounds are alike has changed. Understanding of the etiology of the wound is essential for appropriate care. Local wound care products as well as supportive care must be individualized for the particular wound. For example, a venous stasis ulcer might require a highly absorptive dressing as well as the necessary compression therapy. A variety of layered bandages beyond the classic "Unna boot" are now used. Checking for ankle-brachial index and pulses using a Doppler has become a standard part of the total care of a patient with a peripheral vascular ulcer. However, compression therapy should never be used on an arterial ulcer.

Using wound healing biology to select treatment

An example of increased understanding of the "biology" of wound healing and technology is the use of growth factors. Growth factors are now available either derived from a patient's own platelets or in a drug form dispensed in a tube to apply to diabetic wounds. Research continues as to what combination, what quantity, and when growth factors will best enhance wound healing. Yet another way technology is providing new options for wound management is in the use of tissue-engineered skin equivalents for healing chronic wounds.

Moist wound therapy and dressing options

The essential role and function of a wound dressing is to provide the right environment to enhance and promote wound healing. Research over the last 40 years has lead to the generally accepted phenomena that moist wound dressings create an optimal environment for wounds to heal faster and with less scar formation. The work of Orland[17] and Winter[1] led to the development of moist wound dressings as a clinical intervention to treat wound.

George Winter is often cited as the father of moist wound healing. His laboratory work comparing air drying to occlusive dressings, effect on epithelialization in the animal model is generally considered to be a landmark study.[18] Fear of increasing infection with occlusive therapy slowed the development of the first moist wound therapy dressing. Sixteen years passed before the development of what is considered the first moist wound therapy dressing, Opsite. Continued research, clinician experiments, and interest in wounds in general, has led many companies to develop a potpourri of moist wound treatment dressings. This has created a challenge for health care providers, who struggle to keep up with the ever-increasing number of new products.

The following synopsis will review the major dressing categories, with helpful practice points on what, when, and how, to use these dressings.

Transparent film dressings
Transparent film dressings, so named for their see-through properties, are thin polyurethane membranes. They are coated with an adhesive that allows them to adhere to the wound margins without sticking to the actual wound, as shown below.

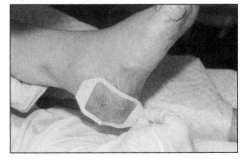

(Text continues on page 144.)

Wound care products

Numerous categories and classifications of wound dressings have been published. The chart below summarizes some of the most commonly used wound dressings.

No one product is a panacea for care. Dressing choices must be made in conjunction with the wound assessment and the principles of wound care. Wound dressings should be changed to meet the characteristics of the wound bed. Manufacturer instructions and recommendations found on the dressing package regarding frequency of dressing change and application method should be read and followed.

Use this chart to select the dressing most appropriate for the patient, the wound, and the site.

Dressing category	Description and composition	Trade name		
WOUND CARE PRODUCTS				
Transparent film	Polyurethane or co-polymer with porous adhesive layer that allows oxygen to pass through the membrane and moisture vapor to escape	Bioclusive Blister Film CarraFilm ClearCell Clear Site Mefilm	Opsite Opsite Plus Suresite Polyskin II Polyskin MR ProCyte	Tegaderm Tegaderm HP Suresite Transeal UniFlex
Hydrocolloid	Hydrophilic colloid particles bound to polyurethane foam; impermeable to bacteria and other contaminants; minimal to moderate absorptive properties; contact layer may differ	CarraSmart CombiDerm ACD CombiDerm nonadhesive Comfeel Plus Comfeel Triad Curaderm Cutinova Hydro Duoderm CGF	Duoderm Extra Thin & Paste Exuderm Exuderm LP Exuderm RCD Hydrocol Hyperion MPM Excel NU-DERM Procol	RepliCare RepliCare Thin Restore Restore CX Restore Plus Sorbex SignaDres Tegasorb Tegasorb Thin Ultec Ultec Pro
Hydrogel	Water- or glycerin-based, non-adherent, crossed-linked polymer (Variable absorptive properties; contains 80% to 99% water.)	AquaSite Aqua Flo Biolex CarraDres CarraSmart Carrasyn Carrasyn Gel Curafil Gel Curagel Curasol Gel	Derma-Gel Dermagran Elasto-Gel, Plus Elta Hypergel Iamin Hydrating Gel IntraSite Gel FlexiGel MPM Hydrogel	Normlgel Nu-Gel Purilon Gel Restore Gel Skintegrity SoloSite TenderWet Gel Tegagel Vigilon XCell

Indications	Advantages and benefits	Disadvantages
• Primary or secondary dressing • Partial-thickness wounds • Stage I or II pressure ulcers • Superficial burns • Donor sites	• Wound inspection • Impermeable to fluids and bacteria • Conformable • Promotes autolytic debridement • Prevents or reduces friction • Change daily or if leakage noted • Numerous sizes available	• Nonabsorptive • May adhere to some wounds • Not for draining wounds • Fluid retention may lead to maceration of the periwound area
• Primary or secondary dressing • Partial- and full-thickness wounds • Pressure ulcers • Dermal ulcers • Under compression wraps • Granular wounds • Necrotic wounds • Use as a preventive dressing • Use as a secondary dressing or under taping procedures	• Facilitates autolytic debridement • Self-adherent (some may adhere to wound bed) • Impermeable to fluids and bacteria • Conformable • Reduction of pain • Thermal insulation • Minimal to moderate absorption • Long wear time: most, 3 to 5 days; some, up to 7 days; decreases frequency of dressing changes • Numerous sizes, shapes, forms, thicknesses, and adhesive properties available	• Some are opaque • Not recommended for heavily draining wounds, sinus tracts, tunnels, or fragile skin • Some are contraindicated for full-thickness wounds and infection • Some may be difficult to remove and may leave a residue • Leakage can be a problem if not applied correctly • Odor noted with removal can be confused with infection; some may leave a residue in the wound bed
• Stage II to stage IV pressure ulcers • Partial- and full-thickness wounds • Dermabrasion • Painful wounds • Dermal ulcers • Skin tears • Minor burns • Radiation burns • Donor sites • Necrotic wounds	• Nonadherent • Trauma-free removal • Rehydrates the wound bed • Minimal to moderate absorption • Can be used with topical medications, in infected wounds, and in cavities or tunnels • Softens and loosens necrosis and slough to aid autolytic debridement • Numerous sizes and forms (gels, sheets, strips, with gauze) available	• Some require secondary dressing to secure • May macerate periwound skin • Not recommended for heavily draining wounds, check absorptive ability • Daily dressing changes may be needed

(continued)

Wound care products *(continued)*

Dressing category	Description and composition	Trade name		
WOUND CARE PRODUCTS *(continued)*				
Foam	Hydrophilic polyurethane/polymer or gel-film-coated foam; nonocclusive, nonadherent, absorptive wound dressing	3M Foam Adhesive and Nonadhesive Dressing Allevyn Allevyn Cavity Biatain CarraSmart	Curafoam Cutinova Flexzan Hydrasorb Lyofoam Mepilex Mitraflex Optifoam	Polyderm Polymem PolyWic Sof-Foam Tielle Tielle Plus VigiFoam
Calcium alginate	Nonwoven composite of fibers from calcium alginate, a cellulose-like polysaccharide (Highly absorptive dressing manufactured from brown seaweed; forms a soft gel when mixed with wound fluid.)	Algiderm AlgiSite CarraGinate Carrasorb Comfeel Seasorb Curasorb Cutinova Alginate	Kaltostat Polymem Alginate Maxorb CMC Melgisorb NU-DERM Alginate	NutraStat Restore CalciCare Sorbsan Tegagen HI & HG Alginate
Composites	Combination of two or more physically distinct products manufactured as a single dressing that provides multiple functions (Features may include a bacterial barrier, absorptive layer, foam, hydrocolloid, or hydrogel; available in semiadherent or nonadherent.)	Alldress CompDress Island Covaderm Plus Epigard	Medipore + MPM Multi-layer Repel Stratasorb Tenderwet	Telfa Island Tegaderm Absorbent Pad Viasorb
Collagens	Major protein of the body (Stimulates cellular migration and contributes to new tissue development and wound debridement.)	Catrix Fibracol hyCure	Kollagen-Medifil Particles/Gel/Pads	Kollagen-Skin Temp Sheets Promogran Matrix

Indications	Advantages and benefits	Disadvantages
• Partial- and full-thickness wounds with minimal to heavy drainage • Stage II to stage IV pressure ulcers • Surgical wounds • Dermal ulcers • Under compression wraps or stockings • Infected and noninfected wounds (varies, check product package insert) • Tunneling and cavity wounds (varies, check product package insert)	• Nonadherent • Trauma-free removal • Conformable • Fluid management: absorptive, minimal to moderate heavy drainage; some wicking action • Easy to apply and remove • Frequency of dressing change depends on the amount of drainage—up to 7 days • Available in numerous sizes, shapes, pads, sheets, and cavity dressings; with adhesive borders and without	• Not recommended for non-draining wounds • Not recommended for dry eschar • Not all foams recommended for infected wounds and for use in tunnels and tracts (check product package insert) • May require secondary dressing or tape to secure • May macerate periwound area if not changed appropriately
• Partial- and full-thickness wounds • Moderate to heavy draining wounds • Stage III to stage IV pressure ulcers • Dermal wounds • Surgical incision/dehisced wounds • Postoperative wounds for hemostasis • Sinus tracts, tunnels, or cavities • Infected wounds • Donor sites	• Highly absorbent and nonocclusive • Trauma-free removal • Can be used on infected wounds with tunneling or undermining • Hemostatic properties for minor bleeding • Reduced frequency of dressing changes • Facilitates autolysis • Available in sheets, ropes, and within other composite-type dressings	• Contraindicated for dry eschar, third degree burns, surgical implantation, and heavy bleeding • May require secondary dressing to secure • Gel may have odor during dressing change • Can desiccate the wound bed if not changed appropriately • Some forms can leave fibers in the wound bed if drainage not sufficient to gel product
• Primary and secondary dressings for partial- and full-thickness wounds • Stage I to stage IV pressure ulcers; varies according to product • Minimal to heavy draining wounds • Dermal ulcers • Surgical incisions	• Facilitates autolytic or mechanical debridement • Conformable • Multiple sizes and shapes available • Easy to apply and remove • Most include adhesive border • Frequency of dressing change dependent on wound type (check product package insert)	• Adhesive borders may limit use on fragile skin • Some contraindicated for stage IV ulcers (check product package insert) • Not all composites provide moist wound therapy; may desiccate the wound bed (check product package insert)
• Partial- and full-thickness wounds • Stage III and some stage IV pressure ulcers (check product package insert)	• Absorbent, nonadherent • Conforms well, easy to apply • Change in 1 to 7 days; daily if infection present	• Contraindicated for dry wounds, third degree burns, and sensitivities to collagen/bovine products *(continued)*

Wound care products (continued)

Dressing category	Description and composition	Trade name		
WOUND CARE PRODUCTS *(continued)*				
Collagens *(continued)*				
Contact layers	Single layer of a woven net (polyamide); acts as a low-adherence material when applied to wound surface (Wound drainage is wicked to secondary dressing.)	Conformant 2 Dermanet Mepitel	N-Terface Profore Wound Contact Layer	Telfa Clear Tegapore
Gauze dressings	Manufactured in many forms; woven and nonwoven, impregnated, and nonadherent (Not all gauze is appropriate for wound application.)	**Manufacturers and distributors:** Derma Sciences DeRoyal Industries	Johnson & Johnson MPM Medline	Molnycke Kendall Smith & Nephew
Antimicrobial dressings	Antimicrobial dressing may contain Cadeoxmer iodine, silver, or polyhexamethylene	Acticoat AcryDerm Silver Arglaes Arglaes Powder	Aquacel AG Contreet Iodosorb Gel	Iodoflex SilverSorb Silverlon
Drugs	Prescription drugs	Accuzyme Cloderm Cream	Granulex Panafil	Prudoxin Cream
ADVANCED WOUND CARE PRODUCTS				
Tissue-engineered skin (human skin equivalents)	Bilayered skin substitute grown in the laboratory; developed from human neonate foreskin cells and collagen	Apligraf	Dermagraft	

Indications	Advantages and benefits	Disadvantages
• Infected wounds • Tunneling wounds • Dermal ulcers • Donor sites • Skin grafts • Surgical wounds	• May be used in combination with topical agents and other dressings • Available in numerous sizes, pads, sheets, and rope	• Not recommended for necrotic wounds • Requires secondary dressing to secure • May require rehydration
• Primary dressing • Full-thickness wounds, minimal to heavy drainage • Donor sites	• Protection of wound base from dressing change trauma • May be applied with topical medications, fillers, or gauze dressings • Available in pads, sheets, and rolls	• Contraindications vary by product (check product package insert) • May not be recommended for tunneling wounds, stage I pressure ulcers, clean or debriding wounds, or third-degree burns
Indications vary with individual gauze products. • Partial- and full-thickness wounds • Draining wounds • Wounds requiring debridement, packing, or management of tunnels, tracts, or dead space • Surgical incisions • Postoperative wounds • Burns • Dermal ulcers • Pressure ulcers	• Readily available in many sizes and forms • Conformable, easy to apply, requires secondary dressing or tape to secure • Can be used on infected wounds and in combination with other topical products • Effective as a packing agent in tracts, tunnels, and undermined areas • Some absorptive and have wicking action • Some impregnated with other topical products • Mechanical debridement	• May disrupt wound healing if allowed to dry out or if changed inappropriately • Fibers may shed and adhere to wound bed • Usually requires secondary dressing • Not recommended for effective moist wound therapy treatment • Frequent dressing changes required • Not all gauze is absorbent, some may cause pooling of fluid and drainage leading to periwound maceration
• Infected wounds	• Controls bacteria bioburden • Effective against a broad spectrum of microorganisms	• Patient hypersensitivity to product contents (silver, iodine) • No magnetic resonance imaging when using silver dressings
• Varies by product	• See package insert for use	• Prescription needed
• Partial- and full-thickness wounds • Venous ulcers • Granular wounds	• Growth factors present in dermal skin equivalent • Decrease wound healing time	• Physician has to apply • Costly • Has to be stored properly • Wound has to be granular

(continued)

Wound care products *(continued)*

Dressing category	Description and composition	Trade name			
ADVANCED WOUND CARE PRODUCTS *(continued)*					
Extracellular matrix	Extracellular matrix material derived from the submucosal layer of porcine small intestines	Oasis Wound Matrix			
Growth factors	Platelet-derived wound healing formula created from the patient's own platelets	Autologous platelet GF, PDGF, TGFβ, b-FGF, ECF			
Becaplermin gel	Genetically engineered endogenous platelet derived growth factors produced in yeast and then formulated into a gel (Promotes proliferation of cells and granulation tissue.)	Regranex			
COMPRESSION THERAPY					
Compression therapy (2-, 3-, or 4-layer)	Used to manage edema and promote the return of venous blood to the heart (Use cautiously in patients with arterial ulcers.) *2-layer:* Zinc-oxide–impregnated bandaging system that provides realistic compression; usually provides 18 to 25 mm Hg compression *3- and 4-layer:* Sustained graduated compression bandages; usually provides 30 to 40 mm Hg compression *Elastic wraps*	Unna boot: • Primer • Tendrwrap • Unna-flex CircAid system 2-layer: • Conco • Medicopaste	3-layer: • Dynaflex • Profore Lite 4-layer: • Conco • Profore	Elastic wraps: • Comprilan • Setopress • Dyna-Flex • Flex Wrap • Soft Wrap • SurePress • Tubigrip	
ALTERNATIVE WOUND CARE THERAPIES					
Negative pressure therapy	Noninvasive active therapy using localized negative pressure to promote healing (Removes interstitial fluids from the wound.)	VAC device Provant Wound Closure			

Indications	Advantages and benefits	Disadvantages
• Diabetic wounds • Partial- and full-thickness injuries • Second-degree burns • Graft sites	• Biological dressing • Strength and flexibility	• Patient hypersensitivity to porcine- or bovine-derived products
Dependent on particular growth factor being used; may include: • Chronic, nonhealing wounds • Diabetic ulcers • Arterial ulcers • Venous ulcers	• Adjuncts to promote wound healing environment • Research ongoing	• Costly • No reimbursement • Continued research needed to demonstrate effectiveness
• Diabetic ulcers • Neuropathic ulcers • Granular ulcers	• Increases growth of new tissue and promotes cell division and movement of protein • Once daily	• Contraindicated for infected wounds, necrotic wounds, and for patients with poor lower extremity blood supply • Secondary dressing needed • Must be refrigerated • Costly
• Venous ulcers	• Can stay on for up to 1 week • Maintains compression for 1 week • Minimal cost due to less frequent need for dressing changes	• Contraindicated for use with arterial disease • Ankle-brachial index must be performed prior to use • Training is needed for proper application
• Granular draining wounds • Full-thickness wounds • Venous, arterial, diabetic, and pressure ulcers • Surgical wounds • Flaps, grafts • Acute traumatic wounds	• Removes excess interstitial fluid • Decreases edema and bacterial colonization • Increases blood supply and granular tissue formation • Enhances epithelial and cell migration	• Needs special supplies, training • Not reimbursed in acute or long-term care • Can increase pain in wounds • Not for infected, necrotic, malignant, or osteomyelitis wounds or fistulas *(continued)*

Wound care products *(continued)*

Dressing category	Description and composition	Trade name
ALTERNATIVE WOUND CARE THERAPIES *(continued)*		
Normothermic therapy	Noncontact radiant heat system delivered by a semiocclusive, moisture retentive dressing that warms wounds toward normothermia	Warm Up Therapy
Electrical stimulation	Electrical currents delivered into a wound and periwound skin through two electrodes applied directly to a patient's skin (Stimulates tissue growth.)	

Note: This chart isn't all-inclusive. No inferences should be made regarding the inclusion or exclusion of products on this list. Always read manufacturer's recommendations for appropriate use.

Adapted with permission from Baranoski, S.; McIntosh, A.; Barkauskas, C.; and Galvan, L. Lecture, Symposium on Advances in Skin and Wound Care, Dallas, Tex., September 2001.

Transparent films have no absorptive capacity but do transmit moisture vapor and are semipermeable to gases. These dressings imitate the outer skin layer to provide a moist environment, similar to a blister. This covering allows epithelial cells to migrate over the surface of the wound. Fluid may accumulates under these dressings. This fluid is sometimes mistaken for pus, a sign of infection. The fluid is a useful adjunct to create an autolytic environment, thereby inducing a cleaner wound surface. When excess fluid accumulates or leaks out from the sides of the dressing, it needs to be changed. Maceration of periwound skin can occur if not changed in a timely manner.

The dressings provide a valuable protective barrier against outside contaminates, fluid, and bacteria. Transparent films also provide protection from friction and aid in autolytic debridement and pain control. Film makes an excellent secondary dressing, as well. Most films can be left on for up to 7 days. Transparent films can be used on a variety of wound types, such as stages I and II pressure ulcers, superficial wounds, minor burns, lacerations; over sutures, catheter sites, donor sites, and superficial dermal ulcers; and for protection of the skin against friction.

Indications	Advantages and benefits	Disadvantages
• Partial- and full-thickness wounds • Stage III to stage IV pressure ulcers • Venous ulcers • Arterial ulcers • Diabetic ulcers • Surgical wounds	• Noncontact layer doesn't disturb wound bed when removed • Length of treatment 1 hour 3 times per day • Protects wound from trauma and contamination • May be used on infected wounds with concurrent antibiotic therapy	• Can't be used on third-degree burns • Caution with fragile skin • Reimbursement not yet available (pending) • Need to train staff on appropriate use
Chronic wounds, including: • Pressure ulcers • Diabetic ulcers • Arterial ulcers • Venous ulcers • Donor sites • Flaps • Burns	• Can be used on infected wounds • Decreases bacteria and wound pain • Increases oxygen perfusion and tensile wound strength	• Reimbursement issues • Length of treatment: 1 hour every day, for 5 to 7 days per week • Can't be used with osteomyelitis

Practice essentials

• Apply transparent film dressings to healthy skin; use with caution on aging and fragile skin. These dressings aren't recommended for infants and small children.

• These dressings may be used on dry to minimally moist wounds.

• Don't use transparent film dressings on exudating wounds.

• Transparent film dressings make excellent secondary dressings.

• Don't use film dressings on infected wounds.

• Change the dressing every 7 days, when fluid reaches the dressing margin, or as needed.

• When removing the dressing, lift the corner and pull the film toward the outside of the wound to break the adhesive barrier.

• Avoid roughness when pulling the film off; gently stretch the dressing and support the skin as you're removing the dressing.

• Skin protective wipes and sprays can be used on the periwound area before applying the dressing. Skin wipes also provide an additional seal to prevent the dressing edges from rolling.

• Always read the package insert before applying the dressing because product usage may vary.

• Numerous sizes and shapes are available.

Economic considerations for nurses

- Clean rather than sterile dressings can usually be used in the home with chronic wounds (refer to your facility's policy).
- Saline solution can be made at home by adding 8 teaspoons of salt to 1 gallon of boiling water.[16]
- Dressings shouldn't be left at the patient's bedside.
- Cost of product selected and resources available for financial assistance should be considered.
- Frequency of dressing changes and cost-effective use of materials affect economy.
- Fistula management may use pouching versus dressing.
- Hydrogen peroxide, povidone-iodine, hypochlorite solution, and acetic acid should be avoided as wound cleansers. All contribute to delayed healing of wounds.[16]

Adapted with permission from Baranoski, S. "Wound Dressings: Challenging Decisions," *Home Healthcare Nurse* 17(1):19-25, January 1999.

Hydrocolloid dressings

Hydrocolloid dressings were introduced in the 1980s. These new wafer-shaped dressings, as shown below, became the

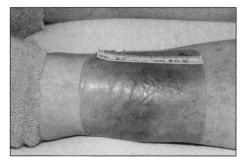

mainstay for wound management for many years. Hydrocolloids are impermeable to gases and water vapor.[19] They are composed of opaque mixtures of adhesive, absorbent polymers, pectin gelling agents, and sodium carboxmethyl cellulose. Hydrophilic particles within the dressing react with the wound fluid to form a soft gel over the wound bed. According to Choucair,[19] some hydrocolloid dressings provide an acidic environment and some act as a bacterial or viral barrier. Their translucent appearance allows for viewing of the amount of exudate absorbed and fluid accumulation under the dressing.

Hydrocolloid dressings may have a noticeable odor during dressing changes. This is normal in the absence of clinical signs of infection. Some hydrocolloids may also leave residue in the wound bed.

Hydrocolloid dressings have evolved into a shape to fit most wounds and locations. They're available in wafers, sheets, pastes, powders, and numerous sizes. Adhesive properties and ability to absorb exudate vary by product. Because the dressings are adhesive, care must be taken when using on fragile skin. Correct application requires the dressing to be bigger then the actual wound size. For optimal dressing adherence, the dressing must extend at least 1″ (2.5 cm) onto the healthy skin surrounding the wound. The dressing should be changed as recommended by the manufacturer. This could be from 3 to 7 days and often depends on the amount of exudate. Many of the newer hydrocolloids may also have other absorptive ingredients added, such as alginate, or have tapered borders or film adhesive edges.

Hydrocolloids are indicated for minimally to moderately heavy exudating wounds, abrasions, skin tears, lacerations, some pressure ulcers, dermal wounds, granular, or necrotic wounds and under compression wraps. They also provide a moist environment conducive to autolytic debridement. Excessive granulation (hypergranulation tissue) and maceration can occur if dressing isn't changed appropriately. Hydrocolloids are often used as a preventive dressing on high-risk areas and around surgical wounds to protect the skin from frequent tape removal. Hydro-colloids shouldn't be used on clinically infected wounds or those with heavy exudate.

Practice essentials
• Change the dressing every 3 to 7 days, or before it reaches its maximal absorption or when fluid reaches within 1″ (2.5 cm) of the edge.
• Don't use hydrocolloid dressings on infected wounds.
• These dressings aren't recommended for undermining, tunnels, or sinus tracts.
• Hydrocolloid dressings may be cut to fit the wound area, such as an elbow or heel.
• These dressings may be used as primary or secondary dressing, or over other wound filler products.
• Remove the dressing by starting at a corner and gently rolling it off the wound; don't pull to remove.
• Flush out any residue with saline.
• Skin protective wipes or sprays may be used on the periwound area to enhance adherence.
• Picture-framing with tape may prevent the dressing edges from rolling.

Hydrogel dressings

Hydrogel dressings, as shown below, have provided clinicians with a viable means to hydrate dry wound beds.

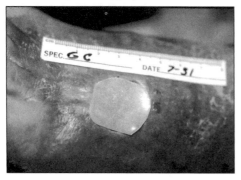

Amorphous hydrogel dressings, as shown below, are water in a gel form or matrix. Their unique cross-linked polymer structure entraps water and reduces the temperature of the wound bed by up to 5° C.[19,20] The moist environment created facilitates autolysis and removal of devitalized tissue.

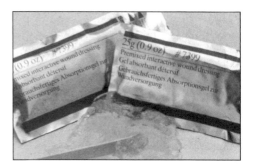

The main application for hydrogels is hydrating dry wound beds and softening and loosening slough and necrotic wound debris. Hydrogels have a limited absorptive capacity due to their high water concentration. Some hydrogels have other ingredients, such as alginates, collagen, or starch, to enhance their absorptive capacity and will absorb low to moderate amounts of exudate. Absorptive capability varies by product and type of gel. They can be used for many types of wounds, including pressure ulcers, partial- and full-thickness wounds, and vascular ulcers. The soothing and cooling properties also make them excellent choices for use in skin tears, dermabrasion, dermal wounds, donor sites, and radiation burns.

Maceration can be a concern for clinicians. Periwound skin areas need to be protected from excess hydration. Protective barriers are often recommended. One of the benefits of a hydrogel is the ability to be used with topical medications or antibacterial agents. Hydrogels are packaged as sheets, tube gels, sprays, and impregnated gauze pads or strips for packing tunneling and undermined areas within the wound bed. Some require a secondary dressing to secure the hydrogel, new versions have adhesive borders.

Practice essentials
• Don't use hydrogel with heavily draining wounds or on intact skin.
• Daily dressing changes may be necessary due to evaporation of the hydrogel. Some sheet hydrogels may last for several days. Check daily to maintain a moist environment.
• Protect the surrounding skin with a skin barrier ointment, wipe, or spray.

Foam dressings

Foam dressings, as shown below, are highly absorbent and are usually made from a polyurethane base with a heat- and pressure-modified wound contact layer.[21] Foam dressings are permeable to both gases and water vapor. The hydrophilic properties allow for absorption of exudate into the layers of the foam.

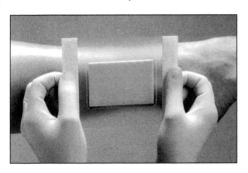

Foam dressings are some of the most adaptable dressings for wound care. They are indicated for wounds with moderate to heavy exudate, prophylactic protection over bony prominences or friction areas, partial and full thickness wounds, granular or necrotic wound beds, skin tears, donor sites, under compression wraps, surgical or dermal wounds, in combination with other primary dressings and wounds of any etiology. They can also be used on infected wounds if changed daily.[22]

Foams shouldn't be used on dry eschar wound beds. They could cause further desiccation of the wound site. Foams may be used in combination with topical treatments and or enzymatic debriders. Foams are available in many sizes and shapes, and as cavity (pillow type) dressings. Many foams don't have an adhesive border, so they'll need to be secured with tape. However, new foam products have emerged with adhesive borders. Caution with fragile skin may be warranted.

Practice essentials
• Not all foams have FDA approval for use on infected wounds — be sure to check the package insert.
• Foam dressings can be left in place for up to 7 days, depending on the amount of exudate absorption.
• Removal of these dressings is trauma-free.
• Foam dressings can be cut to fit the size of the wound.
• Skin wipes or sprays can be used to protect the periwound area from maceration.
• Nonadhesive border dressings will require taping or wraps to secure.

Calcium alginate dressings

Calcium alginate dressings, as shown below, provide yet another choice for clinicians. Alginates have greatly impacted the wound care market. Clinicians need-

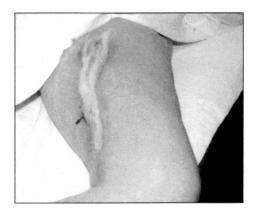

ed a dressing for managing highly exudative wounds. Alginate dressings are absorbent, nonadherent, biodegradable, nonwoven fibers derived from brown seaweed, composed of calcium salts of alginic acid and mannuronic and guluronic acids.[19-21]

When alginate dressings come in contact with sodium-rich solutions such as wound drainage, the calcium ions undergo an exchange for the sodium ions, forming a soluble sodium alginate gel. This gel maintains a moist wound bed and supports a therapeutic healing environment. Alginates can absorb 20 times their weight; this may vary based on product. They are extremely beneficial in managing large draining cavity wounds, pressure ulcers, vascular ulcers, surgical incisions, wound dehiscence, tunnels, sinus tracts, skin graft donor sites, exposed tendons, and infected wounds. Alginates are contraindicated for dry wounds, eschar covered wounds, surgical implantation or third-degree burns. Additionally, their hemostatic and absorptive properties make them useful on bleeding wounds.

Alginates are available in sheet, pad, and rope formats and in numerous sizes. They are usually changed daily or as indicated by the amount of drainage. Early wound care interventions may warrant more frequent dressing changes due to high volume of drainage. As fluid management is attained, the frequency of dressing changes can be decreased.

Practice essentials
• Calcium alginate dressings provide easy application and trauma-free removal.
• These dressings are a good choice for undermined or tunneled, draining wounds.
• These dressings require a secondary dressing.

• Calcium alginate dressings provide no bacterial barrier unless combined with another occlusive-type product.
• These dressings may leave fiber residue; flush with saline to remove.
• Calcium alginate dressings facilitate autolytic debridement.
• These dressings are cost-effective if used appropriately.

Composite dressings

A combination of materials makes up a single layered composite dressing. These dressings provide multiple functions. Features of these dressings include a bacterial barrier, an absorptive layer other than an alginate, foam, hydrocolloid, or hydrogel.[21] Additionally, they must have an adhesive border, and semiadherent or nonadherent properties. Not all composite dressings provide a moist environment; many are used or created with a secondary dressings. They are also referred to as island dressings. These dressings are conformable and are available in numerous sizes and shapes.

Practice essentials
• Use composite dressings with caution when treating a patient with fragile skin.
• Composite dressings are easy to apply.
• These dressings may be used on infected wounds and with topical products.
• They may facilitate autolytic or mechanical debridement.
• Frequency of dressing change depends on the wound type and manufacturers' recommendations.
• These dressings may adhere to wound bed; use caution when removing.

Collagen dressings

Collagen is a major protein of the body and is necessary for wound healing and repair. Collagen dressings are derived from bovine hide (cowhide). Collagen dressings are either 100% collagen or may be combined with alginates or other products. They are a highly absorptive hydrophilic moist wound dressing.

Seaman[22] suggests that collagen powders, particles, and pads are useful in treating highly exudating wounds. If the wound has low to moderate exudate, use sheets. If the wound is dry, use gels. Collagen dressings can be used on granulating or necrotic wounds and partial or full thickness wounds.[22]

A collagen dressing should be changed a minimum of every 7 days. If wound infection is present, then daily dressing change is recommended. Collagen dressings require a secondary dressing for securement.

Practice essentials
• Use collagen dressings with caution when treating patients with fragile skin if adhesive secondary dressings are also being used.
• These dressings are contraindicated for patients sensitive to bovine products.
• Don't use these dressings on dry wounds or third-degree burns.
• Collagen dressings are easy to remove.
• Their gel properties prevent these dressings from adhering to the wound bed.
• These dressings facilitate a moist wound environment and may be used with other topical products.
• Change collagen dressings daily if used on infected wounds.

Contact layer dressings

Contact layer dressings are a single layer of a woven net that acts as a low adherence material when applied to wound surfaces.[21] A contact layer dressing is applied directly to the wound. It acts as a protective interface between the wound and the secondary dressings. Their main purpose is to allow exudate to pass through the contact layer and into the secondary dressing. They are often used with ointments, creams, or other topical products such as growth factors or tissue engineered skin substitutes. Contact layer dressings aren't recommended for dry wounds or third-degree burns. Check the package insert for clarification as to which wounds the product can be used. Various sizes and shapes are available. Frequency of change of dressing is dependent on the etiology of the wound and the amount of exudate.

Practice essentials
• Contact layer dressings aren't recommended for dry wounds or third-degree burns.
• Contact layer dressings are easy to apply and are secured with a secondary dressing.
• They provide protection of wound bed during dressing changes.

Gauze dressings

Gauze dressings have been used in wound care for many years. They were once considered a standard of care. Gauze still remains one of the most widely used dressings. Numerous variations of woven and nonwoven gauze products are available. Many are used as packing agents, primary and secondary dressings, wound infections and for mechanical debridement. Woven gauze may leave lint fibers in the wound bed contributing to inflammation and possible infection. Nonwoven gauze is absorbent and doesn't leave fibers in the wound. Should gauze be included in the wound dressing list of products? Yes, but not as a moist wound therapy intervention but as a secondary dressing when used with other moist wound products. Gauze doesn't create an optimal moist healing environment, even if moistened with saline. Gauze impedes healing, increases the risk of infection, requires numerous dressing changes, and is a substandard of care in today health care environment.[6] The benefits of gauze dressings are over-shadowed by the disadvantages.

Practice essentials
• Gauze dressings are easy to apply.
• They don't provide an adequate moist wound environment.
• Gauze dressings require frequent changes; check your facility's policy for guidelines.
• These dressings may traumatize the wound bed when being removed.
• Woven gauze may leave lint fibers in the wound bed.
• Gauze dressings are labor-intensive.

Antimicrobial dressings

Antimicrobial dressings have added a new dimension to the wound dressing arena. Clinicians now have several choices of dressings when dealing with wound infections. These new dressings are different than topical antibiotic therapy. They provide the benefit of an antimicrobial effect against bacteria and a moist environment for healing. The active ingredient may be silver ions, cadexomer iodine, or polyhexamethylene biguanide. Antimicrobial dressings provide an adjunct in treating wound infections. They may not replace the need for systemic antibiotic therapy. As research continues and new products become available, this classification of wound dressing will expand. Antimicrobial dressings are available in a variety of forms: transparent dressings, gauze, island dressings, foams, and absorptive fillers. Some of these dressings can remain in place for 7 days.

Practice essentials
• Antimicrobial dressings are an adjunct in treating wound infections.

• Frequency of dressing change varies among antimicrobials.

Tissue-engineered skin substitutes

New technology has spawned a new generation of materials to advance wound healing and provide all of the characteristics of natural skin. Tissue engineering involves the development of materials that combine novel materials with living cells to yield functional tissue equivalents, such as skin substitutes.[22] Currently, two tissue-engineered products containing living cells are approved for use in the United States. Apligraf and Dermagraft both contain living cells derived from neonatal foreskin. A single foreskin can produce over 200,000 units of the product.[18] Apligraf is a bilayered skin product consisting of a dermal equivalent composed of type I bovine collagen that contains living human dermal fibroblasts as an overlying cornified epidermal layer of living human keratinocytes. Apligraf doesn't contain Langerhans' cells, melanocytes, or endothelial cells, perhaps explaining why it isn't clinically rejected. Dermagraft is a living dermal replacement made of mesh Vicryl and human neonatal foreskin-derived fibroblasts and their products. It contains only human fibroblasts and is extensively tested for infectious agents.

Tissue-engineered skin has been approved for use on venous ulcers, diabetic ulcers, and burns. Additional applications will most likely be available in the future. Skin substitutes are surgically applied by a physician in the outpatient setting. Several applications may be needed for "take" to occur. Prior to application the wound bed preparation process needs to be strictly followed. Wounds are debrided, moisture balance maintained, and infection monitored. If infection does occur, it can be successfully handled with various topical medications. The graft site must be protected from injury; the secondary dressing is changed without disturbing the graft site. Tissue engineered skin holds a promising future for wound care clients.

Practice essentials
• Skin substitutes will only adhere to a clean wound bed.
• Watch for signs and symptoms of infection.
• Don't allow graft site to adhere to secondary dressing.

Compression therapy dressings

Compression therapy is the foundation for completed vascular management of venous ulcers. Compression therapy wraps are used to manage edema and promote sufficient return of venous blood to the heart. Several types of compression wraps are available and instructions on their application technique vary. Some are applied in a spiral fashion while others are wrapped in a figure eight configuration. The degree of compression ranges from high to low and short stretch to long stretch. Clinicians need to be proficient at applying the correct techniques based on the product they select. Detailed package inserts describe how to apply these products. Their effectiveness is well documented in managing venous ulcer patients. Compression therapy dressings aren't recommended for arterial ulcer patients. If the patient presents with a mixed etiology, he should be aggressively monitored to be sure vascular compromise isn't occurring.

Practice essentials
• Vascular assessment and a Doppler study are recommended prior to the use of compression therapy dressings.
• Application techniques vary according to product; read package insert before applying.

Negative pressure wound therapy

Negative pressure wound therapy (NPWT) was developed in the early 1990s. Negative pressure therapy applies subatmospheric pressure, or suction, to the wound bed via a computerized unit attached to an open-celled foam sponge that's placed in the wound and secured with an adhesive drape. The adhesive drape provides a semiocclusive environment that supports moist wound healing. The drape is vapor permeable to facilitate gas exchange, an important consideration when treating wounds infected with anaerobic organisms.[25] The suction effect removes excess fluid from the wound bed via a tubing system attached to a canister. Removal of interstitial fluid allows for enhanced circulation and disposal of cellular waste from the lymphatic system. Stagnant wound fluid has been shown to contain elements that delay wound healing by suppressing proliferation.[26]

The NPWT guidelines for appropriate wounds are acute and traumatic wounds; surgical dehiscence; pressure ulcers; diabetic, arterial and venous ulcers; fresh flaps; and any compromised flap. Dressing changes vary between 48 hours and 72 hours. Untreated infected wounds should have the dressing changed every 12 hours. Two types of foam densities are utilized for different types of wounds. The black, sterile, polyurethane foam has large pores and is more effective for stimulating granulation tissue and wound contraction. The white, sterile, polyvinyl alcohol soft foam is denser with smaller pores and is recommended when growth of granulation tissue is less needed or when patient can't tolerate the polyurethane foam due to pain. Negative pressure wound therapy has greatly enhanced the ability of clinicians to deal with many complex and difficult to management wounds.

Practice essentials

Dressing changes should be performed between 48 and 72 hours, or if seal is broken.

Normothermic therapy

Normothermic therapy is a sterile, non-contact thermal wound dressing that covers and protects and actively warms the wound bed. The device consists of a power supply and battery charger, a control unit, a warming insert and a dressing that supports the warming insert and protects the wound.[27] Normothermic therapy increases blood flow to the wound, which in turn increases subcutaneous oxygen tension and delivery of growth factors to the wound bed. This assists the body's own healing process by maintaining warmth and humidity in the periwound area. The system maintains appropriate levels of temperature and moisture in and around the wound. Normothermic therapy is used on partial- and full-thickness wounds including venous, arterial, diabetic, and pressure ulcers. Currently, Medicare doesn't reimburse for normothermic therapy. More research is needed to determine the efficacy of normothermic therapy.

Practice essentials
• Use cautiously in patients with infected wounds. Concurrent antibiotic therapy is recommended.
• Normothermic therapy is contraindicated for third-degree burns.

Electrical stimulation

Electrical stimulation (ES) is the use of electrical current to transfer energy to a wound by capacitative coupling of an applied surface electrode through a wet electrolytic current.[28] High voltage pulsed current (HVPC) has increasingly been used for wound treatments in the last decade. This wound management treatment is performed by trained physical therapists and recommended for wounds that have been unresponsive to other treatments. According to Myer,[28] HVPC has a waveform of paired short-duration pulses with a long interpulse interval. It's a pulsed or interrupted monophasic waveform. The duration of treatment is usually 45 to 60 minutes, 5 to 7 times per week. ES is contraindicated in wounds with osteomyelitis, malignancy, and wounds containing heavy metals. Patients with demand-type cardiac pacemakers, or who are pregnant shouldn't use ES.

Practice essentials
• Don't place electrodes over the carotid sinus, close to the heart, or near the laryngeal musculature.
• Electrical stimulation should be an adjunct treatment and use in combination with other moist wound therapy interventions.

Growth factors

Growth factors are proteins (polypeptides) that naturally occur in the body. Growth factors are primarily found in platelets and macrophages. Various types of growth factors are being researched: epidermal growth factors, platelet derived growth factor, transforming growth factors, and fibroblast growth factors, to list a few. The types of growth factors used in research can be categorized into two major groups: single growth factors manufactured through recombinant DNA technology, and multiple growth factors secured from human platelet releasate.[24] PDGF is the most widely recognized growth factor today. It has been found to be efficacious in the management of diabetic ulcers and in granulating wounds. Although growth factor research is still in its infancy, it holds a promising future for wound care patients.

Summary

This chapter strives to convey a comprehensive and current understanding of the important characteristics of wound dressing products. The concepts of moist wound healing and the significance of clinical treatment decisions regarding wound care dressing options described herein are essential elements of your wound care arsenal. Helpful practice points, tables, figures, and a product algorithm guide you through the milieu of product alternatives. Improving technology and evolving research into wound care dressings will continue to create new and challenging opportunities for all of us.

Show what you know

1. Wound dressings have evolved into a new concept of:

A. dry gauze.
B. moist wound therapy.
C. open to air.
D. wet to dry.

ANSWER: B. A, C, and D are all old concepts of wound management.

2. The following are categories of moist wound care dressings, except:

A. hydrogel dressing.
B. calcium alginate dressing.
C. roller gauze dressing.
D. foam dressing.

ANSWER: C. Gauze is a form of dry dressing therapy. A, B, and D are moist wound therapy dressings.

3. Wound dressing selection should be based on the characteristics of the wound. All of the following should be considered when selecting dressings except:

A. size of dressing.
B. nurse preference.
C. moist or dry wound bed.
D. drainage.

ANSWER: B. Nurse preference shouldn't be a parameter of dressing selection. A, C, and D are appropriate dressing parameters.

4. A disadvantage of transparent film is that it:

A. is nonabsorptive.
B. is conformable.
C. allows wound inspection.
D. is impermeable to bacteria.

ANSWER: A. Transparent film doesn't absorb fluid. B, C, and D are all advantages of transparent film use.

5. The acronym "MEASURES" is a useful tool for remembering the principles of wound care.

A. True
B. False

ANSWER: A

6. The following dressing is a dermal skin substitute:

A. Accuzyme.
B. Tegaderm.
C. Allevyn.
D. Apligraft.

ANSWER: D. Apligraft is a bilayered skin substitute. A, B, and C are all moist wound therapy dressing choices.

7. Alternative wound care therapies are helpful adjuncts to care. Which of the following isn't considered an alternative option?

A. Negative pressure therapy
B. Normothermic therapy
C. Electrical stimulation
D. Collagen dressing

ANSWER: D. Collagen isn't an alternative therapy. A, B, and C are alternative therapy choices

References

1. Winter, G.D. "Formation of the Scab and the Rate of Epithelialization of Superficial Wounds in the Skin of Young Domestic Pigs," *Nature* 193:293-94, 1962.
2. Hinman, C.D., and Maibach, H.I. "Effect of Air Exposure and Occlusion on Experimental Human Skin Wounds," *Nature* 200:377, 1963.
3. Baranoski, S. "Wound Dressings: Challenging Decisions," *Home Healthcare Nurse* 17(1):19-26, January 1999.
4. Hatz, R.A., et al. Wound Dressings, Wound Healing and Wound Management: A Guide for Private Practice. Washington, D.C.: Springer-Verlag New York, 1994.
5. Field, C., and Kerstein, M. "Overview of Wound Healing in a Moist Environment," *American Journal of Surgery* 167(suppl 1A):2S-5S, January 1994.
6. Ovington, L.G. "Hanging Wet-to-dry Dressings Out to Dry," *Advances in Skin & Wound Care* 15(2):79-86, March-April 2002.
7. Pieper, B., et al. "Wound Prevalence, Types, and Treatments in Home Care," *Advances in Skin & Wound Care* 12(3):117-26, May-June 1999.
8. Lim, J.K., et al. "Normal Saline Wound Dressing—Is It Really Normal?" *British Journal of Plastic Surgery* 53(1):42-45, January 2000.
9. Hedman, L.A. "Effect of a Hydrocolloid Dressing on the Pain Level from Abrasions on the Feet during Intensive Marching," *Military Medicine* 153(4):188-90, April 1988.
10. Nemeth, A.J., et al. "Faster Healing and Less Pain in Skin Biopsy Sites Treated with an Occlusive Dressing," *Archives of Dermatology* 11:1679-83, November 1991.
11. Thomas, S. *Wound Management and Dressing,* London: The Pharmaceutical Press, 1990.
12. Lawrence, J.C. "Dressings and Wound Infection," *American Journal of Surgery* 167(suppl 1A):1S-24S, January 1994.
13. Hutchinson, J.J. "Prevalence of Wound Infection under Occlusive Dressings: A Collective Survey of Reported Research," *Wounds* (1):123-33, 1989.
14. Hutchinson, J.J. "A Prospective Clinical Trial of Wound Dressings to Investigate the Rate of Infection under Occlusion," in *Proceedings of the First European Conference on Advances in Wound Management.* Edited by Harding, K. London: Macmillan, 1993.
15. Baranoski, S. "Wound Assessment and Dressing Selection," *Ostomy Wound Management* 41(suppl 7A):7S-14S, August 1995.
16. Rodeheaver, G. "Wound Cleansing, Wound Irrigation, Wound Disinfection," in *Chronic Wound Care,* 2nd ed. Edited by Krasner, D., and Kane, D. Wayne, Pa.: Health Management Publications, Inc., 1997.
17. Orland, G. "The Fine Structure of the Interrelationship of Cells in the Human Epidermis," *Journal of Biophysical and Biochemical Cytology* 4:529-35, 1958.
18. Eaglstein, W.H. "From Occlusive to Living Membranes," *Journal of Dermatology* 25(12):766-74, December 1998.
19. Choucair, M., and Phillips. "Wound Dressings," in *Dermatology in General Medicine.* Edited by Fitzpatrick. New York: McGraw-Hill Book Co., 2954-2958, 2000.
20. Ovington, L.G. "The Well-dressed Wound: An Overview of Dressing Types," *Wounds* 10:1A-11A, 1998.
21. Hess, C.T. *Clinical Guide: Wound Care,* 4th ed. Springhouse, Pa.: Springhouse Corp., 2002.
22. Seaman, S. "Dressing Selection in Chronic Wound Management," *Journal of the American Podiatric Medical Association* 92(1):24-33, January 2002.
23. Sefton, M.V., and Woodhouse, K.A. "Tissue Engineering," *Journal of Cutaneous Medicine and Surgery* 3(suppl 1):S1-18, December 1998.
24. Fylling, C.P. "Growth Factors: A New Era in Wound Healing." In Krasner, D., and Kane, D., *Chronic Wound Care,* 2nd ed. Wayne, Pa.: Health Management Publications, Inc. 344-47, 1997.
25. Mendez-Eastman, S. "Guidelines for Using Negative Pressure Wound Therapy," *Advances in Skin & Wound Care* 14(6):314-22, November-December 2001.
26. Falanga, V. "Growth Factors and Chronic Wounds: The Need to Understand the Microenvironment," *Journal of*

Dermatology 19(11):667-72, November 1992.

27. Bello, Y.M., and Phillips, T.J. "Therapeutic Dressings," *Advances in Dermatology* 16:253-71, November 2000.

28. Myer, A. "The Role of Physical Therapy in Chronic Wound Care," in Krasner, et al., eds., *Chronic Wound Care: A Clinical Source Book for Healthcare Professionals*, 3rd ed. Wayne, Pa.: Health Management Publications, Inc., 2001.

CHAPTER 10

Nutrition and wound care

Mary Ellen Posthauer, RD, CD, LD
David R. Thomas, MD

OBJECTIVES

After completing this chapter, you'll be able to:

- describe the process of screening to identify nutritional problems/concerns

- identify the parameters involved in completing a nutritional assessment

- describe the role of nutrients in wound prevention and healing

- define the role of nutrition management for malnutrition.

Nutritional concerns

Nutrition plays a key role in the prevention and treatment of wounds. The goal in preventing pressure ulcers is to screen and identify individuals at risk for ulcer development. A nutritional assessment should be completed both for individuals at high risk for pressure ulcer development and for those currently with wounds. Data derived from the assessment is then used to develop a nutritional care plan.

Based on the assessment, nutrition interventions are selected that are most appropriate to manage the current condition. These interventions are based on standard protocols that should be reviewed as new research data becomes available.

Role of nutrients in healing

There are six major classes of nutrients: carbohydrates, proteins, fats, vitamins, minerals, and water. Through the process of metabolism, organic nutrients are broken down to yield energy, rearranged to build body structures, or used in chemical reactions for body processes.

Carbohydrates

Carbohydrates provide energy and prevent gluconeogenesis from protein stores. Carbohydrate calories should comprise 50% to 60% of the patient's total caloric needs. An inadequate supply of carbohydrates results in muscle wasting (when the body is forced to convert protein stores for energy use), loss of subcutaneous tissue, and poor wound healing. Complex carbohydrates are encouraged rather than simple sugars.

Protein and amino acids

Protein is the only nutrient containing nitrogen in addition to carbon, hydrogen, and oxygen; some protein also contains sulfur and phosphorus. These elements combine to form amino acids, the smallest molecular units of protein. Protein is responsible for repair and synthesis of enzymes involved in wound healing, cell multiplication, and collagen and connective tissue synthesis. Protein is a component of antibodies needed for immune system function; 20% to 25% of calories should be obtained from protein sources.

The protein requirement for patients with pressure ulcers is debatable, but it's higher than the adult recommendation of 0.8 g/kg per day. Current recommendations for dietary intake of protein in stressed elderly patients ranges between 1.2 and 1.5 g/kg per day. Many chronically ill elderly people can't maintain nitrogen balance at this level. Increasing protein intake beyond 1.5 g/kg per day may not increase protein synthesis and may cause dehydration.[1] While the optimum protein intake for this population hasn't been established, the range is probably between 1.5 and 1.8 g/kg per day.[2]

The association of dietary protein intake with wound healing has led to investigation of specific amino acids. Glutamine is essential for immune system function, but supplemental glutamine hasn't shown noticeable effects on wound healing.[3]

Arginine enhances immune function and wound collagen deposition in healthy elderly people.[4,5] One study tried to determine the level of oral arginine supplementation required, how it's metabolically tolerated, and its effectiveness in enhancing immune function in elderly patients with pressure ulcers. Study conclusions were that pharmacologic doses of arginine were well tolerated but didn't enhance lymphocyte proliferation or interleukin-2 production in nursing home residents with pressure ulcers.[6] Enteral formulas supplemented with arginine are often recommended or ordered for elderly patients. This study concluded that elderly patients with normal renal function and appropriate fluids could tolerate the increased nitrogen loads. Additional research is needed to show the effect of arginine supplementation and pressure ulcer healing.

Fats and fatty acids

Fat is the most concentrated source of energy and provides a reserve source of energy in the form of stored triglycerides in adipose tissue. Fat calories should comprise 20% to 25% of the total calories.

Vitamins

Vitamins are organic compounds that the body requires in small amounts for proper functioning. Since the body doesn't produce vitamins, they must be obtained from food and beverages or synthetic supplements.

Fat-soluble vitamins

Fat-soluble vitamins A, D, E, and K remain in the liver and fat tissue of the body until used. Because the body doesn't excrete excess fat-soluble vitamins, the risk of toxicity from overdose exists.

PRACTICE POINT

Look for signs and symptoms of overdose toxicity from fat-soluble vitamins A, D, E, and K if the patient is receiving supplements.

Vitamin A is responsible for epithelium maintenance. It also stimulates cellular differentiation in fibroblasts and collagen formation. Vitamin A deficiency, which is uncommon, results in delayed wound healing and increased susceptibility to infection.[7] Vitamin A supplementation has been shown to be effective in counteracting delayed healing in patients on corticosteroids.[8] Patients receiving high-dose steroids are often administered oral supplementation of 25,000 IU per day for 10 days.[9,10]

Vitamin E is an antioxidant and is responsible for normal fat metabolism and collagen synthesis. Vitamin E deficiency doesn't appear to play an active role in wound healing,[11] and it impedes the absorption of vitamin A by reducing the rate of hepatic retinyl ester hydrolysis.[12]

Water-soluble vitamins

Water-soluble vitamins C and B play a role in wound healing. Vitamin C is essential for collagen synthesis. Collagen and fibroblasts compose the basis for the structure of a new wound bed. A deficiency of vitamin C prolongs the healing time and contributes to reduced resistance to infection. There's no clinical evidence that wound healing is improved by providing doses of vitamin C above the recommended daily allowance (RDA) of 60 mg per day.[13] In a multicenter, blinded trial, 88 patients with pressure ulcers were randomized to either 10 mg or 500 mg twice daily of vitamin C. The trial failed to demonstrate any improved healing or closure rate between groups.[14] Supertherapeutic doses of vitamin C haven't been shown to accelerate wound healing.[15] Patients who consume diets deficient in vitamin C sources — fruits, vegetables, and juices — and those with severe wounds may benefit from a supplement.

Coenzymes (B vitamins) are necessary for the production of energy from glucose, amino acids, and fat. Pyridoxine (B$_6$) is important for maintaining cellular immunity and forming red blood cells. Thiamine and riboflavin are needed for adequate cross-linking and collagenation.

Minerals

Zinc, a cofactor for collagen formation, also metabolizes protein, liberates vitamin A from storage in the liver, interacts with platelets in blood clotting, and assists in immune function. Deficiency can occur rapidly through wound drainage or excessive GI fluid loss or from long-term poor dietary intake. No clinical evidence exists to support supplementation (such as with zinc sulfate 200 to 300 mg daily). In a small study of patients with pressure ulcers, no effect on ulcer healing was seen at 12 weeks in zinc-supplemented versus non–zinc-supplemented patients.[16] High serum zinc levels may inhibit healing, impair phagocytosis, and interfere with copper metabolism.[17-19] The RDA for zinc is 12 to 15 mg, but most elderly people consume 7 to 11 mg of zinc per day,[20] chiefly from meats and cereals.

Copper is responsible for collagen cross-linking and erythropoeisis; the daily requirement for adult men and women is 900 mcg per day.

Iron is a constituent of hemoglobin, collagen transport, and oxygen transport; the daily requirement for adult men and women ages 50 to 70 is 8 mg per day.

Water

Water, which constitutes about 60% of the adult body weight, may be the most important nutrient of all. It's distributed

Signs of dehydration

Sufficient hydration is essential for all patients, and no less so for the patient with a wound. Use the following guidelines to prevent dehydration — and to recognize and treat it should it occur.
- If the patient can drink independently, keep water or other beverages at bedside so that they're easily accessible and in a container the patient can handle easily.
- If the patient doesn't consume fluids on his own, offer water at least every 2 hours.

If you suspect dehydration, look for:
- dry skin
- cracked lips
- thirst (often diminished in the elderly)
- poor skin turgor (The pinch test for skin turgor may be an unreliable indicator for dehydration in the elderly. If you use this test, use only the skin on the forehead or sternum, and pinch gently. If well-hydrated, the skin goes back into place in 2 seconds.)
- fever
- appetite loss
- nausea
- dizziness
- increased confusion
- laboratory values (Serum creatinine, hematocrit, blood urea nitrogen, potassium, chloride, and osmolarity are increased. Sodium can be increased, normal, or low, depending on the underlying cause of dehydration.)
- decreased blood pressure
- increased pulse rate
- constipation (Recent diarrhea may explain the dehydrated state, and constipation is common when dehydration exists.)
- concentrated urine.

in the body in three fluid compartments (intracellular, interstitial, and intravascular). Water serves many vital functions in the body:
- It aids in hydration of wound sites and in oxygen perfusion.
- It acts as a solvent for minerals, vitamins, amino acids, glucose, and other small molecules and enables them to diffuse into and out of cells.
- It transports vital materials to cells as well as waste away from cells.

Patients with draining wounds, emesis, diarrhea, elevated temperature, or increased perspiration need additional fluids. Patients on air-fluidized beds require 500 ml of additional fluids daily. The dehydrated patient has weight loss (2%, mild; 5%, moderate; and 8%, severe), dry skin and mucous membranes, rapid pulse, decreased venous pressure, subnormal body temperature, low blood pressure, and altered sensation.

Patients who are at risk of dehydration require careful monitoring. (See *Signs of dehydration.*) Daily body weight assessment can indicate large fluid losses as well as gains. For example, a weight loss of 2 kg in 48 hours indicates a corresponding loss of 2 L of fluid. Elderly patients, whose sense of thirst often declines, should prompt health care providers to offer hydration more frequently.

The Centers for Medicare and Medicaid Services (CMS) has distributed nutrition care alerts to long-term-care facilities, listing warning signs and recommending strategies for dehydration, weight loss, and pressure ulcers. (See *CMS nutrition care alerts.*)

Nutritional intervention may occur at two levels. (See *Staging nutritional intervention*, page 163.)

Daily caloric requirements

Daily caloric requirements range from 25 kcal/kg per day for sedentary adults

PRACTICE POINT

CMS nutrition care alerts

The chart below sets out the Centers for Medicare and Medicaid Services (CMS) warning signs and interventions for unintended weight loss, dehydration, and pressure ulcers.

Warning signs	Interventions
UNINTENDED WEIGHT LOSS	
The following are some signs that a patient may be at risk of or suffer from unintended weight loss:	Below are some action steps to increase food intake, create a positive dining environment, and help patients get enough calories:
• Needs help to eat or drink • Eats less than half of meals and snacks served • Has mouth pain • Has dentures that don't fit • Has a hard time chewing or swallowing • Coughs or chokes while eating • Has sadness, crying spells, or withdrawal from others • Is confused, wanders, or paces • Has diabetes, COPD, cancer, HIV, or other chronic disease	• Report observations and warning signs to nurse and dietitian! • Honor food likes and dislikes. • Offer many kinds of foods and beverages. • Provide oral care before meals. • Position the patient correctly for feeding. • Encourage the patient to eat. • Notify nursing staff if the patient has trouble using utensils. • Help the patient who has trouble feeding himself. • Allow enough time to finish eating. • Record meal and snack intake. • If the patient has had a loss of appetite or seems sad, ask what's wrong.
DEHYDRATION	

The following are some signs that a patient may be at risk of or suffer from dehydration:
• Drinks less than 6 cups of liquids daily
• Has one or more of the following:
  – Dry mouth
  – Cracked lips
  – Sunken eyes
  – Dark urine
• Needs help drinking from a cup or glass
• Has trouble swallowing liquids
• Has frequent vomiting, diarrhea, or fever
• Is easily confused or tired
	Most patients need at least 6 cups of liquids to maintain hydration. Below are some action steps to help patients get enough fluids:
	• Report observations and warning signs to nurse and dietitian!
	• Encourage the patient to drink every time you see him.
	• Make sure pitcher and cup are near enough and light enough for the patient to lift.
	• Offer the appropriate assistance as needed if the patient can't drink without help.
	• Offer 2 to 4 oz of water or liquids frequently.
	• Offer ice chips frequently (unless patient has a swallowing problem).
	• Check swallowing precautions, then, if appropriate, offer sips of liquid between bites of food at meals and snacks.
	• Drink fluids with the patient, if your facility permits you to do so.
	• Be sure to record fluid intake and output.

(continued)

PRACTICE POINT ▬▬▬
CMS nutrition care alerts (continued)

Warning signs	Interventions
PRESSURE ULCERS	

The following are some signs that a patient may be at risk of or suffer from pressure ulcers:
• Is incontinent
• Needs help:
  – moving arms, legs, or body
  – turning in bed
  – changing position when sitting
• Has weight loss
• Eats less than half of meals and snacks served
• Is dehydrated
• Has discolored, torn, or swollen skin over bony areas
	Below are some action steps to help patients who are at risk of or suffer from pressure ulcers:
	• Report observations and warning signs to nurse and dietitian!
	• Check and change linens as appropriate.
	• Handle and move the patient carefully to avoid skin tears and scrapes.
	• Reposition the patient frequently and properly.
	• Use unintended-weight-loss action steps so the patient receives more calories and protein.
	• Use dehydration action steps so the patient gets more to drink.
	• Record meal and snack intake.

Reprinted with permission from the Nutrition Screening Initiative, a project of the American Academy of Family Physicians and the American Dietetic Association, funded in part by a grant from Ross Products Division, Abbott Laboratories, Inc. HCFA Pub No. 10177.

to 40 kcal/kg per day for elderly patients under moderate stress. Various formulas, including the Harris-Benedict equation, can be used to predict caloric requirements, but controversy exists over accuracy in obese or severely undernourished individuals.[21] Other formulas have been adjusted for severely stressed hospitalized subjects.[22]

Nutritional screening

As defined by the American Dietetic Association (ADA), a nutritional screening is the process of identifying characteristics known to be associated with nutritional problems. It's purpose is to pinpoint individuals who are malnourished or at nutritional risk. Intervention takes place after screening occurs.

A screening can be completed by a member of the health care team, such as the dietitian, dietetic technician, nurse, physician, or other qualified health professional.[23] (See *Nutritional screening algorithm,* page 164.)

The screening process should identify risk factors for the development of pressure ulcers as well as identify those individuals who are malnourished or at risk of malnutrition:

• Significant weight loss: 5 lbs or more in 1 month; 5% in 30 days; 10% in 180 days
• Disease states and conditions: diabetes, dementia, malnutrition, pulmonary disease, cancer, renal disease, obesity
• Immobility and inactivity: hip fracture, spinal cord injury (SCI), stroke
• Chewing and swallowing problems: dysphagia, stroke, Parkinson's disease, cerebral palsy
• Poor food and fluid intake
• Medication adverse effects.

Staging nutritional intervention

Level I

1. Estimate nutritional needs.
2. Monitor ability to self-feed; consider use of finger foods, adaptive utensils, refeeding programs, increased time, or feeding assistance.
3. Pay attention to food preferences and tolerances; optimize the eating environment by individualizing meal times and patterns as much as possible; ensure good food quality and variety.
4. Monitor food and fluid intake.
5. Consider an interdisciplinary assessment of chewing and swallowing ability.
6. Add medical nutritional products to supplement intake.
7. Limit the use of unsupplemented liquid diets or other restrictive diets.

8. Routinely reassess nutritional status and response to nutritional intervention.
9. Document and reevaluate the care plan.

Level II

1. Institute tube feedings to meet nutritional needs if this is compatible with overall goals of care.
2. Take precautions to prevent pulmonary aspiration and other complications.
3. Monitor nutritional intake through counting calories.
4. Routinely reassess nutritional status and response to nutritional interventions.
5. Document and reevaluate the care plan.

Reprinted with permission from S.M. Campbell. *Pressure Ulcer Prevention and Intervention: A Role for Nutrition.* May 1994. © Ross Products Division, Abbott Laboratories, Inc., Columbus, Ohio.

Significant weight loss without any known medical condition places a patient at risk for malnutrition. Functional limitation, such as difficulty chewing or swallowing, affects the ability of the patient to ingest adequate calories and fluids. Immobility affects a patient's ability to either prepare meals or travel to a dining room for meals. Hip fracture and SCI restrict mobility, often resulting in increased pain, thereby interfering with eating. Poor hearing and vision compromise the patient's communication skills, often resulting in poor intake at meals. Altered mental status often limits patients' abilities to feed themselves or to comprehend the importance of consuming a balanced diet. Advanced dementia often results in weight loss, dysphagia, malnutrition, and pressure ulcers. When patients become incapable of responding to caregivers' assis-

tance to nourish them, the probability of developing pressure ulcers increases.

Disease states and conditions can increase the risk of pressure ulcer development. Patients with chronic obstructive pulmonary disease (COPD) often have poor intake leading to anorexia and muscle wasting due to cytokine-induced inflammation and sarcopenia. In 1993, Ryan and colleagues studied ten patients with stable COPD with undernutrition (defined as < 85% ideal body weight), resting energy expenditure was 94% ± 16% of that predicted by the Harris-Benedict equation. When patients were randomly assigned to receive either nocturnal enteral feeding or to be sham-fed for a mean of 16 ± 3 days, resting energy expenditure didn't change significantly during inpatient refeeding. A large meal caused substantial increases in energy expenditure, carbon dioxide production,

Nutritional screening algorithm

This algorithm illustrates the nutritional screening process.

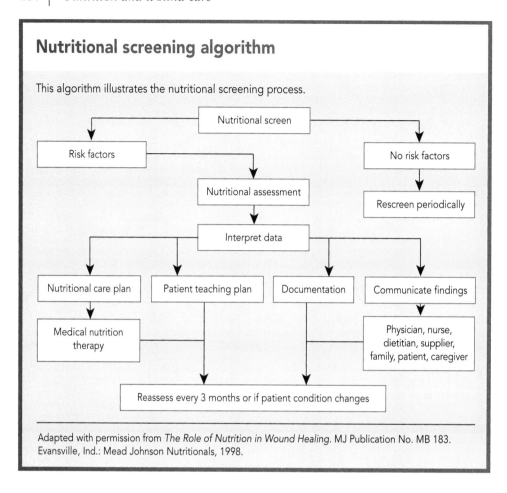

Adapted with permission from *The Role of Nutrition in Wound Healing*. MJ Publication No. MB 183. Evansville, Ind.: Mead Johnson Nutritionals, 1998.

and oxygen consumption. Based on this study, stable undernourished COPD patients consume adequate calories to meet average energy requirements and don't have an increased resting energy expenditure. Nocturnal enteral feedings resulted in weight gain, but the thermogenic affect of a large meal caused a metabolic and ventilatory load that could precipitate acute respiratory failure.[24]

Diabetes with chronic hyperglycemia may both cause and affect poor wound healing. High levels of glucose compete with transport of ascorbic acid into the cells, which is necessary for deposition of collagen.

Obese patients—those whose body weight is > 130% of the ideal body weight—usually have excessive weight

placed on bony prominences; in addition, moisture often collects between skin folds, leading to skin impairment. Patients with renal disease often have multiple medical conditions, such as diabetes or heart disease, which complicates the nutrient parameters of their diet. For example, a renal diet limited in calories, protein, potassium, phosphorus, sodium, and fluid often results in poor dietary intake that doesn't meet the patient's needs.

Drug therapy can often cause adverse effects, such as nausea and gastric disturbances, that curtail a patient's food and fluid intake. Corticosteroids increase the risk of wound complications such as infection and inhibit protein synthesis. Corticosteroids cause depletion of vitamin A from the liver, plasma, adrenals,

Definition of high risk for pressure ulcer development

The Centers for Medicare and Medicaid Services (CMS) has identified the following risk factors for the development of pressure ulcers:
- impaired mobility or transfer
- end-stage renal disease
- malnutrition
- coma.
  Clinical conditions that are the primary risk factors for developing pressure sores include, but aren't limited to, resident immobility and:
1. The resident has two or more of the following diagnoses:
- Continuous urinary incontinence or chronic voiding dysfunction
- Severe peripheral vascular disease
- Diabetes
- Severe COPD

- Chronic bowel incontinence
- Paraplegia
- Quadriplegia
- Sepsis
- Terminal cancer
- Chronic end-stage renal, liver, or heart disease
- Disease- or drug-related immunosuppression
- Full body cast.
2. The resident receives two or more of the following treatments:
- Steroid therapy
- Radiation therapy
- Chemotherapy
- Renal dialysis
- Head of bed elevated most of the day due to medical necessity.

Reprinted from F tag 314; Procedures: 483.25(c): Federal Register, Vol 56, No 187, Sept 1991.

and enzymes, and interfere with collagen synthesis and resistance to infection.[25]

The CMS, which regulates long-term-care facilities, has targeted pressure ulcers, inadequate nutrition, and inadequate hydration as key survey issues. The development of a pressure ulcer in a person who was a low risk is automatically considered a sentinel event. CMS has established a definition to identify those at high risk for pressure ulcer development. (See *Definition of high risk for pressure ulcer development*.)

Nutritional assessment

Nutritional assessment is a comprehensive approach, completed by a registered dietitian, that defines nutritional status using medical, nutritional, and medication histories; physical examination; anthropometric measurements; and laboratory data. It includes interpretation of data from the screening process. The assessment process includes a review of data from other disciplines (such as physical therapy and occupational therapy) that may affect the assessment process. Nutrition assessment precedes a care plan, intervention, and evaluation.[23]

As part of the nutritional assessment, the dietitian reviews the screens and assessments from the various disciplines. Observation during mealtime provides the health care professional the opportunity to determine if the patient has chewing or swallowing problems that may require the services of either a speech therapist or occupational therapist. Adequate intake of food and fluid is a concern for those with swallowing problems, and this in turn places them at risk for pressure ulcers. The speech therapist

Severity of weight loss

Weight loss may be categorized as significant or severe. Significant weight loss consists of:
- 10% in 6 months
- 7.5% in 3 months
- 5% in 1 month
- 2% in 1 week.
  Severe weight loss consists of:
- >10% in 6 months
- >7.5% in 3 months
- >5% in 1 month
- >2% in 1 week.

© 1998, American Dietetic Association. *Nutrition Care of the Older Adult.* Used with permission.

defines the diet texture, including the needs for special feeding techniques, which are implemented by the dietary department. As an example, patients may require thickened liquids to prevent dehydration or aspiration. The occupational therapist often determines the need for self-help feeding devices that promote eating independence. Physical therapy sessions often result in the need for both increased calories and fluid, which the dietitian will calculate and arrange provision at appropriate times.

Anthropometric factors

Anthropometry — the measurement of body size, weight, and proportions — is used to evaluate a patient's nutritional status. A change in anthropometric values can signal problems such as wasting or edema, reflecting nutritional excess or deficit. Accurate heights and weights are critical as they are the basis for determining caloric and nutrient requirements. Adjustment or notations should be made for casts and other appliances that alter true weight.

 PRACTICE POINT

Weigh your patient each time on the same scale, at the same time of day, and with minimal clothing.

Body mass index (BMI) is used to assess ideal weight in relationship to height. The BMI is a weight-to-height ratio composed of body weight in kilograms divided by the square of the height in meters:

$$BMI = \frac{Weight\ (kg)}{Height\ (m^2)}$$

OR

$$BMI = \frac{Weight\ (lbs)}{Height\ (in^2)} \times 705$$

A normally hydrated person with a BMI ≥ 30 is considered obese.[26] BMI < 19 places the patient at nutritional risk.[27]

Stress as a result of injury, surgery, burn, fracture, or wounds results in depletion of nutrient stores required for healing. Protein stores are used as energy sources if adequate carbohydrate and fat aren't provided.

Ideal body weight, sometimes called recommended body weight or desired body weight, can be approximated using specific calculations. However, any deviation from usual body weight is a more reliable measurement of the severity of malnutrition.

$$\%\ ideal\ weight = \frac{Actual\ weight \times 100}{Usual\ body\ weight}$$

When evaluating the severity of weight variances, it's important to determine possible causes such as recent surgery, diuretic therapy, or other new treatments that affect weight status. (See *Severity of weight loss* and *Nutritional assessment guidelines.*)

Nutritional assessment guidelines

Use the following formulas and charts to determine a patient's nutritional status and needs. Estimated daily calorie levels are determined by multiplying the patient's basal energy expenditure (BEE) and the appropriate injury and activity factors.

Recommended weight for height
Calculate the appropriate weight for the patient's height using the following formulas:
* Female: 100 lb per 5' + 5 lb per inch > 5'
* Male: 106 lb per 5' + 6 lb per inch > 5'

Basal energy expenditure
Calculate the patient's BEE using the following equations:
Female: 655 + (9.6 × weight in kg) + (1.8 × height in cm) − (4.7 × age in years)
Male: 66 + (13.7 × weight in kg) + (5.0 × height in cm) − (6.8 × age in years)
   Determine estimated daily calorie levels by multiplying the BEE and the appropriate injury or activity factor.

Injury factors
* 1.00 to 1.05 — postoperative (no complications)
* 1.05 to 1.25 — peritonitis
* 1.10 to 1.45 — cancer
* 1.15 to 1.30 — long bone fracture
* 1.20 to 1.60 — wound healing
* 1.25 to 1.50 — blunt trauma
* 1.30 to 1.55 — severe infection; multiple trauma
* 1.50 to 1.70 — multiple trauma with client on ventilator
* 1.60 to 1.70 — trauma with steroids
* 1.75 to 1.85 — sepsis

Burns
* 1.00 to 1.50 — 0% to 20% total body surface burned
* 1.50 to 1.85 — 20% to 40% total body surface burned
* 1.85 to 2.05 — 40% to 100% total body surface burned

Activity factors
* 1.2 — patient confined to bed
* 1.3 — ambulatory patient
* 1.5 to 1.75 — normally active person
* 2.0 — extremely active person

(continued)

Nutritional assessment guidelines (continued)

Protein needs for adults

	Albumin level	Prealbumin level	Protein requirements
CONDITION			
Normal nutrition	3.5 gm/dl	19 to 43 mg/dl	0.8 gm/kg/day
Mild depletion	2.8 to 3.5 gm/dl	10 to 15 mg/dl	1.0 to 1.2 gm/kg/day
Moderate depletion	2.1 to 2.7 gm/dl	5 to 10 mg/dl	1.2 to 1.5 gm/kg/day
Severe depletion	2.1 gm/dl	< 5 mg/dl	1.5 to 2.0 gm/kg/day
COPD			100 to 125 gm protein/day total
EXCEPTIONS			
Renal failure			
• Nondialyzed			0.5 to 0.6 gm/kg/day
• Hemodialyzed			1.0 to 1.2 gm/kg/day
• Peritoneal-dialyzed			1.2 to 1.5 gm/kg/day
Hepatic failure			0.25 to 0.5 gm/kg/day
Pulmonary compromise			1.2 to 1.9 gm/kg/day (maintenance)
			1.6 to 2.5 gm/kg/day (repletion)

Alternative method for determining protein needs

Calorie to nitrogen ratio is used to determine protein needs, especially for enteral and parenteral feedings. Adequate energy is needed to support the use of protein for anabolism. Calculate the ratio of nonprotein calories (kcal) to grams of nitrogen (N). Example: 6.25 g protein = 1 g N.

Patient conditions	Ratio of nonprotein kcal: 1 g N
Adult medical	125 to 150:1
Minor catabolic	125 to 180:1
Severe catabolic	150 to 250:1
Hepatic or renal failure	250 to 400:1

Fluid status

Normal fluid status is 25 to 30 cc/kg of body weight. In patients with heart failure or edema, it's 25 cc/kg of body weight.
• 1 ml/kcal (often used when calculating tube feedings)
• To calculate: 100 ml/kg for the first 10 kg body weight + 50 ml/kg for the second 10 kg body weight + 15 ml/kg for remaining body weight
• Shortcut method: (kg body weight − 20) x 15 + 1,500 ml

Adapted with permission from Childester, J.C., and Spanger, A.A. "Fluid Intake in the Institutionalized Elderly," *Journal of the American Dietetic Association* 97:23-28, 1997.

Signs of malnutrition

Assess the patient's skin condition, checking for loss of subcutaneous fat as evidenced by loose skin in the extremities. Observe for muscle wasting and the presence of peripheral edema, in the absence of cardiac disease or circulatory disorder. Dull, dry, sparse hair can be a possible protein energy deficiency. Does the patient appear listless? For further signs, see *Physical signs of malnutrition,* page 170.

The older adult is particularly prone to pressure ulcers as a result of decreased mobility, multiple comorbid conditions, poor nutrition, and loss of muscle mass. Nutritional factors that contribute to skin breakdown include: protein deficiency, which creates a negative nitrogen balance; anemia, which inhibits the formation of red blood cells; and dehydration, which causes dry, fragile skin.

In addition, immune function declines with age, increasing the risk of infection and delayed wound healing.[6] With advancing age also comes decreased skin response to temperature, pain, and pressure. This affects the skin's elasticity and the healing process.

Biochemical and laboratory values

Biochemical tests are evaluated as part of the nutrition assessment process. (See *Laboratory screening for hydration status,* page 171, and *Guide to anemias,* pages 172 and 173.)

Protein status can be evaluated through a nitrogen-balance study, visceral protein blood levels, and tests of immune function such as total lymphocyte counts.

The albumin level is dependent upon hepatocyte function. The half-life of albumin is 12 to 21 days, so significant changes in liver function specific to albumin synthesis may go undetected. This long half-life makes albumin a poor indicator of early malnutrition. Infection will decrease the level of albumin. Acute stress such as surgery or cortisone excess reduces albumin even when protein intake is adequate. Edema and dehydration affect levels. When albumin levels are low, serum calcium levels are low. Decreases in serum albumin may reflect the presence of inflammatory cytokine production or comorbidity rather than nutritional status.[28] (See *Nutrition markers linked to pressure ulcers,* pages 174 and 175.)

Pre-albumin (transthyretin and thyroxine-binding albumin) has a half-life of 2 to 3 days. Pre-albumin is a sensitive indicator of protein deficiency and of improvement in protein status with refeeding. Levels aren't greatly affected by mild liver or renal disease or fluid changes. (See *Laboratory values for nutritional assessment,* pages 176 and 177.)

Treatment

Medications have an influence on nutrients. Drugs may either inhibit or induce metabolism of a nutrient or increase the excretion of a nutrient. Medications designed to calm and reduce agitation may in turn reduce mobility and activity levels and place patients at risk for pressure ulcer development. Drugs may increase or decrease appetite, alter sense of taste or smell, or cause gastric disturbances. Radiation therapy, chemotherapy, and renal dialysis can result in increased nausea and vomiting as well as decreased activity, placing the patient at risk. Medications have been identified as a cause of weight loss.[29] (See *Prescription drugs linked to anorexia,* page 178.)

Physical signs of malnutrition

Signs	Possible causes
HAIR	
• Dull, dry, lack of natural shine	• Protein-energy deficiency
• Thin, sparse, loss of curl	• Zinc deficiency
• Color changes, depigmentation, easily plucked	• Manganese, copper, other nutrient deficiencies
EYES	
• Small, yellowish lumps, white rings around eyes	• Hyperlipidemia
• Pale eye membranes	• Vitamin B_{12}, folic acid, or iron deficiency
• Night blindness, dry membranes, dull or soft cornea	• Vitamin A or zinc deficiency
• Redness and fissures of eyelid corners	• Niacin deficiency
• Angular inflammation of eyelids	• Riboflavin deficiency
• Ring of fine blood vessels around cornea	• Generally poor nutrition
LIPS	
• Redness and swelling	• Niacin, riboflavin, iron, or pyridoxine deficiency
GUMS	
• Spongy, swollen, red; bleed easily	• Vitamin C deficiency
• Gingivitis	• Vitamin A, niacin, or riboflavin deficiency
MOUTH	
• Cheilosis, angular scars	• Riboflavin or folic acid deficiency
TONGUE	
• Swollen, scarlet, raw; sores	• Folic acid or niacin deficiency
• Smooth with papillae (small projections)	• Riboflavin, vitamin B_{12}, or pyridoxine deficiency
• Glossitis	• Iron or zinc deficiency
• Purplish	• Riboflavin deficiency
TASTE	
• Diminished	• Zinc deficiency
TEETH	
• Grey-brown spots	• Increased fluoride intake
• Missing or erupting abnormally	• Generally poor nutrition
FACE	
• Skin color loss, dark cheeks and eyes, enlarged parotid glands, scaling of skin around nostrils	• Protein-energy deficiency, specifically niacin, riboflavin, or pyridoxine deficiency
• Pallor	• Iron, folic acid, vitamin B_{12}, or vitamin C deficiency
• Hyperpigmentation	• Niacin deficiency
NECK	
• Thyroid enlargement	• Iodine deficiency
• Symptoms of hypothyroidism	

Reprinted with permission from *Nutrition Care of the Older Adult*, Consultant Dietitians in Health Care Facilities, the American Dietetic Association, 1998.

Laboratory screening for hydration status

This chart lists the laboratory tests most commonly used to evaluate a patient's hydration status.

Lab test	Normal values	Dehydration	Overhydration
Osmolality	Adults: 285 to 295 mOsm/kg H_2O	> 295 mOsm/kg H_2O	< 285 mOsm/kg H_2O
Serum sodium	135 to 150 mEq/L	> 150 mEq/L	< 130 mEq/L
Albumin	3.5 to 5.0 g/dl	Higher than normal	Lower than normal
Blood urea nitrogen (BUN)*	7 to 23 mg/dl	Elevated	Lower than normal
BUN - creatinine ratio	10:1	> 25:1	< 10:1
Urine specific gravity	1.035 to 1.003	> 1.010	< 1.003

* BUN is only useful in the absence of renal disease

Reprinted with permission from *Nutrition Care of the Older Adult,* Consultant Dietitians in Health Care Facilities, the American Dietetic Association, 1998.

Nutritional interventions

Does nutritional status influence the incidence, progression, and severity of pressure sores? A review of several epidemiological studies supports this concept.[30,31]

Research supports the finding that undernourishment on admission to a health care facility increases a person's likelihood of developing a pressure ulcer. In one prospective study, high-risk patients who were undernourished (17%) on admission to the hospital were twice as likely to develop pressure ulcers as adequately nourished patients (9%).[32] Similarly, one study found that 59% of residents were undernourished and 7.3% were severely undernourished on admission to a long-term care facility. Pressure ulcers occurred in 65% of these severely undernourished residents, while no pressure ulcers developed in the mild-to-moderately undernourished or well-nourished residents.[33]

Epidemiological studies in the long-term care setting have correlated development of pressure ulcers with poor dietary intake. Studies revealed that residents with lower protein intake developed pressure ulcers. No other nutritional variable was significant for predicting ulcer development, including total intake of calories, vitamins A and C, iron, and zinc.[34] The use of pharmacologic agents to stimulate appetite, or orexigenic agents, has demonstrated weight gain, chiefly in patients with cancer or acquired autoimmune deficiency disease. Clinical studies using oxandrolone have shown weight gain in similar populations. While it has been hypothesized that weight gain in undernourished persons with wounds would lead to better outcomes in terms of wound healing, there are no published studies yet that test the value of these agents in pressure ulcers or other chronic wounds.[35]

Effects of undernutrition

Undernutrition, or protein-energy malnutrition (PEM), is defined as "a wasting

Guide to anemias

This chart lists the tests most commonly used to evaluate microcytic anemias, macrocytic anemias, and anemias of chronic diseases.

Normal values	Iron deficiency	Megaloblastic anemia (folate)	Pernicious anemia (B_{12})	Anemia of chronic disease
HEMOGLOBIN (Hb)				
12 to 16 g/dl (female) 14 to 16 g/dl (male)	< 12 g < 14 g	< 12 g < 14 g	< 12 g < 14 g	< 12 g < 14 g
HEMATOCRIT (HCT)				
33% to 43% (female) 39% to 49% (male)	< 33% < 39%	< 33% < 39%	< 33% < 39%	< 33% < 39%
MEAN CORPUSCULAR VOLUME (MCV)				
80 to 95 μm^3	< 80 μm^3	> 95 μm^3	> 95 μm^3 or normal	Normal
MEAN CORPUSCULAR HEMOGLOBIN (MCH)				
27 to 31 pg	< 27 pg	> 31 pg	> 31 pg	Normal
MEAN CORPUSCULAR HEMOGLOBIN CONCENTRATION (MCHC)				
32 to 36 g/dl	< 32 g/dl	Normal	Normal	Normal
SERUM IRON (FE)				
60 to 190 mcg/dl	< 60 mcg/dl	> 190 mcg/dl	> 190 mcg/dl	< 60 mcg/dl
TOTAL IRON BINDING CAPACITY (TIBC)				
250 to 420 mcg/dl	> 420 mcg/dl			< 250 mcg/dl
FERRITIN: M				
12 to 300 ng/ml	< 12 ng/ml	> 300 ng/ml	> 300 ng/ml	Normal or elevated
FERRITIN: F				
10 to 150 ng/ml	< 10 ng/ml	> 150 ng/ml	> 150 ng/ml	Normal or elevated
SERUM B_{12}				
100 to 1,300 pg/ml	Normal	Decreased	Decreased	Normal
B_{12} (SCHILLING TEST)				
8% to 40%		> 8%	> 8%	Normal or decreased

Guide to anemias *(continued)*

Normal values	Iron deficiency	Megaloblastic anemia (folate)	Pernicious anemia (B_{12})	Anemia of chronic disease
FOLATE				
5 to 20 mcg/ml		< 5 mcg/ml	> 20 mcg/ml	Normal or decreased
HEMOCYSTEINE (HCY)				
7 to 22 μmol/L		Increased	Increased	Normal
METHYL MALONIC ACID (MMA)				
19 to 76 ng/ml		Normal	Increased	Normal

Note: Serum ferritin is only useful in the absence of acute infection, chronic inflammatory conditions (such as rheumatism) or chronic renal disease. The same is true of iron. The total iron binding capacity is only useful in the absence of liver disease.

Reprinted with permission from *Nutrition Care of the Older Adult*, Consultant Dietitians in Health Care Facilities, the American Dietetic Association, 1998.

and excessive loss of lean body mass resulting from too little energy being supplied to body tissues." Functional deficits, such as impaired mobility, severe visual losses, poor dentition, and difficulty chewing, can predispose persons to PEM.[36] PEM has been associated with changes in immune function, increasing susceptibility to infection, and delayed recovery from illness. (See *Consequences of protein-energy malnutrition,* page 179.)

The three types of PEM are marasmus, kwashiorkor, and marasmic kwashiorkor. Marasmus results from severe deprivation or impaired absorption of protein, energy, vitamins, and minerals. Typically, the person has weight loss, but the visceral protein stores (serum albumin, pre-albumin, and transferrin) remain normal. Cancer and COPD are common causes of marasmus.

Kwashiorkor, or hypoalbuminemic malnutrition, is more difficult to detect because the person's muscle mass is preserved. The person may even appear well nourished, especially if edema is present. Serum albumin and cellular immunity are impaired, resulting in infection, poor wound healing, skin breakdown, and pressure ulcers.

Marasmic kwashiorkor, a combination of both types of malnutrition, is associated with the highest risk of morbidity and mortality.[37]

Increasing knowledge of the complexity of wound healing has led to the hypothesis that providing hypercaloric feeding in the form of nutritional supplements to patients at risk for undernutrition might reverse undernutrition and prevent the development of pressure ulcers. Despite epidemiological association, results of nutritional intervention trials in the prevention of pressure ulcers have been disappointing. No nutritional

(Text continues on page 177.)

Nutrition markers linked to pressure ulcers

This chart lists the nutritional markers that are — and aren't — associated with development of pressure ulcers.

First author	Clinical setting	Markers associated with presence of pressure ulcer	Markers not associated with presence of pressure ulcer
Allman [a]	Acute care	Albumin	Weight, hemoglobin, TLC, nutritional assessment
Gorse [b]	Acute care	Albumin	Nutritional assessment score
Inman [c]	Acute care, intensive care unit	Albumin (measured at 3 days)	Serum protein, hemoglobin, weight
Abbasi [d]	Acute care	Body mass index (BMI), total lymphocyte count (TLC)	Albumin, triceps skinfold thickness (TSF), arm circumference, weight loss, hemoglobin, nitrogen balance
Hartgrink [e]	Acute care, orthopedic	—	Nocturnal enteral feeding
Anthony [f]	Acute care	Albumin < 32 g/dl	—
Moolten [g]	Long-term care	Albumin < 3.5 g/dl	—
Pinchcofsky-Devin [h]	Long-term care	Severe malnutrition by biochemical markers	Mild-to-moderate malnutrition or normal nutrition
Berlowitz [i]	Long-term care	Impaired nutritional intake	Albumin, serum protein, hemoglobin, TLC, BMI/weight
Bennett [j]	Long-term care	—	Weight, BMI, weight gain
Brandeis [k]	Long-term care	Dependency in feeding	BMI/weight, TSF
Trumbore [l]	Long-term care	Albumin, cholesterol	—
Breslow [m]	Long-term care	Albumin, hemoglobin	Serum protein, cholesterol, zinc, copper, transferrin, weight, BMI, TLC
Bergstrom [n]	Long-term care	Dietary protein intake 93% of recommended daily allowance, dietary iron	Serum protein, cholesterol, zinc, copper, transferrin, weight, BMI, TLC
Ferrell [o]	Long-term care	—	Albumin, serum protein, BMI, hematocrit

Nutrition markers linked to pressure ulcers (continued)

First author	Clinical setting	Markers associated with presence of pressure ulcer	Markers not associated with presence of pressure ulcer
Bourdel-Marchasson[p]	Long-term care	—	Oral nutritional supplement (26% vs. 20% incidence)
Guralnik[q]	Community	—	Albumin, BMI, impaired nutrition, hemoglobin

[a] Allman, R. "Pressure Sores: A Randomized Trial," *Annals of Internal Medicine* 107:641-48, 1987.

[b] Gorse, G.J., and Messner, R.L. "Improved Pressure Sore Healing with Hydrocolloid Dressings," *Archives of Dermatology* 123:766-71, 1987.

[c] Inman, K.J., et al. "Clinical Utility and Cost-effectiveness of an Air Suspension Bed in the Prevention of Pressure Ulcers," *JAMA* 269:1139-43, 1993.

[d] Abbasi, A.A., and Rudman, D. "Undernutrition in the Nursing Home: Prevalence, Consequences, Causes, and Prevention," *Nutrition Reviews* 52(4):113-22, April 1994.

[e] Hartgrink, H.H., et al. "Pressure Sores and Tube Feeding in Patients with a Fracture of the Hip: A Randomized Clinical Trial," *Clinical Nutrition* 17:287-92, 1998.

[f] Anthony, D., et al. "An Investigation into the Use of Serum Albumin in Pressure Sore Prediction," *Journal of Advanced Nursing* 32:359-65, 2000.

[g] Moolten, S.E. "Bedsores in the Chronically Ill Patient," *Archives of Physical Medicine & Rehabilitation* 53:430-38, 1972.

[h] Pinchcofsky-Devin, G., and Kaminski, M. "Correlation of Pressure Sores and Nutritional Status," *Journal of the American Geriatric Society* 34:435-40, 1986.

[i] Berlowitz, D.R., and Wilking, S.V. "Risk Factors for Pressure Sores: A Comparison of Cross-sectional and Cohort-derived Data," *Journal of the American Geriatric Society* 37:1043-50, 1989.

[j] Bennett, R.G., et al. "Air-fluidized Bed Treatment of Nursing Home Patients with Pressure Sores," *Journal of the American Geriatrics Society* 37:235-42, 1989.

[k] Brandeis, G.H., et al. "Epidemiology and Natural History of Pressure Ulcers in Elderly Nursing Home Residents," *JAMA* 264:2905-09, 1990.

[l] Trumbore, L.S., et al. "Hypocholesterolemia and Pressure Sore Risk with Chronic Tube Feeding," *Clinical Research* 38:760A, 1990.

[m] Breslow, R.A., et al. "Malnutrition in Tubefed Nursing Home Patients with Pressure Sores," *Journal of Parental and Enteral Nutrition* 15:663-68, 1991.

[n] Bergstrom, N., and Braden, B. "A Prospective Study of Pressure Sore Risk Among Institutionalized Elderly," *Journal of the American Geriatrics Society* 40:747-58, 1992.

[o] Ferrell, B.A., et al. "A Randomized Trial of Low-air-loss Beds for Treatment of Pressure Ulcers," *JAMA* 269:494-97, 1993.

[p] Bourdel-Marchasson, I., et al. "Prospective Audits of Quality of PEM Recognition and Nutritional Support in Critically Ill Elderly Patients," *Clinical Nutrition* 18:233-40, 1999.

[q] Guralnik, J.M., et al. "Occurrence and Predictors of Pressure Sores in the National Health and Nutrition Examination Survey Follow-up," *Journal of the American Geriatrics Society* 36:807-12, 1988.

Laboratory values for nutritional assessment

This chart contains additional laboratory value information to use in the nutritional assessment process.

Test	Normal values	Some implications
Albumin	3.5 to 5.0 g/dl 35 to 50 g/L (SI units)	• **Function:** Maintains colloidal osmotic pressure; transport molecule for ions, hormones, some drugs, enzymes, fatty acids, amino acids, bilirubin, and pigments • **Site of synthesis:** Liver • **Half-life:** 12 to 18 days • **Increased:** Dehydration • **Decreased:** Overhydration, liver disease, severe burns, malnutrition, pre-eclampsia, malabsorption, heart failure, nephritic syndrome, infection, stress, advanced malignancies, protein-losing enteropathies, thyroid disease, renal disorders, pregnancy, vasculitis, ulcerative bowel disease, trauma, sepsis, pernicious anemia, spinal cord injury, decubitus ulcer, cystic fibrosis, excessive administration of I.V. glucose in water, starvation, burns, surgery, myocardial infarction (MI), cytokine-induced inflammatory states, patient age 70 or older
Blood urea nitrogen	10 to 20 mg/dl 3.6 to 7.1 mmol/L	• **Function:** Detoxified product of protein metabolism, indicates recent protein intake • **Site of synthesis:** Liver • **Increased:** Dehydration, increased protein intake, urinary obstruction, renal failure/insufficiency, increased catabolism of protein due to infection, tumors, starvation, stress, trauma, myocardial infarction, diabetes mellitus, increased age, steroid therapy, gastrointestinal bleeding, heart failure, shock, GI hemorrhage, chronic gout, burns, sepsis • **Decreased:** Overhydration, liver damage or advanced cirrhosis, low-protein diet, malnutrition, pregnancy, impaired absorption
Cholesterol, total	< 200 g/dl < 5.20 mmol/L	• **Function:** Used to form bile salts, hormones, and cell membranes • **Site of synthesis:** Liver • **Increased:** Cardiovascular disease, atherosclerosis, myocardial infarction, hypothyroidism, uncontrolled diabetes mellitus, biliary cirrhosis, pregnancy, hyperlipoproteinemia, nephritic syndrome, biliary obstruction, high cholesterol or saturated fat diet, hypertension • **Decreased:** Hyperthyroidism, malnutrition, malabsorption, liver disease, anemia, stress, severe infection, cancer, pernicious anemia, cytokine-induced inflammatory states

Laboratory values for nutritional assessment (continued)

Test	Normal values	Some implications
Creatinine	Male: 0.6 to 1.2 mg/dl 53 to 106 mmol/L Female: 0.5 to 1.1 mg/dl 44 to 97 mmol/L	• **Function:** Nitrogenous byproduct in breakdown of muscle creatine phosphate due to energy metabolism • **Site of synthesis:** N/A • **Increased:** Impaired renal function, shock, diabetic nephropathy, heart failure, acute MI, some cancers, dehydration, chronic nephritis, urinary tract obstruction, muscle disease, nephrotoxic drugs, gigantism, acromegaly, rhabdomyolysis • **Decreased:** Overhydration, muscular dystrophy, pregnancy, eclampsia, sarcopenia or muscle wasting, severe wasting
Prealbumin	15 to 36 mg/dl 150 to 360 mg/L	• **Function:** Transports thyroxine, complexes with retinol-binding protein for vitamin A transport • **Site of synthesis:** Liver • **Half-life:** 2 to 3 days • **Increased:** Renal failure, dehydration, Hodgkin's lymphoma, pregnancy • **Decreased:** Liver disease, malnutrition, catabolic states, metabolic stress, inflammation, surgical trauma, hyperthyroidism, overhydration, protein-losing enteropathy, infection, inflammations, cytokine-induced inflammatory states
Total lymphocyte count	3,000 to 3,500 cells/μl	• **Increased:** Leukemia, infectious bacterial diseases, leukocytosis • **Decreased:** Corticosteroid therapy, cancer, chemotherapy, radiotherapy, surgery, lymphopenia, malnutrition • **Degrees of depletion:** Mild = 1,500 to 1,800; moderate = 900 to 1,500; severe < 900

Adapted with permission from *Pocket Resource for Nutrition Assessment*, 2001 rev., Consultant Dietitians in Health Care Facilities, the American Dietetic Association.

intervention has shown effectiveness in the prevention of pressure ulcers.[38,39]

Providing nutritional support

Nutritional support is the variety of techniques available for use when a person can't meet his nutritional needs by normal ingestion of food. Nutritional support options include such strategies as providing additional liquid nutritional supplements or various snack foods to the person's oral diet, feeding via a tube placed into the GI tract or — the most invasive method — giving nutrients via the venous system as total parenteral nutrition when the GI tract isn't functional.

Nutritional support is used to place the patient into positive nitrogen balance (the body maintains the same amount of protein in its tissues from day to day), according to the goals of care and

Prescription drugs linked to anorexia

This list of commonly prescribed medications have anorexia as a major adverse effect, which may lead to weight loss.

* Amlodipine (Norvasc)*
* Ciprofloxacin (Cipro)
* Cisapride (Propulsid)*
* Conjugated estrogens (Premarin)
* Digoxin (Lanoxin)
* Enalapril maleate (Vasotec)
* Famotidine (Pepcid)
* Fentanyl transdermal system (Duragesic)*
* Furosemide (Lasix)
* Ipratropium bromide (Atrovent)
* Levothyroxine sodium (Synthroid)
* Narcotic analgesics (Propacet)
* Nifedipine (Procardia XL)
* Nizatidine (Axid)*
* Omeprazole (Prilosec)*
* Paroxetine hydrochloride (Paxil)*
* Phenytoin (Dilantin)
* Potassium replacement (K-Dur)
* Ranitidine (Zantac)
* Risperdone (Risperdal)*
* Sertraline (Zoloft)
* Warfarin (Coumadin)

* Indicates drugs with fastest growing usage.

whether it's compatible with the patient's and family's wishes. Enteral feeding (tube feeding) may be initiated when the ability to chew, swallow, and absorb nutrients through normal gastrointestinal route is compromised. This occurs in conditions such as stroke, Parkinson's disease, cancer, and dysphagia, or when patients can't meet their nutritional needs orally. Most enteral tube feeding formulas are nutritionally complete and are designed for a specific purpose. Parenteral nutrition is the delivery of nutrient solutions directly into a vein, bypassing the intestine. It's necessary in patients when enteral tube feeding is contraindicated, is insufficient to maintain nutritional status, or has led to serious complications. (See *Nutritional assessment and support,* page 180.)

Does providing enteral feedings prevent pressure ulcers? The answer may lie in the limited number of studies that have been completed involving the use of tube feedings in persons with pressure ulcers. No difference in the number or healing of pressure ulcers was found in 49 residents with pressure ulcers in a long-term care facility who received enteral feedings for 3 months.[40] While pressure ulcers occur frequently in patients with hip fractures, randomized clinical trials of enteral nutrition in this population haven't been successful in preventing pressure ulcer development.[41] It's possible that poor tolerance of the feedings may have contributed to this result. In another study of 135 long-term-care residents with severe cognitive impairment, provision of tube feedings didn't increase survival or have an apparent effect on the prevalence of pressure ulcers.[42]

Ways to enhance nutritional intake

Our bodies need adequate fluid. Many elderly people are chronically dehydrated. Assuring adequate oral fluid intake can be challenging. Use creative ways to encourage daily fluid intake. For example, in warm climates use frozen Popsicles, while in cooler climates hot soup would be a good approach. While it may be tempting to think any liquid will increase the person's fluid intake, this may not be true. Avoid beverages with caffeine, alcohol, or high glucose content, as they will act as diuretics and actually cause fluid loss.

Rather than just relying on supplemental shakes to increase calories and nutrients, consider adding powdered milk to foods the patient is already eating, such as pudding or yogurt. Offer small, frequent meals and snacks, such as high-calorie snacks, bars, and other forms of nutrient rich products. The adage that you must individualize feedings based on the person's preferences is so true. Sometimes making a contract with your patient to eat or drink some portion or percentage of his meals in return for something he loves that doesn't have as much nutritional value, might enhance his overall food and nutrient intake.

Exploring why a patient isn't eating is the first step in helping him meet his nutritional needs. For example, is there an emotional or physical reason why eating is a problem? Find out if something is bothering the patient that's preventing him from eating. Provide a social environment that, for example, reduces noxious smells that decrease appetite while increasing aromas such as food being prepared or other such pleasant smells like cinnamon. A quiet, unhurried eating environment with frequent cueing is particularly helpful for cognitively impaired persons. Similarly, in evaluating physical ability to eat, consider the following questions:

• How much time does it take the patient to eat? Fatigue or fear of choking may cause him to eat slowly.

• Does the patient have the physical ability to bring the food to his mouth? Can he handle eating utensils? Neuromuscular impairments, fatigue, or decreased endurance can interfere with the patient's ability to feed himself. Consider use of assistive devices and consultation from an occupational therapist. Some

Consequences of protein-energy malnutrition

Immunologic
- Impaired cell-mediated and humoral immunity
- Nosocomial infections (such as tuberculosis, *Helicobacter pylori*, or *Clostridium difficile*)

Integumentary
- Skin breakdown and development of pressure ulcers
- Delayed wound healing
- Sparse, dry, easily plucked hair
- Dermatitis

Musculoskeletal
- Decreased physical activity causing decreased muscle strength
- Recurrent falls
- Reduced ADLs

Cardiac
- Loss of cardiac muscle leading to decreased cardiac output

Pulmonary
- Impaired diaphragmatic movement
- Impaired clearance of secretions
- Increased susceptibility to aspiration

Gastrointestinal
- Atrophy of mucosal cells

Adapted with permission from *Nutrition Management and Restorative Dining for Older Adults*, Consultant Dietitians in Health Care Facilities, the American Dietetic Association, 2001.

patients may prefer "finger" foods. Even with appropriate utensils, consider if the patient has the coordination to make

Nutritional assessment and support

This algorithm can be used to determine when to consider enteral and parenteral feeding.

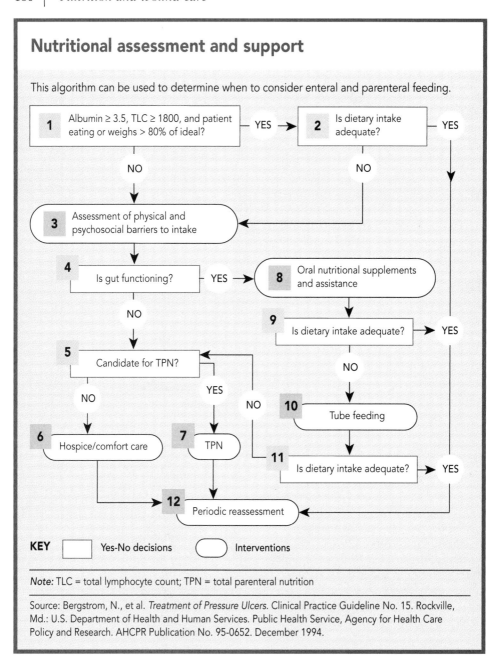

KEY ☐ Yes-No decisions ⬭ Interventions

Note: TLC = total lymphocyte count; TPN = total parenteral nutrition

Source: Bergstrom, N., et al. *Treatment of Pressure Ulcers.* Clinical Practice Guideline No. 15. Rockville, Md.: U.S. Department of Health and Human Services. Public Health Service, Agency for Health Care Policy and Research. AHCPR Publication No. 95-0652. December 1994.

sure the food reaches his mouth and not land on his lap or the floor.
• Can the patient see the food on his tray? Changes in visual fields from stroke, cataracts, glaucoma, or diabetes may alter ability to see food on all or part of the tray. Arrange food so the patient can see and reach it.
• Can the patient chew? Check on the condition of his oral cavity. Provide appropriate mouth care to optimize taste buds and stimulate appetite. Evaluate his

oral hygiene and proper fitting or use of any dentures.

• Can the patient swallow? Cranial nerve and other neurologic conditions can cause swallowing difficulties. Evaluate the patient for any signs of abnormal swallowing. Teach the patient and family members to direct food to the unaffected side of the patient's mouth. Consultation from a speech therapist for management of swallowing difficulties and recommendations about food textures can be very helpful.

PRACTICE POINT

Evaluating if a person can swallow is critical for preventing aspiration. Signs of abnormal swallowing include: drooling, collection of food in the cheeks, frequent coughing, gagging, or clearing the throat during the meal, and leakage of fluid from the nose after swallowing.

Involuntary weight loss, reduced appetite, and severe undernutrition are common in the geriatric population, and often go unexplained.[43] A common cause may be loss of appetite due to a variety of psychological, GI, metabolic, and nutritional factors.[44] Loss of appetite may initiate a vicious cycle of weight loss and increasing undernutrition.

Cytokine-induced cachexia rather than simple starvation may be the reason that hypercaloric feedings in patients with pressure ulcers aren't effective. Hypercaloric feeding has positive results in all but the terminally undernourished patients. Cytokine-induced cachexia is remarkably resistant to hypercaloric feeding.[45,46]

Cytokine-mediated anorexia and weight loss are common in those who develop pressure ulcers. (See *Associations between cytokines, undernutrition, and chronic wounds.*) Serum interleukin (IL)-1∃ is elevated in patients with pressure ulcers.[47] Levels of IL-1∀ are elevated in pressure ulcers but low in acute wound fluid.[48] Circulating serum levels of IL-6, IL-2, and IL-2R are higher in patients with spinal cord injuries compared to normal controls, and highest in patients with pressure ulcers. The highest concentration of cytokines were in patients with the slowest healing pressure ulcers.[49] In other studies, IL-6 serum levels were increased in patients with pressure ulcers but IL-1 and tumor necrosis factor were not elevated.[50]

Documentation in medical record

Medical nutrition therapy documentation in the medical record should include:

Associations between cytokines, undernutrition, and chronic wounds

Proinflammatory cytokines
• Suppressed appetite
• Promotion of or interference with wound healing

Undernutrition
• Poor wound healing
• Increased risk of infection
• Increased incidence of pressure ulcers

Chronic wounds
• Source of cytokines
• Increased association with undernutrition
• Increased serum levels of cytokines

Monthly medical nutrition therapy pressure ulcer progress note

NAME: _____

TARGET WEIGHT _____ lbs. HEIGHT: _____

GENDER: ❏ M   ❏ F

AGE: _____ years

DIET ORDER: _____ FLUID INTAKE: _____ _____ % intake _____ ml	DIET ORDER: _____ FLUID INTAKE: _____ _____ % intake _____ ml
SUPPLEMENT TYPE: TIME: _____ _____ % intake	SUPPLEMENT TYPE: TIME: _____ _____ % intake
FORTIFIED FOODS:	FORTIFIED FOODS:
TUBE FEEDING: FLUSH:	TUBE FEEDING: FLUSH:
FEEDING ABILITY Dependent ❏ Independent ❏ Limited assist ❏ Set-up only ❏ Self-help devices ❏ Type _____	FEEDING ABILITY Dependent ❏ Independent ❏ Limited assist ❏ Set-up only ❏ Self-help devices ❏ Type _____
NUTRIENT NEEDS: BEE _____ Activity factor _____ Injury factor _____ Total calories _____ Protein ____ gm/kg Total protein _____ Fluid _____ cc/kg Total fluids _____ ml	NUTRIENT NEEDS: BEE _____ Activity factor _____ Injury factor _____ Total calories _____ Protein ____ gm/kg Total protein _____ Fluid _____ cc/kg Total fluids _____ ml
CURRENT WEIGHT_____ (lb) ___ % change ❏ 30 days ❏ 90 days ❏ 180 days	CURRENT WEIGHT_____ (lb) ___ % change ❏ 30 days ❏ 90 days ❏ 180 days
PRESSURE ULCER(S) STAGE: 1 2 3 4 LOCATION: _____ SIZE: _____ Exudate: Light Moderate Heavy Pressure Ulcer Scale for Healing (PUSH) score:____	PRESSURE ULCER(S) STAGE: 1 2 3 4 LOCATION: _____ SIZE: _____ Exudate: Light Moderate Heavy Pressure Ulcer Scale for Healing (PUSH) score:____
PRESSURE ULCER(S) STAGE: 1 2 3 4 LOCATION: _____ SIZE: _____ Exudate: Light Moderate Heavy Pressure Ulcer Scale for Healing (PUSH) score:____	PRESSURE ULCER(S) STAGE: 1 2 3 4 LOCATION: _____ SIZE: _____ Exudate: Light Moderate Heavy Pressure Ulcer Scale for Healing (PUSH) score:____
RECOMMENDATIONS:	RECOMMENDATIONS:
RD SIGNATURE: _____	RD SIGNATURE: _____

- amount of food consumed in both quantity and quality or type of food related to amount needed
- average fluid consumed daily (ml), related to amount required
- ability to eat — assisted, supervised, or independent
- acceptance or refusal of diet, meals, or supplements
- current weight and percentage gained or lost
- new conditions affecting nutritional status, such as introduction of thickened liquids or new diagnosis
- new medications affecting nutritional status
- current laboratory results (previous 3 months)
- wound condition and stage
- current calorie, protein, or fluid requirements
- recommendation for care plan.
(See *Monthly medical nutrition therapy pressure ulcer progress note.*)

Summary

Nutrition is an important consideration when treating the patient with pressure ulcers because it not only facilitates healing, but also improves or stabilizes the patient's quality of life. Unfortunately, there's no nutritional "magic bullet" that can be used to accelerate wound healing. Instead, focus on optimal nutrition for each patient. For some patients, optimal nutrition may be achieved by a diet that includes supplements and allows the patient to enjoy his favorite foods. For others, enteral and parenteral nutritional support might be necessary. The amount and type of nutritional support provided to patients with pressure ulcers should be consistent with medical goals and the patient's wishes.[51,52]

Show what you know

1. *A patient who is 68" tall and weighs 188 lb has a body mass index of:*

  A. 20.5.
  B. 28.6.
  C. 27.1.
  D. 25.

ANSWER: B. weight (188lb) ÷ height $(68")^2 \times 705 = 28.6$

2. *A patient who weighs 125 lb with a stage IV pressure ulcer, poor appetite, and a pre-albumin level of 25 mg/dl has a recommended daily protein requirement of:*

  A. 57 to 118 g.
  B. 68 to 107 g.
  C. 85 to 113 g.
  D. 68 to 86 g.

ANSWER: D. $125 \div 2.2 = 57$ kg $\times$ 1.2 − 1.5 = 68.4 g to 85.5 g.

3. *Clinical signs of kwashiorkor include:*

  A. well-nourished appearance, edema.
  B. decreased energy intake, normal serum protein.
  C. decreased protein intake, infections.
  D. A and C.
  E. All of the above.

ANSWER: D.

4. *Recommendations for a severely stressed patient with a stage IV pressure ulcer whose nutritional status is compromised include:*

  A. calories of 30 to 35 g/kg of body weight; protein 1.5 g/kg per day; zinc sulfate 220 mg per day; 6 to 8 cups fluid per day.
  B. calories of 20 to 30 g/kg of body weight; protein 1.5 g/kg per day; multivitamin; 6 to 8 cups fluid per day.

C. calories of 40 to 35 g/kg of body weight; protein 1.5 g/kg per day; ascorbic acid supplements 500 mg per day; 6 to 8 cups fluid per day.

D. calories of 30 to 35 g/kg of body weight; protein 1.5 g/kg per day; multivitamin; 6 to 8 cups fluid per day.

ANSWER: D. There's no evidence to prove supplementation of zinc or ascorbic acid benefits healing unless there's a deficiency. Calories, protein and fluid requirements are increased in stressed patients.

References

1. Long, C.L., et al. "A Physiologic Basis for the Provision of Fuel Mixtures in Normal and Stressed Patients," *Journal of Trauma* 30(9):1077-86, September 1990.

2. Gersovitz, M., et al. "Human Protein Requirements: Assessment of the Adequacy of the Current Recommended Dietary Allowance for Dietary Protein in Elderly Men and Women," *American Journal of Clinical Nutrition* 35(1):6-14, January 1982.

3. McCauley, R., et al. "Effects of Glutamine Infusion on Colonic Anastomotic Strength in the Rat," *Journal of Parenteral and Enteral Nutrition* 15(4):437-39, July-August 1991.

4. Barbul, A., et al. "Arginine Enhances Wound Healing and Lymphocyte Immune Response in Humans," *Surgery* 108(2):331-37, August 1990.

5. Kirk, S.J., et al. "Arginine Stimulates Wound Healing and Immune Function in Aged Humans," *Surgery* 114(2):155-60, August 1993.

6. Langkamp-Henken B., et al. "Arginine Supplementation is Well Tolerated but Doesn't Enhance Mitogen-induced Lymphocyte Proliferation in Elderly Nursing Home Residents with Pressure Ulcers," *Journal of Parenteral and Enteral Nutrition* 24(5):280-87, September-October 2000.

7. Hunt, T.K. "Vitamin A and Wound Healing," *Journal of the American Academy of Dermatology* 15(4 Pt.2):817-21, October 15, 1986.

8. Ehrlich, H.P., and Hunt, T.K. "Effects of Cortisone and Vitamin A on Wound Healing," *Annals of Surgery* 167(3):324-28, March 1968.

9. Levenson, S.M., and Demetriou, A.A. "Metabolic factors," in Cohen, I.K., et al., eds. *Wound Healing: Biochemical and Clinical Aspects*. Philadelphia: W.B. Saunders Co., 248-73 1992.

10. "Wound Healing," in Gottschlich, M.M., et al., eds. *Nutrition Support Dietetics Core Curriculum*, 2nd ed. Silver Spring, Md.: Aspen Pubs., Inc., 1993.

11. Waldorf, H., and Fewkes, J. "Wound Healing," *Advances in Dermatology* 10:77-96, 1995.

12. Clark, S. "The Biochemistry of Antioxidants Revisited," *Nutrition in Clinical Practice* 17(1):5-17, February 2002.

13. Rackett, S.C., et al. "Diet and Dermatology. The Role of Dietary Manipulation in the Prevention and Treatment of Cutaneous Disorders," *Journal of the American Academy of Dermatology* 29(3):447-61, September 1993.

14. Riet, G., et al. "Randomized Clinical Trial of Ascorbic Acid in the Treatment of Pressure Ulcers," *Journal of Clinical Epidemiology* 48(12):1453-60, December 1995.

15. Vilter, R.W. "Nutritional Aspects of Ascorbic Acid: Uses and Abuses," *Western Journal of Medicine* 133(6):485-92, December 1980.

16. Norris, J.R., and Reynolds, R.E. "The Effect of Oral Zinc Sulfate Therapy on Decubitus Ulcers," *Journal of the American Geriatric Society* 19:793, 1971.

17. Goode, P., and Allman, R. "The Prevention and Management of Pressure Ulcers," *Medical Clinics of North America* 73(6):1511-24, November 1989.

18. Thomas, D.R. "The Role of Nutrition in Prevention and Healing of Pressure Ulcers," *Clinics in Geriatric Medicine* 13(3):497-511, August 1997.

19. Reed, B.R., and Clark, R.A.F. "Cutaneous Tissue Repair: Practical Implications of Current Knowledge II," *Journal of the American Academy of Dermatology* 13(6):919-41, December 1985.

20. Gregger, J.L. "Potential for Trace Mineral Deficiencies and Toxicities in the

Elderly," in *Mineral Homeostasis in the Elderly.* Edited by Bales, C.W. New York: Marcel Dekker, 1989.

21. Choban, P.S., et al. "Nutrition Support of Obese Hospitalized Patients," *Nutrition in Clinical Practice* 12(4):149-54, August 1997.

22. Ireton-Jones, C.S. "Evaluation of Energy Expenditures in Obese Patients," *Nutrition in Clinical Practice* 4(4):127-29, August 1989.

23. Posthauer, M.E., et al. "ADA's Definition for Nutrition Screening and Nutrition Assessment," *Journal of the American Dietetic Association* 94(8):838-39, August 1994.

24. Ryan, C.F., et al. "Energy Balance in Stable Malnourished Patients with Chronic Obstructive Pulmonary Disease," *Chest* 103(4):1038-44, April 1993.

25. Maklebust, J., and Sieggreen, M. *Pressure Ulcers: Guidelines for Prevention and Management,* 3rd ed. Springhouse, Pa.: Springhouse Corporation, 2001.

26. Report of the Dietary Guidelines Advisory Committee on the Dietary Guidelines for Americans 2000.

27. Niedert, K. *Pocket Resource for Nutrition Assessment. Consultant Dietitians in Health Care Facilities.* Chicago: American Dietetic Association, 2001.

28. Friedman, F.J., et al. "Hypoalbuminemia in the Elderly is Due to Disease not Malnutrition," *Clinical Experimental Gerontol* 7:191-203, 1985.

29. Morley, J.E., and Kraenzle, D. "Causes of Weight Loss in a Community Nursing Home," *Journal of the American Geriatric Society* 42(6):583-85, June 1994.

30. Thomas, D.R. "Nutritional Factors Affecting Wound Healing," *Ostomy/ Wound Management* 42(5):40-49, June 1996.

31. Thomas, D.R. "Improving Outcome of Pressure Ulcers with Nutritional Interventions: A Review of the Evidence," *Nutrition* 17(2):121-25, February 2001.

32. Thomas, D.R, et al. "Hospital Acquired Pressure Ulcers and Risk of Death," *Journal of the American Geriatric Society* 44(12):1435-40, December 1996.

33. Pinchcofsky-Devin, G.D., and Kaminski, M.V., Jr. "Correlation of Pressure Sores and Nutritional Status," *Journal of the Amerian Geriatric Society* 34(6):435-40, June 1986.

34. Bergstrom, N., and Braden, B. "A Prospective Study of Pressure Sore Risk Among Institutionalized Elderly," *Journal of the American Geriatric Society* 40(8):747-58, August 1992.

35. Demling, R.H., and DeSanti, L. "Oxandrolone, an Anabolic Steroid, Significantly Increases the Rate of Weight Gain in the Recovery Phase After Major Burns. *Journal of Trauma-Injury Infection & Critical Care* 43(1):47-51, July 1997.

36. Rubenstein, L.Z. "An Overview of Aging-demographics, Epidemiology and Health Services," in Morley, J.E., et al., eds. *Geriatric Nutrition: A Comprehensive Review.* New York: Raven Press; 1990.

37. Curtas, S., et al. "Evaluation of Nutritional Status," *Nursing Clinics of North America.* 2(2):301-11, June 1989.

38. Bergstrom, N. "Lack of Nutrition in AHCPR Prevention Guideline," *Decubitus* 6(3):4-6, May 1993.

39. Thomas, D.R. "Improving the Outcome of Pressure Ulcers with Nutritional Intervention: A Review of the Evidence," *Nutrition* 17(2):121-25, February 2001.

40. Henderson, C.T., et al. "Prolonged Tube Feeding in Long-term Care: Nutritional Status and Clinical Outcomes," *Journal of the American College of Clinical Nutrition* 11(3):309-25, June 1992.

41. Hartgrink, H.H., et al. "Pressure Sores and Tube Feeding in Patients with a Fracture of the Hip: A Randomized Clinical Trial," *Clinical Nutrition* 17(6):287-92, December 1998.

42. Mitchell, S.L., et al. "The Risk Factors and Impact on Survival of Feeding Tube Placement in Nursing Home Residents with Severe Cognitive Impairment," *Archives of Internal Medicine* 157(3): 327-32, February 10, 1997.

43. Thompson, M.P., and Merria, L.K. "Unexplained Weight Loss in Ambulatory Elderly," *Journal of the American Geriatric Society* 39(5):497-500, May 1991.

44. Morley, J.E., and Thomas, D.R. "Anorexia and Aging: Pathophysiology," *Nutrition* 15(6):499-503, June 1999.

45. Souba, W.W. "Drug Therapy: Nutritional Support," *New England Journal of Medicine* 336(1):41-48, January 1997.

46. Atkinson, S., et al. "A prospective, Randomized, Double-blind, Controlled Clinical Trial of Enteral Immunonutrition in the Critically Ill," *Critical Care Medicine* 26(7):1164-72, July 1998.

47. Matsuyama, N., et al. "The Possibility of Acute Inflammatory Reaction Affects the Development of Pressure Ulcers in Bedridden Elderly Patients," *Rinsho Byori-Japanese Journal of Clinical Pathology* 47(11):1039-45, November 1999.

48. Barone, E.J., et al. "Interleukin-1" and Collagenase Activity are Elevated in Chronic Wounds," *Plastic & Reconstructive Surg* 102:1023-27, 1998.

49. Segal, J.L., et al. "Circulating Levels of IL-2R, ICAM-1, and IL-6 in Spinal Cord Injuries," *Archives of Physical Medicine & Rehabilitation* 78(1):44-47, January 1997.

50. Bonnefoy, M., et al. "Implication of Cytokines in the Aggravation of Malnutrition and Hypercatabolism in Elderly Patients with Severe Pressure Sores," *Age & Ageing* 24(1):37-42, January 1995.

51. Thomas, D.R., et al. "Nutritional Management in Long-term Care: Development of a Clinical Guideline. Council for Nutritional Strategies in Long-Term Care" *Journals of Gerontology Series A-Biological Sciences & Medical Sciences* 55(12):M725-34, December 2000.

52. Thomas, D.R. "The role of Nutrition in Prevention and Healing of Pressure Ulcers," *Clinics in Geriatric Medicine* 13(3):497-511, August 1997.

CHAPTER 11

Seating, positioning, and support surfaces

David M. Brienza, PhD
Mary Jo Geyer, PhD, PT, CWS, CLT
Stephen Sprigle, PhD, PT

OBJECTIVES

After completing this chapter, you'll be able to:

- demonstrate an understanding of tissue biomechanical properties, their measurement, and their relationship to soft tissue-loading tolerance

- identify support surface characteristics related to the maintenance of tissue integrity

- demonstrate an understanding of the categories, functions, and limitations of various support surfaces

- outline an assessment process for selecting an appropriate support surface (seat cushion or horizontal support) and related interventions (positioning).

Preventing skin breakdown

Among other interventions, the essential care for maintaining tissue integrity includes managing loads on the skin and associated soft tissue. A comprehensive care plan should include tissue load management strategies for individuals while in bed and when seated. Properly chosen support surfaces, adequate periodic pressure relief, protection of especially vulnerable bony prominences such as the heels, and consideration of special patient needs are all essential components of such a plan.

Unless specifically identified as either a seat cushion or a horizontal support surface (overlay, mattress, or specialty bed), in the context of this chapter the term "support surface" refers to both products. Achieving a good match between the patient's needs and the performance capabilities of the support surface has a profound, positive impact on patients' health and well-being. Conversely, a poor match has an equally negative impact. Support

Support surface performance parameters

Nine parameters must be considered when evaluating the characteristics of a support surface for the patient with a wound:

- Redistribution of pressure
- Moisture control
- Temperature control
- Friction control (between patient and product)
- Infection control
- Flammability
- Life expectancy
- Fail safety
- Product reputation.

Adapted with permission from Krouskop, T., and van Rijwijk, L. "Standardizing Performance-Based Criteria for Support Surfaces," *Ostomy/Wound Management* 41(1):34-44, January-February 1995.

---

cient to replace good clinical decision-making and follow-up evaluations. Furthermore, existing clinical recommendations need to be updated regularly to reflect new research, technology, and treatment strategies as they become available.

Knowledge of a product's composition and contents is a necessary part of the selection process. While describing the material components of support surface technology may be informative, it isn't always instructive. In terms of selecting a product, the information on the function or performance of the surface is most critical, regardless of composition. Krouskop and van Rijswijk[1] focused on performance parameters when they identified nine key support surface characteristics. (See *Support surface performance parameters.*)

Unfortunately, the information from clinical validation studies necessary for function- and performance-based categorization of seat cushions and support surfaces isn't yet available. The best we can do now is to group the devices according to the technologies and materials used in their construction and relate the characteristics of these technologies to the factors believed to have significant affects on the prevention and healing of pressure ulcers.

surfaces counteract the body's weight and protect the tissue while providing for proper body alignment, comfort and, as part of a seating system, may provide postural control during functional movement. These effects frequently conflict. Clinical decision-making commonly requires a compromise between protective and functional goals.

In a perfect world, we would be able to choose the "right" surface by using a tried and true algorithm to input an individual's characteristics, conditions, environment, and desires and produce a prescription for an ideal, personalized support surface. Unfortunately, the world isn't perfect and the research in this area has failed to produce strong evidence to justify the selection of one product over another for any given situation. Some guidance is available, but it isn't suffi-

Soft tissue biomechanics

Human soft tissues consist of a variety of macrostructures including skin, fat, muscle, vessels, nerves, ligaments, and tendons. The relative amounts and arrangement of the tissue macromolecules of the skin and supporting soft tissues are adapted to their specific functions and dictate their biomechanical properties.

In most connective tissue, fibroblasts secrete the macromolecules that make up the extracellular matrix. The matrix is made up of two main classes of macro-molecules:

• polysaccharide chains of a class called glycosaminoglycans, which are usually found covalently linked to protein in the form of proteoglycans

• fibrous proteins that are either primarily structural (for example, collagen and elastin) or primarily adhesive (for example, fibronectin and laminin).

Glycosaminoglycans and proteoglycans form a highly hydrated, gel-like "ground substance" in which the proteins are embedded. The ground substance is analogous to glue that fills the lattice of collagen and elastin fibers, providing lubrication and shock absorbing qualities. The polysaccharide gel resists compressive forces on the matrix while the collagen fibers along with elastin fibers provide tensile strength and resilience.

Tissue mechanical properties

In general, soft tissues are anisotropic, incompressible biosolid, biofluid mixtures.[2] Because soft tissue is largely incompressible, it tends to move slowly from areas of greater pressure to areas of lesser pressure. This slow movement of ground substance and interstitial fluid is responsible for the time-dependent (viscoelastic) behavior of the soft tissue manifested as four phenomena: stress relaxation, creep, hysteresis, and pseudoelasticity (preconditioning).[3]

These phenomena may be graphically represented as stress-strain curves. Stress is represented as the deforming force on the *y* axis and the tissue strain (deformation) is plotted on the *x* axis. When soft tissue is suddenly deformed (strained) and the strain is thereafter kept constant, the corresponding stress induced in the tissue decreases over time. This phenomenon is known as stress relaxation. (See *Stress-relaxation phenomenon.*) Alternatively, creep describes the progressive tissue de-

Stress-relaxation phenomenon

The stress vs. strain curve, shown below, illustrates the stress-relaxation phenomenon. With the compression of tissue (strain) held constant, the force (stress) generated in the tissue as a result of that compression reduces over time. The degree of stress relaxation—that is, the amount of reduction in the holding force—can be determined by measuring the distance along the vertical axis between the time when the load is first applied to the time when it reaches steady-state (downward sloping ends).

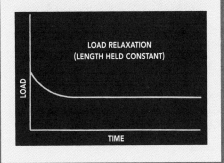

formation that occurs over time when stress remains constant. (See *Creep phenomenon,* page 190.) During cyclic loading such as that produced by a dynamic, or alternating pressure, mattress, the stress-strain relationship demonstrated during the loading phase is different from that of the recovery or unloaded portion of the cycle. This effect is known as hysteresis. Finally, pseudo-elasticity is the term associated with an increase in the repeatability and predictability of a tissue's stress-strain relationship following a defined period of repetitive cyclic loading.

Creep phenomenon

Creep reflects the ability of tissue to resist deformation over time when the force causing the deformation remains constant. The creep phenomenon shown here indicates that the tissue progressively deforms over time without any additional force being applied. If creep were zero, the curve would be a flat line, indicating that deformation was constant over time.

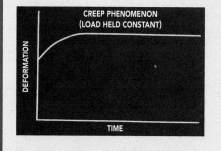

Tissue loading and pressure ulcer formation

Body weight resting on bony prominences such as the scapula, sacrum, greater trochanters, ischial tuberosities, and heels can cause significant concentrations of pressure at the skin's surface and in the underlying soft tissue. The pressure peaks and the pressure gradients surrounding these peaks can put the soft tissue at risk of breakdown. However, high pressure alone usually isn't a sufficient condition for the development of a pressure ulcer. Research has clearly demonstrated that the damaging effects of pressure are related to both its magnitude and duration. Simply stated, tissues can withstand higher loads for shorter periods of time. (See *Guidelines for sitting duration.*)

Limitations of interface pressure as a predictor of tissue damage

Tissue interface pressure is the force per unit area that acts perpendicularly between the patient's body and the support surface.[4] It's measured noninvasively by placing a pressure sensor between the patient's skin and the support surface. This measurement is believed to provide an approximation of the pressure on the tissue test site or surrounding area. Single sensors have been used to measure local pressure over a single bony prominence; multiple sensors integrated into a mat may be used to "map" the entire body area in contact with the support surface.

Interface pressure has been used extensively as a tool for predicting the clinical effectiveness of various support surfaces and for comparing products. Many research efforts have been directed toward establishing an interface pressure threshold beyond which pressure ulcers would form. However, research has failed to identify a specific threshold at which loads can be deemed harmful across either subject populations or various tissue body sites. This is because a tissue's loading tolerance varies according to its composition, condition, location, age, hydration, and metabolic state. Therefore, while interface pressure may aid in comparing one surface to another for a specific individual based on that individual's relative responses, interface pressure alone isn't sufficient to evaluate the efficacy of a particular device or class of devices.

More recent research has gone beyond assuming that tissue necrosis is a result of ischemia due to external pressure alone. In fact, all of the well-known extrinsic pressure ulcer risk factors (pressure, shear, friction, temperature, and moisture) tend to influence the tissue's ability to withstand loading. Therefore, current investigations are focusing on a variety of physiological, biochemical, and biomechanical tissue responses to loading.

Clinical implications of aging

The gross morphology of the soft tissues undergoes significant changes due to aging, including decreased moisture content and decreased elasticity manifested as rough, scaly skin with increased wrinkling and laxity. Dry, inelastic skin with larger, more irregular epidermal cells leads to decreased barrier function. These changes are reflected in the tissue biomechanical properties and have been associated with increased risk of tissue injury.

At the microscopic level, flattening of the dermal-epidermal junction (rete ridges) has been observed with the height of the dermal papillae declining by 55% from the 3rd to 9th decades of life. As the space between the well-vascularized dermis and epidermis increases, several functional changes occur. Decreases have been reported in the area available for nutrient transfer, the number of cells within the stratum basale, and the skin's resistance to shearing. A 30% to 50% decrease in epidermal turnover during the 3rd to the 8th decades of life has also been reported. This diminution in repair rate has been quantified as both decreased collagen deposition and diminished wound tensile strength. The loss of subcutaneous fat with aging decreases the protection from injury due to pressure and shearing forces between the bony prominences and the support surface. Moreover, decreased sensory perception increases the risk of injury by mechanical forces such as pressure and the more rigid, less elastic, drier nature of the skin of elderly people results in tissue that tears and bleeds more easily.

Guidelines for sitting duration

This graph provides guidelines on sitting tolerance based on the magnitude of localized pressure.

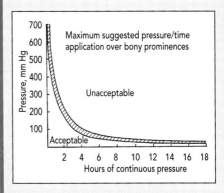

Reprinted with permission from Reswick, J., and Rogers, J. *Experiences at Rancho Los Amigos Hospital with Devices and Techniques to Prevent Pressure Sores. Bedsore Biomechanics.* London: University Park Press, 1976.

Support surface characteristics

Prevention of pressure ulcers is accomplished primarily by managing tissue loads. Support surfaces have been designed to reduce the effects of tissue loading by controlling the intensity and duration of pressure, shear, and friction. Also, attempts have been made to control the physical factors associated with increased risk through elimination of excess moisture and effective dissipation of heat.

Pressure redistribution

The redistribution of pressure reduces the magnitude of pressure and shear forces, both of which can cause excessive tissue distortion and damage soft tissues. Pressure (stress) is defined as force per unit area; the pressure distribution is influenced by mechanical and physical characteristics of the support surface, mechanical properties of the body's tissues, and weight distribution (posture).

Immersion

The fundamental strategy for reducing pressure near a bony prominence is to allow the prominence to be immersed into the support surface. Immersion allows the pressure concentrated beneath a specific bony prominence to be spread out over the surrounding area, including other bony prominences. For example, when a person is sitting on a relatively hard cushion, a disproportionately large portion of his body weight is born by the tissue beneath the ischial tuberocities. On a softer surface, the ischial tuberocities and buttocks may immerse more deeply, even to the level of the greater trochanters. With greater immersion, the body weight divided by a greater surface area results in decreased average pressure. This definition of immersion doesn't distinguish between immersion resulting from compression of the support surface and immersion resulting from the displacement of a support surface's fluid components.

The potential for immersion depends on both the force-deformation characteristics of the cushion and its physical dimensions. For fluid-filled support surfaces, immersion depends on the thickness of the surface and the flexibility of the cover. For elastic and viscoelastic support surfaces, immersion depends on their stiffness and thickness. Consider how the thickness of a seat cushion might limit the potential for immersion. If the seat cushion is 1.5″ (3.8 cm) and the vertical distance between the ischial tuberosities and greater trochanters is 2″ (5 cm), the potential for immersion isn't enough to unload the ischial tuberosities.

Envelopment

Envelopment is a support surface's ability to deform around irregularities on the surface without causing a substantial increase in pressure. Examples of irregularities are creases in clothing, bedding, or seat covers, and protrusions of bony prominences. A fluid support medium would envelop perfectly. However, surface tension plays an important role in envelopment. A fluid-filled support surface such as a waterbed doesn't envelop as well as water alone. The membrane containing the water has surface tension, which has a hammocking effect on irregularities of the interface. Poorly enveloping support surfaces may cause high local peak pressures, thereby potentially increasing the risk of tissue break down.

Pressure gradient

Pressure gradient, also known as pressure differential, is defined as the change in pressure over a distance. Although various distances have been reported in the literature, it's expressed most commonly as change in millimeters of mercury (mm Hg) per square centimeter or square inch. When the pressure across a surface is plotted on a graph, the slope of the curve is the pressure gradient. Since the skin and other soft tissues at risk of breakdown consist of a mixture of interstitial fluid and ground substance into which structural elements are embedded, a pressure differential between adjacent regions will result in a slow flow of the tissue's fluid elements from a region of high pressure to one of lesser pressure. This flow is analogous to the movement produced when one compresses the surface of a bucket of wet sand with one's hand.

Several investigators have hypothesized that the flow of interstitial fluid caused by pressure gradients is the primary factor in the development of pressure ulcers.[5,6] The flow of ground substance and interstitial fluids from an area of high pressure is believed to increase the likelihood of intercellular contact, resulting in cellular ruptures.[5,6] This theory is consistent with the classic experimental results of several researchers[7,8] showing a relationship between duration of pressure application and the magnitude of pressure that results in the formation of a pressure ulcer.

Pressure gradient is intimately linked to pressure and is affected by immersion and envelopment in a similar manner. Under certain circumstances, it's possible to have pressure gradients without high pressure, and vice versa. For example, the boundary of the contact area on a support surface necessarily demonstrates a significant pressure gradient where the pressure magnitude transitions from zero outside the area of support to a nonzero value in the supported region. Despite these significant gradients, boundary areas are typically areas of lower risk for pressure ulcer development, suggesting that pressure gradient only becomes an important factor when combined with high pressure. Research is needed to test and investigate this hypothesis.

Shear and friction reduction

The term "shear" is commonly used to refer to the effect of a loading condition in which the skin surface remains stuck to a support surface while the underlying bony structure moves in a direction tangential to the surface. For example, when the head of a bed is raised or lowered, if the skin over the sacrum doesn't slide along the surface of the bed, or the bed doesn't absorb the resulting shear force by deforming in the horizontal direction, the effect will be a shearing of the soft tissue between the sacrum and the support surface. In engineering terms, the resulting shearing or deformation of the soft tissue would be referred to as "shear

strain." The characteristics of the support surface affecting this potentially harmful situation are the coefficient of friction of the surface and the ability of the surface to deform horizontally. Some support surface technologies protect the skin from shear better than others.

Friction refers to the force acting tangential to the interface that opposes shear force. The frictional force prevents one from sliding off the surface. In a static condition (when a person isn't sliding along the surface), the friction force is equivalent to the shear force. (See *Friction and shear forces*, page 194.)

The maximum friction is determined by the coefficient of friction of the support surface and the pressure. This is why surfaces with high coefficients of friction have the potential for producing high shear. Friction and shear are local phenomena and are affected by moisture on the skin. Moist or wet skin usually has a higher coefficient of friction and, as will be discussed below, is more susceptible to damage caused by shearing. Remember, friction is necessary to prevent a person from simply sliding off the bed surface or wheelchair cushion. For optimal prevention of pressure ulcers, the friction necessary to prevent sliding should be applied in low risk regions of the support surface and minimized near high-risk areas surrounding bony prominences.

Temperature control

The role of temperature in pressure ulcer formation hasn't been definitively investigated. The application of repetitive surface loading alone induces an elevated skin temperature of 41° F (5° C) or greater.[9] In addition, peak skin temperatures have been found to be proportional to the magnitude and duration of the applied pressure.[9,10] The conclusions of research vary depending upon the amount and duration of pressure that's simulta-

Friction and shear forces

This illustration shows the friction and shear forces acting on a person lying in bed.

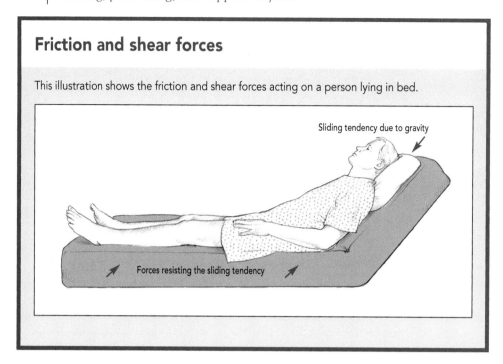

Sliding tendency due to gravity

Forces resisting the sliding tendency

neously applied with varying temperatures.[11,12] However, higher ambient temperatures have been shown to cause an increase in tissue metabolism and oxygen consumption on the order of 10% for every 1.8 F (1° C).[13] Thus, patients with compromised tissue already at risk for pressure ulcers may have increased demands for oxygen in excess of their metabolic capabilities. Any increase in temperature in combination with pressure is believed to increase the susceptibility of the tissue to injury either from ischemia or reperfusion injury when the pressure is relieved.[14]

Increased temperature causes an exponential increase in blood perfusion, which has been associated with either an increase in core body temperature or in local skin temperature.[15,16] In a study of operatively-acquired pressure ulcers, the single greatest predictor of pressure ulcer development was the use of a warming blanket under the patient.[17] These findings clearly indicate the need for additional studies to definitively determine the effects of skin temperature modulation on the development of pressure ulcers. A support surface's heat transfer rate is an objective performance measurement related to the ability of a product to control for temperature effects.

Moisture control

Moisture is another key extrinsic factor in pressure ulcer development. The sources of skin moisture that may predispose the skin to breakdown include perspiration, urine, feces, and fistula or wound drainage. Excessive moisture may lead to maceration.[18] Increases may be due to the slight increase in friction that occurs with light sweating[19] or to the increase in bacterial load resulting when alkaline sources of moisture neutralize the protection provided by the normal acid mantle of the skin.

The detrimental effect of an increase in moisture adjacent to the skin has been demonstrated by tensile tests on excised skin strips in a controlled humidity environment. In Wildnauer's study,[20] the tensile strength of the strips decreased 75% with an increase in relative humidity from 10% to 98%. Skin with such reduced strength may be more prone to mechanical damage from shear stress and could easily be abraded.

Types of support surface systems

The categories for support surfaces described in this section are based on the characteristics of support surface technologies and materials used to reduce the effects of extrinsic factors critical to the development of pressure ulcers, such as pressure redistribution, shear reduction, heat dissipation, and moisture control. These categories include compressive support mediums (elastic foam and viscoelastic foam), fluid-filled and alternating-pressure with two additional categories for horizontal support surfaces only — air-fluidized and low-air-loss.[21] Alternative groupings include foam, viscoelastic foam, gels, and fluid floatation categories.[22] Sprigle[23] adopted Cochran's categories, adding viscoelastic fluid as a separate category. In practice, most products consist of a combination of materials and incorporate multiple therapeutic strategies and features.

Elastic foam

An elastic material deforms in proportion to the applied load; greater loads result in predictably greater deformations, and vice versa. If time is a factor in the load versus deformation characteristic, the response is considered to be viscoelastic, which will be discussed separately. The response of support surfaces made from resilient foam is predominately elastic. Foam support surface products are made from two basic types of foam: open cell or closed cell. Foam is said to have "memory" because of its tendency to return to its nominal shape or thickness.

Foam products typically consist of foam layers of varying densities or combinations of gel and foam. Other products have a series of air-filled chambers covered with a foam structure or are available as multidensity, closed-cell products, 4″ to 10″ (10 to 25.5 cm) deep with deflectable tips. For these types of products, "memory" isn't total because only the foam components will return to their unloaded shape. Several seat cushion products have this construction. Support surfaces with a combination of fluid-filled bladders and resilient foam provide a degree of postural stability with a resilient shell and improved envelopment with a fluid or viscous fluid-filled layer at the interface.

An ideal combination of characteristics for an elastic support surface is resistance that adjusts to the magnitude of compressive forces.[24,25] The support surface should have a high enough compression resistance to fully support the load (prevent bottoming-out) without providing too high a reactive force (memory) so that the interface pressure remains low. Over time and with extended use, foam degrades and loses its resilience. This decreased ability results in higher interface pressures. Krouskop[25] estimates that in approximately 3 years, a foam mattress wears out and the compressive forces are transferred to the underlying supporting structure used to support the foam. In other words, the mattress "bottoms out."

Foams of varying densities may be combined or cut to relieve or conform to bony landmarks to enhance pressure distribution and even reduce shear forces. For example, multidensity, closed-cell foam products with deflectable tips provide some shear protection. Many

Elastic foam seat cushions

These photos show four different types of elastic foam seat cushions.

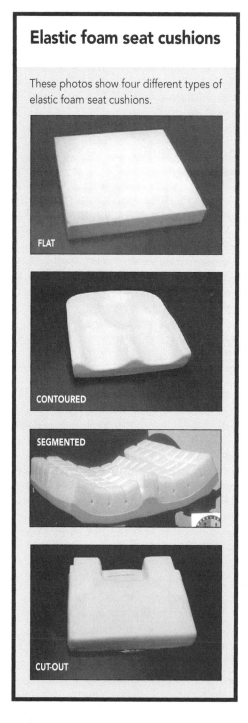

FLAT

CONTOURED

SEGMENTED

CUT-OUT

Foam's stiffness and thickness limit its ability to immerse and envelop; soft foams will envelop better than stiffer foams, but will necessarily be thicker to avoid bottoming out. Foam seat cushions are typically contoured to improve their performance. Precontouring the seat cushion to provide a better match between the buttocks and the cushion increases the contact area and immersion, thereby reducing average pressure and pressure peaks.[26-28] (See *Elastic foam seat cushions.*)

Foam tends to increase skin temperature because foam materials and the air they entrap are poor heat conductors. Moisture doesn't increase as much on foam products with a porous cover because the open cell structure of the cover provides a pathway through which moisture can diffuse. Patient movement can also increase transfer rates. Mean temperature increases of 6.1° F (3.4° C) and a 10.4% increase in moisture at the skin surface have been recorded on foam products after 1 hour of contact.[29]

Viscoelastic foam

Viscoelastic foam products consist of temperature sensitive, viscoelastic open-cell foam. At temperatures near that of the human body, the foam becomes softer, allowing the layer of foam nearest to the body to provide improved pressure distribution through envelopment and immersion when compared to high resilient foam. Viscoelastic foam acts like a self-contouring surface because the elastic response diminishes over time, even after the foam is compressed. However, the desirable temperature and time-sensitive responses of viscoelastic foam may not be realized when the ambient temperature is too low. The properties of viscoelastic foam products vary widely and must be chosen according to the specific needs of the patient for both seat

pressure-reducing mattresses have loose-fitting covers to reduce friction.

and mattress applications. Solid gel products respond similarly to viscoelastic foam products and are included in this category.

Mean temperature increases of 5° F (2.8° C) have been reported for viscoelastic foam.[29] Solid gel products tend to maintain a constant skin-contact temperature or may decrease the contact temperature. (See *Viscoelastic gel seat cushion.*) Gel pads have higher heat flux than foam due to the high specific heat of the gel material. However, in Stewart's study the heat transfer decreased after 2 hours, indicating that the heat reservoir was filling, which suggests that the temperature may increase during longer periods — for example, more than 2 hours — of unrelieved sitting. This further suggests that the temperature may increase during longer periods of unrelieved sitting (more than 2 hours). Moisture increased 22.8% over a 1-hour period.[29] The relative humidity of the skin surface increases considerably because of the nonporous nature of the gel pads.

Fluid-filled products

Fluid-filled products may consist of small or large chambers filled with air, water, or other viscous fluid materials such as silicon elastomer, silicon, or polyvinyl. The fluid flows from chamber to chamber or within a single chamber in response to movement and requires no supplemental power. The term "air-flotation" is sometimes used to describe interconnected multichamber surfaces such as those manufactured by ROHO, Inc. (See *Fluid-filled products*, page 198.)

PRACTICE POINT

Be careful to maintain the correct levels of inflation in air cushions to achieve optimal pressure reduction. Under-inflation causes bottoming out and over-

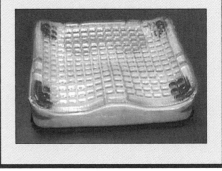

Viscoelastic gel seat cushion

The photo shows a viscoelastic gel seat cushion. Viscoelastic products are also available in other shapes.

inflation increases the interface pressure. For viscous fluid-filled surfaces such as seat cushions, it's important to monitor the distribution of viscous material and manually move it back to the areas under bony prominences if it has moved away from these areas.

Most fluid-filled products permit a high degree of immersion, allowing the body to sink into the surface. The surface conforms to bony prominences, effectively increasing the surface-pressure distribution area and lowering the interface pressure by transferring the pressure to adjacent areas. These products are capable of achieving small to modest deformations without large restoring shear forces. In a direct comparison of interface pressures with air-fluidized (Clinitron, Hill-Rom, Inc.) and low-air-loss (Therapulse, Kinetic Concepts International) beds, the RIK mattress was shown to relieve pressure as effectively as the air-fluidized and low-air-loss surfaces used in the study.[30]

Skin temperature is affected by the specific heat (ability to conduct heat) of the fluid material contained in the support

Fluid-filled products

As the photos demonstrate, fluid-filled products come in a variety of forms.

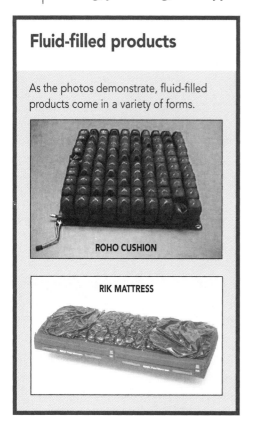

ROHO CUSHION

RIK MATTRESS

encased in a polyester or Gore-Tex sheeting. The granular material takes on the characteristics of a fluid when pressurized air is forced up through them. In some models (FluidAir, KCI), the fluidization feature is variable, permitting individualization based on the patient's needs. These products aid in the reduction of evaporative water loss. Feces and other body fluids flow freely through the sheet; to prevent bacteriologic contamination, the bed must be pressurized at all times and the sheet must be properly disinfected after use by each patient and at least once per week with long-term use by a single patient.[31]

Air-fluidized beds use fluid technology to decrease pressure through the principle of immersion while simultaneously reducing shear. Air-fluidized products permit the highest degree of immersion currently available among support surfaces. The surface conforms to bony prominences by permitting deep immersion into the surface — almost two-thirds of the body may be immersed.[32] The immersion effectively lowers the interface pressure by increasing the surface-pressure distribution area. The greater deformations possible with this technology enable the transfer of pressure to adjacent body areas and other bony prominences. Envelopment and shear force are minimized. A loose but tightly woven polyester or Gore-Tex cover sheet is used to reduce surface tension. Low surface tension enhances envelopment and minimizes shear forces.

The pressurized air in these products is generally warmed to a temperature level of 82.4° to 95° F (28° to 35° C); however, warming may be beneficial or harmful depending on a patient's characteristics. For example, heat may be harmful to patients with multiple sclerosis, but beneficial for patients in pain. The beneficial effects must be balanced

device. Air has a low specific heat and water has a high specific heat. The viscous material used in the RIK mattress also has a high specific heat, and skin temperature decreases have been demonstrated with this product.[30]

Given the large variety of materials used as covers in products falling into the fluid-filled category, it's difficult to generalize on the moisture control characteristics of these products. However, the insulating effects of rubber and plastic used in some fluid-filled products have been shown to increase the relative humidity due to perspiration.[29]

Air-fluidized products

Air-fluidized beds in the late 1960s and were originally developed for use with burn patients. These products consist of granular materials such as silicon beads

Air-fluidized and low-air-loss beds

AIR-FLUIDIZED BED

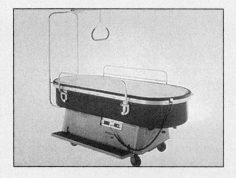

LOW-AIR-LOSS BED

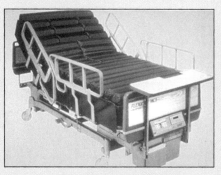

against the increasing metabolic demands of the tissue.

The high degree of moisture-vapor permeability of the air-fluidized system is effective in managing body fluids; in patients with severe burns, air-fluidized beds have been known to cause dehydration. (See *Air-fluidized and low-air-loss beds.*)

PRACTICE POINT

Air-fluidized beds are advantageous for burn patients due to their effectiveness in managing body fluids.

Low-air-loss systems

Low-air-loss systems use a series of connected, air-filled cushions or compartments, which are inflated to specific pressures to provide loading resistance based on the patient's height, weight, and distribution of body weight. An air pump circulates a continuous flow of air through the device, replacing air lost through the surface's pores. The inflation pressures of the cushions vary with patient weight distribution; some systems

have individually adjustable sections for the head, trunk, pelvic or foot areas.[33]

As with other fluid-filled surfaces, the temperature of the skin is affected by the specific heat of the fluid material. Air doesn't have a high specific heat. In addition, the circulating air is warmed. However, the constant air circulation and evaporation tend to keep the skin from overheating.

In low-air-loss systems, the patient lies on a loose-fitting, waterproof cover placed over the cushions. The waterproof covers are designed to let air pass through the pores of the fabric and are usually made of a special nylon or polytetrafluoroethylene fabric with high moisture-vapor permeability. Manufacturers have addressed the problem of skin dehydration by altering the number, size, and configuration of the pores in the covers.[33] The material is very smooth, with a low coefficient of friction; in addition, it's impermeable to bacteria and easy to clean.[32]

In low-air-loss systems, the patient's skin is in contact with the cover. The local tissue environment is a function of the moisture-vapor permeability of the cover and cushion materials, the air flow

Alternating-pressure integrated cushions

The photo shows the characteristics of alternating-pressure integrated cushions.

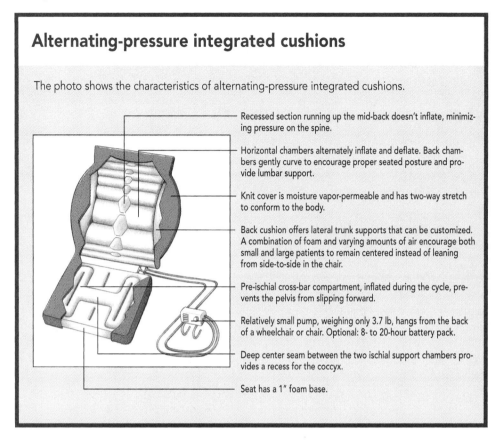

Recessed section running up the mid-back doesn't inflate, minimizing pressure on the spine.

Horizontal chambers alternately inflate and deflate. Back chambers gently curve to encourage proper seated posture and provide lumbar support.

Knit cover is moisture vapor-permeable and has two-way stretch to conform to the body.

Back cushion offers lateral trunk supports that can be customized. A combination of foam and varying amounts of air encourage both small and large patients to remain centered instead of leaning from side-to-side in the chair.

Pre-ischial cross-bar compartment, inflated during the cycle, prevents the pelvis from slipping forward.

Relatively small pump, weighing only 3.7 lb, hangs from the back of a wheelchair or chair. Optional: 8- to 20-hour battery pack.

Deep center seam between the two ischial support chambers provides a recess for the coccyx.

Seat has a 1" foam base.

and porosity of the cover and cushion materials, and the thermal insulation of the cover. The ideal combination of these factors would be a material with a high thermal insulation to prevent excessive loss of body heat, a high moisture vapor permeability to prevent accumulation of excess moisture on the skin, and a moderate airflow to keep the skin from overheating. Low-air-loss devices have been shown to prevent build-up of moisture and subsequent skin maceration.[32]

Alternating pressure

Alternating systems contain air-filled chambers or cylinders arranged lengthwise or in various other patterns. Air or fluid is pumped into the chambers at periodic intervals to inflate and deflate the chambers in opposite phases, thereby changing the pressure distribution. Pulsating pressure differs from alternating therapy in that the duration of peak inflation is shorter and the cycling time is more frequent. Pulsating pressure appears to have a dramatic effect on increasing lymphatic flow.[34]

Rather than increasing the surface area for distribution through immersion and envelopment, alternating pressure devices distribute the pressure by shifting the body weight to a different surface-contact area. This may increase the interface pressure of that area during the inflation phase.

Alternating pressure technology has the same potential as any other fluid-filled support surface to influence temperature at the interface, and care must be taken to maintain the correct levels of inflation. The skin moisture control and temperature control characteristics of alternating pressure surface will also depend on the characteristics of the cover and supporting material. (See *Alternating-pressure integrated cushions.*)

Matching support to patient needs

Although widely used, support surfaces have neither performance standards nor criteria for function that can be tested against clinical outcomes. Indeed, the basis for effective function isn't known, or is poorly understood, for such common products as wheelchair seat cushions and horizontal support surfaces intended for skin protection and healing of wounds. Despite this, clinicians must have some basis for decision-making regarding the selection of these products. The following key questions should be used to guide the decision-making process.

What are the patient's specific load management needs?

An adequate answer to this question must be gleaned from a variety of sources. Regardless of body position, the first step in determining an individualized protective intervention is to perform a general physical assessment and functional evaluation. Much of this information will then be used to assess risk for pressure ulcer development.

General physical examination and functional evaluation

Although patient evaluation is described elsewhere in this text, additional items important to the selection of a horizontal support surface might include assessing the capability of the patient regarding specific bed mobility (movement on the surface, ingress and egress, ability to place supportive devices), the number of available turning surfaces, the time spent in bed per day, and the number of devices or pillows needed for positioning.

For selection of wheelchair cushions, the evaluation is quite extensive because cushions are part of the total seating system that also includes the wheelchair. No cushion can perform effectively if the wheelchair isn't properly fitted. Therefore, it's recommended that the selection of a seat cushion be incorporated into the seating evaluation performed by a trained seating specialist. A longstanding body of knowledge illustrates the effectiveness of seating evaluations in the prevention of pressure ulcers.

The seating evaluation should include a mat exam to determine the functional postural limitations of the spine, pelvis, and extremities and determine appropriate measurements for wheelchair fitting. An extensive functional examination is also required to consider the seating and mobility needs of the individual in the immediate, intermediate, and community environments.[35-37]

Intervention strategies for maintenance of tissue integrity can be extremely complicated for spinal cord-injured, elderly people, and other populations with degenerative neuromuscular conditions or diseases. For example, a person's ability to sit unsupported by gravity can be characterized by the amount of external support needed to maintain a seated posture: hands-free, hands-dependent, or prop-sitting with external support only.[37] This capability has significant implications for compensatory functional postures, ability to reposition, and the method used for intermittent pressure relief.

Assessing risk

The most commonly used risk assessment scales for prediction of pressure ulcer incidence are the Braden, Norton, and Waterlow scales.[38-40] The sensitivity and specificity of these scales varies depending on the population setting and the position of the patient's body. For example, different Braden cut-off scores are associated with different settings (nursing home versus intensive care unit) and in a recent study of risk assessment scales for general inpatients versus wheelchair users, the Waterlow outperformed the Braden.[41,42] Risk assessment scales specifically designed for wheelchair users are currently being developed.

Bergstrom et al.[43] reported that mattress selection based on categorizing patients via a pressure ulcer risk assessment scale produced both efficacious and cost-effective results. Patients of a large tertiary care hospital scoring nine or less on the Braden pressure ulcer risk assessment scale were provided a group 2 support surface (low-air-loss mattress) as a preventative measure. Those scoring above nine were evaluated and provided the most appropriate surface according to patient needs. Results indicated that not only did pressure ulcer incidence and prevalence drop by more than 50%, but costs associated with overlays, replacement mattresses, and low-air-loss beds also decreased.

Similar results have been realized by studies that selected wheelchair cushions from a set of cushion alternatives based upon risk assessment. Krouskop and colleagues[44] described how a seating clinic assigned risk to their clients with spinal cord injury by using gender, interface pressure, lifestyle, and stability. In 80% to 90% of the clients, cushions were selected from three alternatives, with the remaining clients being provided other cushion types.

When assessing risk, remember that proper follow-up is necessary to prevent pressure ulcers regardless of the cushion prescribed, and that skin redness often occurs because of positioning and use and doesn't necessarily indicate that a poor surface choice was made.

Interface pressure-mapping

Pressure mapping — by comparing a patient's relative responses from one surface to another — can be an effective clinical tool to aid in the selection of a support surface for a specific patient. Pressure mapping may also be used to determine the relative effectiveness of modifications to the wheelchair and other positioning devices or to obtain information about pressure relief for patients with spinal cord injuries. For example, Henderson and colleagues used a pressure-mapping system to compare three methods of relieving pressure in seated individuals with spinal cord injuries.[45] The positions studied were tilted back 35 degrees, tilted back 65 degrees, and forward-leaning seated posture; the results indicated that the greatest pressure relief over the ischial tuberosities was seen in the forward-leaning position, followed by the 65-degree backward-tilt position. Observing the change in the pressure distribution on the mapping display allows patients without sensation to observe the effects of various weight-shifting methods and learn to consciously integrate them into their seated behavior.

Using clinical practice guidelines

Clinical practice guidelines offer recommendations, based on scientific evidence and the professional judgment of expert panels, about how health care professionals can provide quality care. The two most commonly referenced clinical practice guidelines in regard to support surface selection are:
- AHCPR Clinical Practice Guideline Number 15, "Treatment of Pressure Ulcers"[46]
- Consortium for Spinal Cord Medicine Clinical Practice Guideline, "Pressure Ulcer Prevention and Treatment Following Spinal Cord Injury."[47]

How does the product function and how well does it perform?

Answers to what the product does and how it performs should be sought from a variety of sources. Sources of information for support surfaces include marketing materials, controlled clinical trials, and objective indirect data from laboratory testing or clinical studies (interface pressure and other physiological responses).

Laboratory testing

What a support surface does has been largely determined by studies using laboratory methods to measure variables believed to be clinically relevant in pressure ulcer formation. For example, Krouskop's[48] study of foam mattress overlays provided the following recommended specifications for selection based on the results of independent laboratory testing:
- a thickness of 3″ to 4″ (7.5 to 10 cm)
- a density of 1.3 to 1.6 lb per cubic foot as an indicator of the amount of foam in the product
- a 25% indentation load deflection (ILD) equal to about 30 lb (the amount of force required to compress the foam to 75% of its thickness as an indicator of the foams compressibility and conformability)
- a modulus of 2.5 or greater (the ratio of 60% ILD to 25% ILD).

Support-surface standards

Few, if any, standards currently exist for support surfaces. Publishing national or international standards for support surfaces requires that uniform test methods be developed to quantify clinically relevant characteristics. Simply stated, to make valid comparisons among products, characteristics and properties need to be measured using the same test and under the same conditions. Testing conditions should model clinically relevant parameters as closely as possible. Standards for terms and definitions, performance parameters, and life expectancy are needed. Seat cushion and support surface standard tests should produce results that can be used to help select and purchase the correct support surfaces.

The results of standard tests often don't include pass-fail criteria. Just as there are valid reasons to purchase an automobile with a big engine that only gets 15 mpg over another with a little engine that gets 25 mpg, so are there reasons to purchase support surfaces with, for example, a low pressure distribution characteristic but high moisture dissipation ability over a product with a high pressure distribution characteristic but low moisture dissipation ability. The primary objectives of the standard tests are to enable the reliable classification of products based on their different functional properties and to permit comparisons of performance among products with similar functions.

Standards for seat cushions are being developed under the auspices of the Rehabilitation Engineering and Assistive Technology Society of North America (RESNA) as an American National Standards Institute accredited standards organization. In June 1998, the RESNA Technical Standards Board authorized the formation of the Standards Subcommittee on Wheelchair and Related Seating to begin work on voluntary wheelchair seating standards. One of the four interrelated working groups focuses on tissue integrity management and is developing test methods from which standards for seat cushions will emerge. The development of standards for seat cushions has been in progress for several years and the tests related to tissue integrity that have been developed include interface pressure measurement, load-deflection and hysteresis, frictional properties, horizontal stiffness, sliding resistance, impact damping, recovery, load contour depth and bottoming, stability of properties with use, determination of heat and water vapor transfer properties, water spillage, biocompatibility, and test report.[49] Related tests for postural support devices include test methods for static strength of postural support devices, test methods for impact strength, and test methods for repetitive loading.[49] In January 2001, the National Pressure Ulcer Advisory Panel formally initiated a similar process to develop standards for horizontal support surfaces.[50]

Patients, clinicians, vendors, manufactures, third-party payers, and researchers all benefit from standard terminology, definitions, and test methods. The range of products on the market places a heavy burden on clinicians to keep abreast of new technology. Clinicians benefit from a mechanism to objectively match a seat cushion or support surface's characteristics to the needs of their patient. Vendors benefit by being able to clearly describe products across manufacturers in a manner understood by clinicians and patients. Testing standards aid manufacturers by guiding new product development and assisting in the redesign of existing products. Standards provide a means of product comparison, thereby targeting gaps in market needs. In addition, standards promote quality assurance within manufacturing processes. The final potential beneficiaries of standards are third-party payers because the seat cushion and support surface market is a payer's market; that is, payer reimbursement drives the market. A validated system to test and objectively characterize support surfaces will give funding agencies an objective means for funding decisions.

Product performance

The effectiveness of a product support service product is measured by two methods: its efficacy in use by patients and in comparison to similar products. Several articles provide an overview of support surface research.[51-54] Rather than basing comparisons on functional classification, most studies compared classes of products based on the product's ability to reduce or relieve pressure.

Considering the limitations ascribed to IP measurement, it may be more useful to categorize devices according to their ability to remove localized pressure (pressure relief) or to redistribute it evenly over the contact surface area (pressure reduction).[55] However, the most common comparison has been the use of IP to compare a product against a "standard" hospital bed or mattress. When reviewing this literature, remember that the "standard" support surface probably varies from study to study. Most studies also vary in the patient population (for example, orthopedic or neurological) and setting studied (for example, acute care, intensive care, long-term care, and home care). All three independent variables (products compared, subject population, setting) affect both outcomes and the interpretation of results. Finally, when comparing performance studies, remember that treatment studies, in which subjects already have ulcers, are fundamentally different from prevention studies.

Prevention effectiveness

Generally, studies have shown that non-powered, constant low-pressure supports (foam, air, gel, and combinations of these materials) are more effective in preventing pressure ulcers than a "standard" hospital mattress. Generalization of the results of studies comparing different pressure redistribution products is difficult. Most comparative studies of various constant low-force products demonstrated no differences in the prevention of pressure ulcers.[56,57]

Conclusions from research investigating the more complex technology, including low-air-loss and alternating-pressure products are similar. Evidence suggests that both low-air-loss and alternating-pressure surfaces are more effective than "standard" mattresses, but comparative studies of the performance of low-air-loss and alternating-pressure are inconsistent regarding the clinical superiority of one over the other. Moreover, comparisons of alternating-pressure to constant low-pressure products haven't produced definitive differences.

Because the evidence isn't definitive, clinicians must carefully read the original study to generalize the results to a specific clinical situation. The characteristics of the population, setting, and products must closely match one's clinical situation and the limitations of the study must be known when considering it's clinical applicability. For example, consider the design of alternating pressure products where variables such as cell height or bladder thickness and cycle timing and frequency can significantly affect product performance. One can't necessarily generalize the performance of one alternating pressure product to another. Similarly, the results of a support surface study within acute care might not produce similar results within home care using the same support surfaces.

Research into the effectiveness of wheelchair cushions is much more limited than research into horizontal support surfaces. Evidence about specific cushions and their respective effectiveness is insufficient. Contradictions exist in the literature regarding the clinical benefits of cushions designed to reduce the risk of sitting-acquired pressure ulcers. Most research has used indirect outcomes such as interface pressure or blood flow. Relatively few studies have measured direct outcomes related to specific types of cushions[21,58-60] but these haven't resulted in definitive findings of efficacy of one product over another. One facility performed two studies targeting elderly wheelchair users. The first study found no difference in the incidence of pressure ulcers in users of flat foam compared to custom contoured foam cushions and a subsequent study found more users of flat foam (41%) developed ulcers compared to users of a contoured foam-viscous fluid cushion (25%), but this difference didn't reach statistical significance. In a study tracking interface pressure and wheelchair cushions in elderly users, Brienza and colleagues[60] found interface pressures were higher for subjects who developed sitting-acquired pressure ulcers compared to those who didn't develop ulcers. No definitive relationship was found between interface pressures and cushion type across these subjects. In fact, the truism for seat cushion research appears to be, no one cushion is best for all people.

Treatment effectiveness

Widely varying subject populations and care settings have complicated the ability to compare results across studies investigating the effectiveness of support surfaces in the treatment for pressure ulcers. Furthermore, a number of treatment outcome measures have been used to judge effectiveness, such as the relative or actual reduction in ulcer size (area or volume), the percentage of ulcers healed within a specified time period, and the time until wound closure. Different operational definitions have also been used for wound status, such as "healed" and "closure." Therefore, generalization of results and comparison across studies are complicated at best.

Generally, studies targeting support surfaces for ulcer treatment have produced results similar to those targeting prevention. Low-air-loss and air-fluidized surfaces have been shown to improve treatment outcomes compared to "conventional" treatment[61,62] and nonpowered foam alternatives.[52,53] Results of alternating pressure surfaces are inconsistent with some studies showing a treatment effect and others showing none. No clinically significant treatment differences have been shown among similar products.

What other patient needs must be met?

To answer this question in regard to managing tissue loads, one must again turn to the available evidence or clinical practice guidelines.

Turning and repositioning schedules

To provide effective pressure relief, both pressure and time must be considered. The frequency of repositioning required to prevent ischemia is variable and unknown, yet regular repositioning is believed to help deter the deleterious effects of pressure by decreasing the duration of exposure. Through the process of repositioning, the body's weight is redistributed and new pressure areas are introduced. In 1961, Kosiak[63] recommended that repositioning be done in intervals of 1 to 2 hours based on the interface readings from healthy subjects. This view has also been endorsed by the Agency for Health Care Research and Quality (AHRQ) in its clinical practice guideline.[4]

Turning schedules have been studied empirically and experimentally. Bliss[64] studied turning schedules in a spinal injury ward and found that 2 hours was adequate for some, whereas others required more frequent and some, less frequent, turning. An important aspect of these findings is that some patients exhibited redness after 2 hours, and that many patients disliked frequent turning. In an experimental study by Knox and colleagues,[65] variables such as temperature, pressure, and redness were monitored while people rested on a mattress for 60, 90, and 120 minutes. Some subjects exhibited redness after each of the intervals, leading the researchers to conclude that a 2-hour turning schedule might not be sufficient.

We have strong theoretical evidence that reducing the duration of loading helps maintain tissue integrity. But we have very limited evidence as to how this theory can drive clinical practice and no real evidence that 2 hours is optimal. Finally, we have no knowledge of how turning schedules should be affected by support surfaces. The best approach is one that's repeated many times in various contexts: each person must be evaluated and reevaluated to best determine an appropriate turning schedule.

Positioning

In addition to the AHRQ guidelines for repositioning and turning, a number of recommendations exist in regard to positioning for management of tissue loads that will be briefly discussed here, including protection of the heels. (See *AHRQ positioning guidelines.*)

The following eight positions are commonly used to reposition patients on horizontal surfaces:
• a prone position with rotation of 30 degrees to the right or left
• a supine position with 30 degrees of rotation to the right or left
• a supine position with slight right or left sacral relief[66]
• a supine position with the head of the bed elevated 30 degrees or less and the feet blocked
• a supine position with the head of the bed elevated 30 degrees or less and the knees flexed with the bed. (See *Horizontal positioning*, page 208.)

The feet are blocked and knees flexed to prevent shear forces created when the patient slides down in bed. In all of these positions, heels must be elevated with pillows or other devices. Note the use of pillows and towels to separate and protect bony prominences.

What's available in this setting?

The question of what's available pertains to the patient's specific health care plan and the availability or access to products in the general marketplace. Availability is linked to broader health policies governing payment for products and services (third-party reimbursement). Reimbursement policies are tied to evidence of clinical effectiveness and cost-effectiveness.

As the need for durable medical equipment increases with the growing population of elderly and disabled individuals, the need for information regarding the effectiveness of support surfaces has become more important. The research needed requires the effective cooperation of multiple disciplines generally found only in academic settings. In general, the public is unaware of the enormous amount of money spent by the government and other third-party payers on products for which there are no standards of performance and, largely, no proof of efficiency. Currently, both useful and worthless products may be reimbursed equally in the absence of useful objective data.

The importance of the role of standards can't be overstated in providing the foundation from which valid and reliable studies of support surfaces may be conducted. The impact from standards development is evident in the new coding policy for wheelchair seat cushions being developed by the Durable Medical Equipment Regional Carriers with assistance from the Statistical Analysis Durable Medical Equipment Regional Carrier. The new policy incorporates a mandate for labeling seat cushions. The

AHRQ positioning guidelines

The Agency for Health Care Research and Quality (AHRQ) 1992 guidelines for positioning include the following:
- Keep the patient's heels protected and elevated off the surface of the bed.
- Maintain the elevation of the head of the bed at 30 degrees or less if medical status permits.
- Turn or reposition the patient's body at least every 2 hours.
- Note that the use of pressure reducing surfaces doesn't replace turning schedules.
- Limit the patient's lateral rotation to 30 degrees from the supine or prone position to avoid direct loading of the greater trochanter.
- Position the patient's body to avoid loading over an existing ulcer or wound.
- Eliminate the use of "donut" type devices.
- Use pillows or wedges to separate bony prominences.

labeling must document the results of performance testing on key indicators. The required testing includes some of the test methods developed and included in the standards for wheelchair seat cushions previously discussed. Thus, all wheelchair users in the United States (1.7 million noninstitutionalized and another 600,000 in nursing homes) will be affected by this policy. As better research becomes available, third-party payers will have an objective means upon which to base reimbursement decisions and wheelchair users will have greater access

Horizontal positioning

The following illustrations show how to position patients properly on horizontal surfaces.

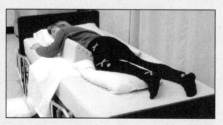 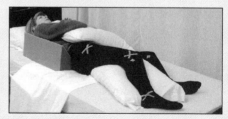

30-degree rotation from prone and supine positions, respectively

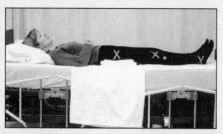 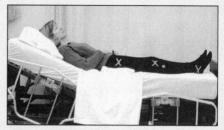

Head of the bed elevated 30 degrees or less with unilateral sacral relief and feet blocked, respectively

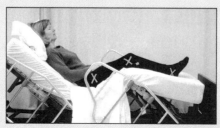

Head of the bed elevated 30 degrees with knees flexed to prevent shearing at the sacrum

to appropriate, safe, and comfortable cushions with proven effectiveness.

How much does it cost?

Technology has produced some treatment products, but costs are high for patients, insurance companies, and hospitals. Prevention is more cost-effective than any other treatment and the technology available today may provide solutions when used correctly. One recent study demonstrated that educated staff can reduce the number of pressure ulcers better than noneducated staff. The same study indicated that the cost of care is significantly less under the supervision of educated staff.[67] The support surface technology currently available is capable of providing higher quality of care and allocation can only be managed effectively if the staff is properly educated in its use. The use of risk-directed strategies to control costs and improve effectiveness has been previously discussed.

The cost of support surfaces varies. Third-party reimbursement, rental versus purchase, and cost-benefit issues need to be carefully evaluated. Some devices are only available on a rental basis. Consideration should be given to the projected number of days that a support surface will be in use. Medicare may provide coverage. More patients are being placed on advanced technology surfaces for considerably longer periods of time. Cost-effectiveness may be measured by relating the cost of the product to its efficacy.

What's practical?

The issue of practicality relates to the overall care plan, the goals of load management (prevention versus treatment), how complicated the product is to use, and whether it will be operated by a health care professional, family member, or the patient. Many hospitals, long-term care facilities, and home care agencies have developed product selection guidelines that are usually presented as an algorithm[4] or graph. These guidelines are typically based on the availability of equipment from previous purchases in accordance with other published guidelines. In addition to guidelines, another common method used in selection and purchasing decisions is the subjective assessment of equipment based on a trial of use in the clinical area. This gives the staff a chance to trial the equipment in a variety of situations and judge its performance.

How easy is the product to use?

Ease of use has been associated with the successful compliance with equipment use. Awkward design or difficult assembly may cause the patient and his family to abandon use of the equipment or increase the likelihood of misuse. Directions must be clear and obvious. For example, if the product is powered, it should have a battery back-up to facilitate transferring patients to other locations as needed.

What are the operational costs of the equipment?

Although reimbursement is an issue in any setting, operational costs are of particular importance if the product is used in the home care setting where costs will be absorbed by the patient.

What service and maintenance is available?

A 24-hour call service with on-site repair or replacement is essential.

What type of alarm system does the product have?

Visual alarms are rarely sufficient, especially if the alarm is obscured under the bed. In the home-care setting, visible alarms are of little value unless there is constant attendance.

Is the equipment easily maintained?

If the equipment must be deflated for storage, reinflation time may be critical as well as the ability to deflate the equipment in the event of a cardiac arrest. If the product isn't a personal use item, one must consider how long it takes to clean and ready the item for subsequent use.

What operating mechanism and space requirements does the product have?

If the product has some form of movement, is cessation possible to facilitate procedures such as bedpan usage and hygiene care? Is the product the correct size for the home or setting where it will be used? Is the floor structure sound and capable of holding the weight of the bed?

PRACTICE POINT

Practical points to consider before purchasing support surfaces include:

- ease of use
- operational costs of the equipment
- service contracts and back-up service
- alarm systems
- daily maintenance
- operating mechanisms and space requirements.

When managing the allocation of specialty mattress and bed systems, a continuous process of evaluation and reevaluation should be employed to assure that patient's needs are reassessed on a regular basis.

Managing tissue loads at the heel

Of all pressure ulcer sites reported in the literature, heel ulcers are especially painful and are among the most difficult to heal.[68] Heel pressure ulcers can have devastating sequelae including infection and, in extreme cases, amputation of the foot. The costs associated with heel pressure ulcers increase proportionally with morbidity and length of hospital stay, adding to the importance of prevention.

The heel presents unique challenges for pressure-reducing interventions. Heel ulcers occur in bedridden individuals as a consequence of pressure applied to a bony prominence over a prolonged period.[7] The heel has a small radius of curvature and only a thin layer of subcutaneous tissue lies between the skin and calcaneal structures.[69] Abu-Own[69] calculated an average interface area 28 mm in diameter in a study of 30 heels at a corresponding interface pressure of 40 mm Hg. Petrie and Hummel[70] found

heel pressures on specialty mattresses ranged from 44.7 to 103.2 mm Hg. This small contact area coupled with a lack of subcutaneous tissue affords minimal protection from the pressure exerted by the weight of the foot and, frequently, a portion of the lower limb. The lower limb is approximately one-sixth of the total body weight, so even if a small proportion of this rests on the heel, high interface pressure may be encountered, even on air support systems.

The Agency for Health Care Policy and Research guideline[4] recommends using pressure-relieving devices on immobile patients' heels. The guideline recommends the use of pillows; however, patients' movements may disrupt proper heel suspension. Diligent nursing care is required to maintain proper positioning and, until recently, few heel pressure-reducing products were available that met the following clinical requirements:

- reducing pressure, friction, and shear
- separating and protecting the ankles
- maintaining heel suspension
- permitting repositioning without increasing pressure in other areas
- preventing footdrop
- enhancing patient comfort
- increasing nursing time-efficiency.

Currently a variety of heel protective devices are commercially available, but, as with support surfaces in general, choosing from the many alternatives is complicated by the lack of information about their performance characteristics and the inconsistent manner in which this information is reported. A lack of uniform terminology, test methods, and reporting requirements limits the internal and external validity of existing studies and makes objective evaluation and matching of a device to the patient's needs difficult.

Evidence for managing heel pressure

Relatively few studies of heel protection devices have been completed in the past decade. The majority of existing studies have examined the pressure distribution capabilities of heel wraps, heel dressings, pillows, water-filled gloves, and various specialty heel products using interface pressure or pressure ulcer incidence as the primary outcomes.

As with other support surfaces, most products consist of a combination of materials and incorporate multiple strategies to optimize their therapeutic function. The distribution of pressure on a heel support surface depends on the relative fit between the heel and the surface, the mechanical properties of the heel tissue and the device, and the distribution of weight in the body part (heel). An ideal pressure distribution is one in which soft tissue shape isn't altered relative to its unloaded condition.

In a study designed to investigate the efficacy of clinically "familiar" heel devices, the preventative use of routine nursing care, hydrocolloid dressings, egg-crate foam, polyester-filled heel boots, and foam footdrop splints were compared in geriatric, orthopedic patients at-risk for pressure ulcers.[71,72] In a similar study, 4″ × 4″ gauze pads in combination with an absorbent pad and gauze roll and a laminated foam boot (Lunax Boot by Bio-Sonics) were compared in at-risk intensive care patients with heel redness.[73] While both studies lacked various aspects of statistical analyses limiting their interpretation, the egg-crate boot and laminated foam boot were more effective in preventing pressure ulcers while other methods either increased incidence or, as in the case of the footdrop splints, were uncomfortable despite their ability to effectively suspend the heel. It's notable that in this study, routine nursing care consisting of heel observation every 2 to 3 hours with subsequent pressure ulcer care as needed (direct pressure relief and repositioning of patients heels) was ineffective in preventing deterioration of the heel tissue. However, a similar study's simultaneous use of heel elevation with a pillow or bath blanket under the calf, the Spenco Silicore quilted heel protector, and prompt reporting of heel discomfort by patients to the nursing staff resulted in zero incidence of pressure ulcers in 30 hip replacement patients.[74]

Using water-filled examination gloves has been suggested as an inexpensive method of decreasing heel pressure (variation in mechanical properties of the device). Measures of mean interface pressure with the heel resting directly on a conventional mattress (126.5 mm Hg) and on a latex glove filled with 260 ml of water (144.6 mm Hg) were compared in a convenience sample of 40 adults.[75] A survey of nurses in this study revealed that 79.4% routinely used water-filled gloves for heel protection. This study emphasizes the need for nursing staff to reevaluate the efficacy of their heel protection interventions. Flemister[76] also examined heel interface pressures with use of both a foam and polyester heel protector (variation in device mechanical properties) in seven patients assessed at moderate to high risk for pressure ulcer development. The foam heel protector marginally reduced heel interface pressures by 1.3 mm Hg and the polyester protector significantly increased the interface pressure.

The pressure distributing ability of six commonly used heel pressure-reducing devices was evaluated by measuring interface pressure at the heel with the subjects in supine and a 30-degree semi-Fowler's position (variation in weight distribution of the body part and mechanical properties of the device).[77] A significant interaction was found between the device and position. For patients in the semi-Fowler's position, the L'Nard Multi-Podus splint yielded 22.9 mm Hg; for patients placed in a supine position, the Lunax laminated foam boot yielded 24.6 mm Hg, the lowest pressures for each position respectively. Pinzur and colleagues[78] compared the effects of five heel protection products on the relative interface pressures of five men with paraplegia and five healthy men (variation in mechanical properties of the heel tissue and the device). Pressure distribution was determined by the ratio between pressure recorded for each device tested and the baseline pressure recorded with the heel in contact with a wooden board. The polyester rug and heel protector were less effective than the foam heel protector and space boot. Not surprisingly, the foam Footdrop Stop was the most effective because it completely suspends the heel. No significant differences in interface pressures were observed between the two groups for any device.

Summary

Understanding the nature of pressure ulcer etiology, the factors affecting pressure redistribution, and other physical factors associated with the use of specific support surface products and heel protection products, and the proper use of such products, is a necessity for nursing and other health care personnel involved with tissue integrity management. As standardized test methods are developed for support surface products, the clinical validation of specialized protective devices and the development of clinical practice guidelines will be possible. Until then, matching products to patient needs is a challenging process and must be based on the available evidence regarding the performance characteristics of existing support surfaces. Continued research in heel protection is needed.

Heels in patients at risk for pressure ulcers require additional protection beyond the use of specialty beds and mattress overlays. Although existing clinical practice guidelines recommend the use of pillows to suspend the heels, pillows don't protect against footdrop, require time and attention to positioning details, and can't protect the heels continuously due to patient movement. To provide continuous heel suspension via heel protective devices, clinicians must consider proper fit, turning schedules and number of turning surfaces, patient position, the presence of additional equipment, and the performance characteristics of the product when selecting heel protection devices.

Show what you know

1. Which one of the following support surfaces isn't classified as fluid-filled?

  A. Air
  B. Water
  C. Viscous fluid
  D. Foam

Answer: D. Air, water, and viscous fluid cushions are filled with substances whose molecules flow freely and have no fixed shape and therefore little resistance to outside stress.

2. Suppose you performed a full-body pressure mapping of a patient to select an appropriate pressure-reducing mattress. Despite a peak pressure reading of 32 mm Hg at the sacrum, the patient developed a pressure ulcer because their capillary closing pressure was less than 32 mm Hg. Which of the following doesn't explain the lack of the support surface's clinical efficacy?

  A. Advanced age
  B. Depression
  C. Low blood pressure
  D. Malnutrition

ANSWER: B. Tissue mechanical properties are affected by advanced age, low blood pressure, and malnutrition, but not depression.

3. Which of the following risk factors for pressure ulcers aren't addressed by support surfaces?

A. Shear and friction
B. Pressure
C. Moisture
D. Immobility

ANSWER: D. Immobility is an intrinsic factor not significantly affected by the support surface characteristics.

References

1. Krouskop, T., and van Rijwijk, L. "Standardizing Performance-Based Criteria for Support Surfaces," *Ostomy/Wound Management* 41(1):34-44, January-February 1995.
2. Cochran, G. *Identification and Control of Biophysical Factors Responsible for Soft Tissue Breakdown.* RSA Progress Report, 1979.
3. Silver-Thorn, M. "In Vivo Indentation of Lower Extremity Limb Soft Tissues," *IEEE Transactions on Rehabilitation Engineering* 7(3):268-77, September 1999.
4. AHCPR. *Pressure Ulcers in Adults: Prediction and Prevention.* AHCPR Clinical Practice Guideline No. 3. Rockville, Md.: Agency for Health Care Policy and Research, Public Health Service, US Department of Health and Human Services. Publication No. 92-0047, 1992.
5. Krouskop, T.A. "A Synthesis of the Factors that Contribute to Pressure Sore Formation," *Medical Hypotheses* 11(2):255-67, June 1983.
6. Reddy, N.G., et al. "Interstitial Fluid Flow as a Factor in Decubitus Ulcer Formation," *Journal of Biomechanics* 14(12):879-81, December 1981.
7. Daniel, R.D., et al. "Etiologic Factors in Pressure Sores: An Experimental Model," *Archives of Physical Medicine and Rehabilitation* 62(10):492-98, October 1981.
8. Reswick, J., and Rogers, J. *Experiences at Rancho Los Amigos Hospital with Devices and Techniques to Prevent Pressure Sores. Bedsore Biomechanics.* London: University Park Press, 1976.
9. Vistnes, L. "Pressure Sores: Etiology and Prevention," *Bulletin of Prosthetic Research* 17:123-25, 1980.
10. Verhonick, P.D., et al. "Thermography in the Study of Decubitus Ulcers," *Nursing Research* 21:233-37, May-June 1972.
11. Patel, S.C., et al. "Temperature Effects on Surface Pressure-Induced Changes in Rat Skin Perfusion: Implications in Pressure Ulcer Development," *Journal of Rehabilitation Research and Development* 36(3):189-201, May-June 1999.
12. Kokate, J.K., et al. "Temperature-Modulated Pressure Ulcers: A Porcine Model," *Archives of Physical Medicine and Rehabilitation* 76(7):666-73, July 1995.
13. Brown, A., and Brengelmann, G. *Energy Metabolism. Physiology and Biophysics.* Philadelphia: W.B. Saunders Co., 1965.
14. Fisher, S.T., et al. "Wheelchair Cushion Effect on Skin Temperature," *Archives of Physical Medicine and Rehabilitation* 59(2):68-72, February 1978.
15. Johnson, J.M., and Park, M. "Reflex Control of Skin Blood Flow by Skin Temperature: Role of Core Temperature," *Journal of Applied Physiology* 47(6):1188-93, December 1979.
16. Johnson, J.M., et al. "Reflex Regulation of Sweat Rate by Skin Temperature in Exercising Humans," *Journal of Applied Physiology* 56(5):1283-88, May 1984.
17. Aronovitch, S. "A Comparative Study of an Alternating Air Mattress for the Prevention of Pressure Ulcers in Surgical Patients," *Ostomy/Wound Management* 45(3):34-44, March 1999.
18. Yarkony, G. "Pressure Ulcers: A Review," *Archives of Physical Medicine and Rehabilitation* 75(8):908-17, August 1994.
19. Sulzberger, M., et al. "Studies on Blisters Produced by Friction: Results of Linear Rubbing and Twisting Techniques," *Journal of Investigational Dermatology* 47(5):456-65, November 1966.
20. Wildnauer, R.H., et al. "Stratum Corneum Biomechanical Properties: Influence of Relative Humidity on Normal and Extracted Human Stratum Corneum," *Journal of Investigational Dermatology* 56(1):72-78, January 1971.

21. Geyer, M.J., et al. "A Randomized Control Trial to Evaluate Pressure-Reducing Seat Cushion for Elderly Wheelchair Users," *Advances in Skin & Wound Care* 14(3): 120-29, May-June 2001.

22. Cochran, G.V., and Palmieri, V. "Development of Test Methods for Evaluation of Wheelchair Cushions," *Bulletin of Prosthetics Research* 33:9-30, Spring 1980.

23. Sprigle, S.L., et al. "Development of Uniform Terminology and Procedures to Describe Wheelchair Cushion Characteristics," *Journal of Rehabilitation Research and Development* 38(4):449-61, July-August 2001.

24. Noble, P.C., et al. "The Influence of Environmental Aging Upon the Load-bearing Properties of Polyurethane Foams," *Journal of Rehabilitation Research and Development* 21(2):31-38, July 1984.

25. Krouskop, T., et al. "Evaluating the Long-term Performance of a Foam-Core Hospital Replacement Mattress," *Journal of Wound, Ostomy, and Continence Nursing* 21(6):241-46, November 1994.

26. Sprigle, S., et al. "Reduction of sitting pressures with custom contoured cushions," *Journal of Rehabilitation Research and Development* 27(2):135-40, Spring 1990.

27. Brienza, D.M., et al. "A System for the Analysis of Seat Support Surfaces Using Surface Shape Control and Simultaneous Measurement of Applied Pressures," *IEEE Transactions on Rehabilitation Engineering* 4(2):103-13, June 1996.

28. Brienza, D.M., and Karg, P.E. "Seat Cushion Optimization: A Comparison of Interface Pressure and Tissue Stiffness Characteristics for Spinal Cord Injured and Elderly Patients," *Archives of Physical Medicine and Rehabilitation* 79(4):388-94, April 1998.

29. Stewart, S., et al. "Wheelchair Cushion Effect on Skin Temperature, Heat Flux and Relative Humidity," *Archives of Physical Medicine and Rehabilitation* 61(5):229-33, May 1980.

30. Wells, J., and Karr, D. "Interface Pressure, Wound Healing and Satisfaction in the Evaluation of a Non-Powered Fluid Mattress," *Ostomy/Wound Management* 44(2):38-54, February 1998.

31. Peltier, G., et al. "Controlled Air Suspension: An Advantage in Burn Care," *Journal of Burn Care Research* 8(6):558-60, November-December 1987.

32. Holzapfel, S. "Support Surfaces and their Use in the Prevention and Treatment of Pressure Ulcers," *Journal of Enterostomal Nursing* 20(6):251-60, November-December 1993.

33. Weaver, V., and Jester, J. "A Clinical Tool: Updated Readings on Tissue Interface Pressure," *Ostomy/Wound Management* 40(5):34-43, June 1994.

34. Gunther, R., and Brofeldt, B. "Increased Lymphatic Flow: Effect of a Pulsating Air Suspension Bed System," *Wounds: A Compendium of Clinical Research and Practice* 8(4):134-40, 1996.

35. Engstrom, B. Seating for Independence. *Ergonomic Seating and Propulsion Improves Performance.* Presentation, Pittsburgh, Pa., August 1997.

36. Waugh, K. *Therapeutic Seating I: Principles and Assessment.* Pittsburgh, PA: RESNA, 1997.

37. Minkel, J. "Seating and Mobility Considerations for People with Spinal Cord Injuries," *Physical Therapy* 80(7):701-09, July 2000.

38. Braden, B.J. and Bergstrom, N. "Clinical Utility of the Braden Scale for Predicting Pressure Sore Risk," *Decubitus* 2(3):44-6,50-1, August 1989.

39. Norton, D. "Norton Scale for Decubitus Prevention," [German] *Krankenpflege* 34(1):16, 1980.

40. Waterlow, J. "Pressure Sores: A Risk Assessment Card," *Nursing Times* 81(48):49-55, November 27-December 3, 1985.

41. Braden, B., and Bergstrom, N. "Predictive Validity of the Braden Scale for Pressure Sore Risk in a Nursing Home Population," *Research in Nursing and Health* 17(6):459-70, December 1994.

42. Anthony, D., et al. "An Evaluation of Current Risk Assessment Scales for Decubitus Ulcer in General Inpatients and Wheelchair Users," *Clinical Rehabilitation* 12(2):136-42, April 1998.

43. Bergstrom, N., et al. "Using a Research-based Assessment Scale in Clinical Practice," *Nursing Clinics of North America* 30(3):539-50, September 1995.

44. Krouskop, T.A., et al. "Custom Selection of Support Surfaces for Wheelchairs and Beds: One Size Doesn't Fit All," *Dermatology Nursing* 4(3):191-94,204, June 1992.

45. Henderson, J.L., et al. "Efficacy of Three Measures to Relieve Pressure in Seated Persons with Spinal Cord Injury,"

Archives of Physical Medicine and Rehabilitation 75(5):535-39, May 1994.

46. AHCPR. "Treatment of Pressure Ulcers," Publication No. 95-0652, 1994.

47. Consortium for Spinal Cord Medicine. *Pressure Ulcer Prevention and Treatment Following Spinal Cord Injury: A Clinical Practice Guideline for Health-Care Professionals.* Washington, D.C.: Paralyzed Veterans of America, 2000.

48. Krouskop, T. "Scientific Aspects of Pressure Relief." IAET Annual Conference, Washington, D.C., 1989.

49. ISO/CD 16840-3: *Wheelchair Seating-Part 3: Postural Support Devices.* Committee draft, International Organization for Standardization, June 2002.

50. National Pressure Ulcer Advisory Panel (NPUAP). NPUAP's Support Surface Standards Initiative (S31), April 2003. *www.npuap.org*

51. Whittemore, R. "Pressure-reduction Support Surfaces: A Review of the Literature," *Journal of Wound, Ostomy, and Continence Nursing* 25(1):6-25, January 1998.

52. Cullum, N. "Evaluation of Studies of Treatment or Prevention Interventions. Part 2: Applying the Results of Studies to Your Patients," *Evidence Based Nursing* 4(1):7-8, January 2001.

53. Cullum, N., et al. "Beds, Mattresses, and Cushions for Pressure Sore Prevention and Treatment," *Nursing Times* 97(19):41, May 10-16, 2001.

54. Thomas, D.R. "Issues and Dilemmas in the Prevention and Treatment of Pressure Ulcers: A Review," *Journals of Gerontology, Series A, Biological Sciences and Medical Sciences* 56(6):328-40, 2001.

55. Rithalia, S.V., and Kenney, L. "Mattresses and Beds: Reducing and Relieving Pressure," *Nursing Times* 96(36 Suppl):9-10, September 7, 2000.

56. Cullum, N., et al. "Preventing and Treating Pressure Sores," *Quality in Health Care* 4(4):289-97, December 1995.

57. Lazzara, D.J., and Buschmann, M.T. "Prevention of Pressure Ulcers in Elderly Nursing Home Residents: Are Special Support Surfaces the Answer?" *Decubitus* 4(4):42-48, November 1991.

58. Lim, R., et al. "Clinical Trial of Foam Cushions in the Prevention of Decubitus Ulcers in Elderly Patients," *Journal of Rehabilitation Research and Development* 25(2):19-26, Spring 1988.

59. Conine, T., et al. "Pressure Ulcer Prophylaxis in Elderly Patients Using Polyurethane Foam or Jay Wheelchair Cushions," *International Journal of Rehabilitation Research* 17(2):123-37, June 1994.

60. Brienza, D.M., et al. "The Relationship Between Pressure Ulcer Incidence and Buttock-seat Cushion Interface Pressure in At-risk Elderly Wheelchair Users," *Archives of Physical Medicine and Rehabilitation* 82(4):529-33, April 2001.

61. Allen, V. et al. "Air-fluidized Beds and Their Ability to Distribute Interface Pressures Generated Between the Subject and the Bed Surface," *Physiological Measurement* 14(3):359-64, August 1993.

62. Munro, B.H., et al. "Pressure Ulcers: One Bed or Another?" *Geriatric Nursing* 10(4):190-92, July-August 1989.

63. Kosiak, M. "Etiology of Decubitus Ulcers," *Archives of Physical Medicine and Rehabilitation* 42(1):19-28, January 1961.

64. Bliss, M.R. "Pressure Sore Management and Prevention," in Brocklehurst, J.C., et al., eds. *Textbook of Geriatric Medicine and Gerontology,* 4th ed. London: Churchill Livingstone, 1992.

65. Knox, D.M., et al. "Effects of Different Turn Intervals on Skin of Healthy Older Adults," *Advances in Wound Care* 7(1):48-56, January 1994.

66. Rappl, L., and Sears, M. "Choosing and Using Seat Support Surfaces for Skin and Wound Management," Symposium on Advanced Wound Care, New Orleans, La., 1997.

67. Moody, B., et al. "Impact of Staff Education on Pressure Sore Development in Elderly Hospitalized Patients," *Archives of Internal Medicine* 148(10):2241-43, October 1988.

68. Versluyen, M. "Pressure Sores: Causes and Prevention," *Nursing* 33(6):216-18, June 1986.

69. Abu-Own, A., et al. "Effects of Compression and Type of Bed Surface on the Microcirculation of the Heel," *European Journal of Vascular and Endovascular Surgery* 9(3):327-34, April 1995.

70. Petrie, L.A., and Hummel, R.S. III. "A Study of Interface Pressure for Pressure Reduction and Relief Mattresses," *Journal of Enterostomal Therapy* 17(5):212-6, September-October 1990.

71. Zernike, W. "Preventing Heel Pressure Sores: A Comparison of Heel Pressure

Relieving Devices," *Journal of Clinical Nursing* 3(6):375-80, November 1994.

72. Zernike, W. "Heel Pressure Relieving Devices: How Effective Are They?" *Australian Journal of Advanced Nursing* 14(4):12-19, June-August 1997.

73. Cheneworth, C.C., et al. "Portrait of Practice: Healing Heel ulcers," *Advances in Wound Care* 7(2):44-8, March 1994.

74. Cheney, A.M. "Portrait of Practice: A Successful Approach to Preventing Heel Pressure Ulcers After Surgery," *Decubitus* 6(4):39-40, July 1993.

75. Williams, C. "Using Water-filled Gloves for Pressure Relief on Heels," *Journal of Wound Care* 2(6):345-48, 1993.

76. Flemister, B.G. "A Pilot Study of Interface Pressure with Heel Protectors Used for Pressure Reduction," *Journal of ET Nursing* 18(5):158-61, September-October 1991.

77. Guin, P., et al. "The Efficacy of Six Heel Pressure Reducing Devices," *Decubitus* 4(3):15-20 passim, August 1991.

78. Pinzur, M.S., et al. "Preventing Heel Ulcers: A Comparison of Prophylactic Body-support Systems," *Archives of Physical Medicine and Rehabilitation* 72(7): 508-10, June 1991.

CHAPTER 12

Pain management and wounds

Linda E. Dallam, MS, APRN,BC, CWCN, GNP
Christine Barkauskas, BS, RN, CWOCN, APN
Elizabeth A. Ayello, PhD, RN, APRN,BC, CWOCN, FAAN
Sharon Baranoski, MSN, RN, CWOCN, APN, FAAN

OBJECTIVES

After completing this chapter, you'll be able to:

- state a definition of pain
- describe types of pain
- describe the relationship between pain and wound types
- state two methods for pain assessment
- discuss pain treatment modalities.

Etiology and definitions of pain

"Pain has an element of blank;
It cannot recollect
When it began, or if there were
A day when it was not."

– Emily Dickinson

As clinicians, we have a tendency to identify certain types of wounds as having a specific type or amount of pain. However, pain is what the patient states it is — not what we believe it to be. Our responsibility as clinicians is to accurately assess the patient's pain and treat it

adequately, without judging the patient or doubting that the pain is as described.

The literature reports numerous definitions of pain. Both the 1979 International Association for the Study of Pain (IASP) Subcommittee on Taxonomy[1] and the Agency for Healthcare Research and Quality (AHRQ, formerly the Agency for Healthcare Policy and Research, or AHCPR)[2] support a common definition of pain. They have defined pain as "an unpleasant sensory and emotional experience associated with actual or potential tissue damage or described in terms of such damage."[1,2]

Another commonly used pain definition is that of McCaffery,[3] who states that "pain is whatever the experiencing person says it is and exists whenever he says it does." McCaffery's definition of pain encompasses the subjective component and acknowledges the patient as the best judge of his own pain experience. Experts in the field of pain have come to accept that the patient's self-reporting of pain, and the characteristics and intensity of the pain, is the most reliable assessment. This belief that the person in pain is the best judge of his pain experience is also accepted as the basis for pain assessment and management by regulatory agencies such as the Joint Commission on Accreditation of Healthcare Organizations (JCAHO)[4] as well as professional organizations such as the American Pain Society.[5]

PRACTICE POINT

Pain is what the person says it is and exists whenever he says it does. The true etiology of pain isn't known. More research is needed to learn its true causes.

Types of pain

Pain can be nociceptive or neuropathic. Nociceptive pain can result from ongoing activation of primary afferent neurons by noxious stimuli. The nervous system is intact. Neuropathic pain is initiated or caused by a primary lesion or dysfunction of the nervous system.[6] The two types of nociceptive pain are somatic and visceral. Somatic pain arises from bone, skin, muscle, or connective tissue. It's usually aching, throbbing, and well-localized. Pressure ulcer pain, for example, is usually of the somatic type.

Visceral pain arises from the visceral organs such as the gut, or from an obstruction of a hollow viscous organ, as occurs with a blockage of the small bow-

el. Visceral pain is poorly localized and is commonly described as cramping. Nociceptive pain (somatic and visceral) responds well to non-opioids and opioids.

In neuropathic pain, the nervous system has been affected. There is abnormal processing of the sensory input by the peripheral or central nervous system. The pain is typically described as burning, stabbing, or electrical. Diabetic ulcer pain and the pain of shingles are examples of neuropathic pain. Neuropathic pain responds more readily to an adjuvant such as anticonvulsants or tricyclic antidepressants. Gabapentin, an anticonvulsant, has been shown to be useful in treating neuropathic pain.[7]

Pain can also be acute or persistent (chronic). Acute pain has a distinct onset, with an obvious cause and short duration; this type of pain subsides as healing takes place. Chronic pain can be from a cancerous or a noncancerous source. It persists for 3 months or more and is usually associated with functional and psychological impairment. Chronic pain can fluctuate in character and intensity.

The American Geriatric Society[8] supports the use of "persistent" pain rather than "chronic" pain to circumvent the negative stereotypes that have been associated with the word "chronic." The AGS Clinical Practice Guideline, "The Management of Persistent Pain in Older Persons" states: "Unfortunately for many elderly persons, chronic pain has become a label associated with negative images and stereotypes commonly associated with long-standing psychiatric problems, futility in treatment, malingering, or drug-seeking behavior. Persistent pain may foster a more positive attitude by patients and professionals for the many effective treatments that are available to help alleviate suffering." [8]

Persistent pain and acute pain can occur at the same time in the same patient;

PRACTICE POINT
Interventions for noncyclic wound pain

- Administer topical or local anesthetics.
- Consider operating room procedure under general anesthesia rather than bedside debridement for large, deep ulcers.
- Administer opioids and nonsteroidal anti-inflammatory drugs before and after procedures.

- Assess and reassess for pain during and after procedures.
- Avoid using wet-to-dry dressings.
- Consider alternatives to surgical/sharp debridement, such as transparent dressings, hydrogels, hydrocolloids, hypertonic saline solutions, or enzymatic agents.[21]

similarly, nociceptive and neuropathic pain may occur at the same time. All types of pain can be associated with functional or psychosocial losses and can affect the quality of life, or the quality of death in patients who are actively dying. Pain can be debilitating and can also cause suffering beyond its physical component.

PRACTICE POINT

Reframing the phrase "patient complains of pain" to "patient reports pain" may help to foster a more positive and objective way for practitioners and caregivers to connect with the patient's experience of pain.

The persistent (chronic) pain experience

Krasner[9-11] has conceptualized pain in chronic wounds as the chronic wound pain experience. Within this model, pain is divided into three subconcepts: noncyclic, cyclic, and chronic pain. *Noncyclic* or *incident* pain is defined as a single episode of pain that might occur, for example, after wound debridement. *Cyclic* or *episodic* pain recurs as the result of repeated treatments, such as dressing changes or turning and repositioning. *Chronic* or *continuous*

pain is persistent and occurs without manipulation of the wound. For example, the patient may feel that the wound is throbbing even when he's lying still in bed and no treatment is being done to the wound. (See *Interventions for noncyclic wound pain*, *Interventions for cyclic wound pain*, page 220, and *Interventions for persistent (chronic) wound pain*, page 221.)

Pain and wound types

The type of pain a patient experiences depends largely on the type of wound. Various wound types, and the types of pain that accompany them, are discussed throughout this chapter.

Pressure ulcer pain

Pain at the site of a pressure ulcer is supported by pressure ulcer experts and anecdotal reports by clinicians, although few studies have been done concerning pressure ulcer pain. The National Pressure Ulcer Advisory Panel (NPUAP) stated at its first conference in 1989 that "pressure ulcers are serious wounds that cause considerable pain, suffering, disability, and even death."[12] Van Rijswijk and Braden[13] reevaluated the AHCPR Treatment of Pressure Ulcer Guidelines in light of studies published after release of the 1994 Guidelines.[14] They reaffirmed

PRACTICE POINT

Interventions for cyclic wound pain

- Perform interventions at a time of day when the patient is less fatigued.
- Provide analgesia 30 minutes prior to dressing change.
- Assess the patient for pain during and after dressing changes.
- Provide analgesia 30 minutes prior to whirlpool.
- If the patient's dressing has dried out, thoroughly soak the wound—especially the edges.
- Observe the wound for signs of local infection.
- Gently and thoroughly irrigate the wound to remove debris and reduce the bacterial bioburden, which can cause contaminated wounds to become infected. Infection will increase the inflammation and pain at the wound site.

- Avoid using cytotoxic topical agents.
- Avoid aggressive packing.
- Avoid drying out the wound bed and wound edges.
- Protect the periwound area with sealants, ointments, or moisture barriers.
- Minimize the number of daily dressing changes.
- Select pain-reducing dressings.
- Avoid using tape on fragile skin.
- Splint or immobilize the wounded area as needed.
- Utilize pressure-reducing devices in bed or chair.
- Provide analgesia as needed to allow positioning of patient.
- Avoid trauma (shearing and tear injuries) to fragile skin when transferring, positioning, or holding a patient.

the AHCPR panel's first recommendation about assessing pressure ulcer patients for pain. Based on the additional evidence from studies supporting reduction of pain with the use of moisture-retentive dressings, van Rijswijk and Braden[13] proposed that the 1994 AHCPR recommendations about pain and pressure ulcers be rewritten.

The etiology of pain in patients with pressure ulcers isn't known. Pieper[15] suggests, based on the work of Rook,[16] that pressure ulcer pain is from "release of noxious chemicals from damaged tissue, erosion of tissue planes with destruction of nerve terminals, regeneration of nociceptive nerve terminals, infection, dressing changes, and debridement."

According to a study by Szors and Bourguignon,[17] pressure ulcer pain depends not only on the stage of the pressure ulcer but also on whether a dressing change is being done at the time the assessment is made. The majority of the patients reported pressure ulcer pain at rest or with dressing changes and stated that the pain ranged from sore to excruciating. Seventy-five percent rated their pain as mild, discomforting, or distressing; 18% rated their pain as horrible or excruciating.

Arterial ulcer pain

Pain associated with peripheral vascular disease can be intermittent claudication; it may occur at night, when the patient's legs are elevated, or at other periods of rest. Intermittent claudication pain results from exercise or activity and has been described as cramping, burning, or aching. Blood flow with exertion is inadequate to meet the needs of tissues; the

PRACTICE POINT

Interventions for persistent (chronic) wound pain

- Utilize all of the interventions listed for noncyclic and cyclic wound pain.
- Control edema.
- Control infection.
- Monitor wound pain while the patient is at rest (at times when no dressing change is taking place).
- Control pain to allow healing and positioning.
- Provide regularly scheduled analgesia, including opioids, patient-controlled analgesia, and topical preparations such as lidocaine gel 2%, depending on the severity of pain.

- Attend to nonwound pain from comorbid pain syndromes such as contractures and diabetes, and iatrogenically induced pain from central lines, venipunctures, catheters, feeding tubes, blood gas drawing, or other equipment or procedures.
- Address the emotional component of the pain or the patient's suffering. For example, find out what the wound represents to him, what the pain means, whether he has associated losses of function, and whether the wound has altered his body image. In addition, determine whether his mental status or behavior has changed related to unrelieved pain.

resultant lack of circulation causes intermittent pain.

Nocturnal pain may have the same symptoms but usually precedes the occurrence of rest pain. Rest pain occurs — even without activity — when blood flow is inadequate to meet the needs of tissues in the extremities. It's described as a sensation of burning or numbness aggravated by leg elevation. It's a constant, intense pain that isn't easily relieved by using pain medications. Pain can sometimes be alleviated by stopping the activity or exercise, and placing legs in a dangling or dependent position.

Venous ulcer pain

The range of venous ulcer pain is extensive; the patient may report mildly annoying pain, a dull ache, or sharp, deep muscle pain. Pain is more intense at the end of the day secondary to edema resulting from the legs being in a dependent position. The pathophysiology of venous disease is related to reduction or

occlusion of blood return to the heart. Thrombus, incompetent valves, gravitational pressure from standing, and venous stasis can produce acute and prolonged pain. Elevating the legs helps to decrease or eliminate the pain; use of support stockings, avoidance of prolonged sitting, weight reduction, and smoking cessation are all clinical management goals.

Neuropathic ulcer pain

Neuropathy is the most common complication of diabetes. The amount of pain present depends on the severity of the neuropathy. The patient may state that the pain interferes with his entire life — especially his ability to sleep. The affected extremity may feel like it's asleep or have the "pins and needles" pain that occurs after a part of the body has "fallen asleep" and starts to wake up. The quality of pain can be aching, burning, sharp, and may include skin sensitivity and itching. True pain relief is primarily accomplished with

PRACTICE POINT

Pain: What we know, what we don't know

McCaffery and Robinson[37] reported on the self-evaluation of nurses about pain.

- Observable changes in vital signs must be relied upon to verify a patient's report of severe pain: False (answered correctly by 88.4%).
- Pain intensity should be rated by the clinician, not the patient: False (answered correctly by 99.1%).
- A patient may sleep in spite of moderate or severe pain: True (answered correctly by 90.6%).
- Intramuscular (I.M.) meperidine is the drug of choice for prolonged pain: False (answered correctly by 85.6%).
- Analgesics for chronic pain are more effective when administered as needed rather than around the clock: False (answered correctly by 92.7%).
- If the patient can be distracted from the pain, he has less pain than he reports: False (answered correctly by 94.7%).
- The patient in pain should be encouraged to endure as much pain as possible before resorting to a pain relief measure: False (answered correctly by 98.4%).
- Respiratory depression (less than 7 breaths per minute) probably occurs in at least 10% of patients who receive one or more doses of an opioid for relief of pain:

False (answered correctly by 60.5%; clinicians tend to exaggerate the risk of respiratory depression with opioid use; according to McCaffery and Robinson, the risk is less than 1%).
- Vicodin (hydrocodone 5 mg and acetaminophen 500 mg) is approximately equal to the analgesia of one-half of a dose of meperidine 75 mg I.M.: False (correctly answered by 48.3%).
- If a patient's pain is relieved by a placebo, the pain isn't real: False (answered correctly by 86.1%).
- Beyond a certain dose, increasing the dosage of an opioid such as morphine won't increase pain relief: False (answered correctly by 57.2%).
- Research shows that promethazine reliably potentiates opioid analgesics: False (correctly answered by 35.1%).
- When opioids are used for pain relief under the following circumstances, what percentage of patients is likely to develop opioid addiction:
  - Patients who receive opioids for 1 to 3 days: Answer is less than 1% (correctly answered by 82.8%).
  - Patients who receive opioids for 3 to 6 months: Answer is less than 1% (correctly answered by 26.7%).

pharmacologic intervention. All pain needs to be adequately assessed to ascertain the most effective treatment modality. If a patient reports excessive pain in a neuropathic limb that hasn't had pain before, an infection may be developing.

PRACTICE POINT

Determining whether pain results from neuropathy or is associated with peripheral vascular disease is extremely important because patients with diabetes have a high incidence of peripheral vascular disease.

Understanding wound pain

Most of our understanding of wound pain comes from literature about diseases.[18] Clinicians are increasingly acknowledging that pain is a major issue for patients suffering from many different types of wounds.[18] (See *Pain: What we know, what we don't know.*)

The European Wound Management Association[19] has developed a position document on wound pain. Of the 3,918 respondents from the United States and 10 countries in western and eastern Europe, pain prevention was the second highest ranking consideration at dressing change, with prevention of trauma being first.[19] Pain from leg ulcers was ranked as the most severe pain among wound types, and dressing removal caused the greatest pain.[19]

Findings of two qualitative studies may provide knowledge about clinicians' understanding of wound pain in patients with pressure ulcers. Hollinworth[18] found that nurses' assessment, management, and documentation of pain after doing wound dressings was inadequate. A qualitative study by Krasner[20] examined the reflections of 42 general and advanced practice nurses after they cared for patients with pressure ulcers and pain. Three patterns — nursing expertly, denying the pain, and confronting the challenge of pain — with eight subsequent themes were identified. They were:

- Nursing expertly
  - Reading the pain
  - Attending to the pain
  - Acknowledging and empathizing with the patient
- Denying the pain
  - Assuming that it doesn't exist
  - Not hearing the cries
  - Avoiding failure
- Confronting the challenge of pain
  - Coping with frustration
  - Being with the patient.[20]

Krasner[10,11,20] suggested that clinicians use this information to provide more sensitive care to patients with pressure ulcer pain.

Few studies (three quantitative and one qualitative) have been done about the pain experience of patients with pressure ulcers. The first study to quantify pain by pressure ulcer stage was done by Dallam and colleagues,[21] who studied perceived intensity and patterns of pressure ulcer pain among hospitalized patients. The study population was diverse, with 66% being white (non-Hispanic) and the remainder being Black (non-Hispanic), Hispanic, or Asian. Of the 132 patients, 44 (33.3%) were respondents and 88 (66.7%) were nonrespondents as they couldn't communicate responses to the instruments. Two different scales were used to measure pain intensity: the Visual Analog Scale and the Faces Pain Rating Scale (FRS). (See the next section for additional discussion of these pain scales.) The authors found a high degree of agreement between the two pain scales. They also noted that the FRS scale was easier to use for patients who were cognitively impaired or for whom English was a second language.

Major findings of this important study by Dallam and colleagues[21] include:
- patients with pressure ulcers have pain (68% of respondents reported some type of pain)
- most patients don't receive analgesics for pain relief; only 2% (*n* = 3) were given analgesics for pressure ulcer pain within 4 hours of pain measurement
- patients who can't express or respond to pain scales may still have pain
- patients with higher stage pressure ulcers had more pain.

Some procedures, such as surgical debridement or wet-to-dry dressings, may increase pain. While the study[21] didn't identify the interventions that might be most effective in controlling pain, patients whose beds had static air mattresses rather than regular hospital bed mattresses, and those whose wounds were dressed with hydrocolloid dressings, had significantly less pain. The study[21] also demonstrated that patients are able to differentiate between ulcer site pain, generalized pain, and other local pain sites such as painful I.V. and catheter sites, and that cognitively impaired patients are able to indicate pain and respond to pain intensity scales.

In another quantitative study, Szors and Bourguignon[17] used a cross-sectional method to examine the pain experience of 32 patients with stage II, III, and IV pressure ulcers at rest and during dressing changes. This study found that a majority of patients had pressure ulcer-related pain. Twenty-eight (87.5%) reported pain at dressing change and 27 (84.4%) reported pain at rest (when dressing changes or other treatments weren't being carried out). Of the nearly 85% of patients reporting pain during dressing changes, 21 (75%) rated their pain as mild, discomforting, or distressing and 5 (18%) described their pain as horrible or excruciating. Twelve (42%) reported their pain as continuous, occurring both at rest and at dressing changes.

Despite the number of patients experiencing pressure ulcer pain at rest and at dressing changes, the study showed that only 6.3% (*n* = 2) received analgesia for their pressure ulcer pain.[17] Both quantitative studies by Dallam et al.[21] and Szors and Bourguinon[17] found that many patients suffer with untreated or undertreated pressure ulcer pain. The first study found that only 2% of patients with pressure ulcer pain received analgesia, while the second study, which occurred 4 years later, found little improvement. Only 6% of patients with pressure ulcer pain had analgesics prescribed to address their pain, although it's well known that pharmacologic man-

agement is the cornerstone of pain treatment regardless of its etiology.

Both studies reflect the need for clinicians to realize the potential for pain from pressure ulcers. Because only 44 of the 132 patients with pressure ulcer pain could respond to pain scales, Dallam and colleagues[21] recommend that pressure ulcer pain should be suspected even when the patient can't report pain. Both studies recommend further research on interventions that can relieve pressure ulcer pain and the suffering it causes.

The Riverside Pressure ulcer study, reported by Franks and Collier,[22] compared 75 home care patients in the United Kingdom who had pressure ulcers with 100 home care patients without pressure ulcers. An interesting finding of this study was that patients with pressure ulcers had less pain than the comparison group. The authors speculated that perhaps pressure ulcer pain might not be the problem, as previously presumed, or that pain control was more effective for these patients.

Langemo and colleagues[23] published the only qualitative phenomenological study about pain and pressure ulcer patients. They interviewed eight adults, half of whom had pressure ulcers at the time of the study and the other half of whom had healed pressure ulcers at that time. Seven themes were identified:

1. perceived etiology of the pressure ulcer
2. life impact and changes
3. psychospiritual impact
4. extreme painfulness associated with the pressure ulcer
5. need for knowledge and understanding
6. need for and effect of numerous, stressful treatments
7. the grieving process.

The fourth theme — extreme pain — was subdivided into three categories: intensity of pain, duration of pain, and analgesic use. Patients commonly referred to the intensity of pain from pressure ulcers with descriptors such as "it burned," "feeling like being stabbed," "sitting on a bunch of needles," or "stinging." Some examples of statements by actual study respondents include a woman with a stage II pressure ulcer who said, "I felt like somebody was getting a knife and really digging in there good and hard." In the words of another male respondent, "They [pressure ulcers] are very painful because no matter what way you put your bottom, it hurts."[23]

Respondents also commented on the duration of the pain, with statements such as "The majority of the time, even when I was lying down, it hurt." Pain continued to be a problem even after the pressure ulcer had healed. As one respondent stated, "Every now and again, it still hurts. But there is nothing there. This time there is nothing really there." The fear of addiction resulting from analgesic use was expressed by some respondents. One respondent with a stage IV pressure ulcer on the buttock commented, "I was constantly in pain and was taking morphine and other types of painkillers to try and ease the pain."

Pain assessment

Despite the American Pain Society's identification of pain as "the fifth vital sign,"[5] it isn't always included in the assessment of a patient's pressure ulcer. Dallam and colleagues[21] urged that pain be added to the assessment of pressure ulcers and that a patient's pain status be assessed during dressing changes as well as when the patient is at rest. (See *Essential pain assessment elements.*) They also cautioned clinicians to remember that absence of response or expression of pain doesn't mean that the patient doesn't have pain.

Essential pain assessment elements

Use the PQRST mnemonic (shown below) to assess your patient's pain.

P = Palliative/provocative factors
- What makes the pain worse?
- What makes it better?

Q = Quality of pain
- What kind of pain are you experiencing?
- Would you describe it as sore, aching, deep, cramping, burning, shooting, or sensitive (or any combination thereof)?
- Do you have other symptoms with the pain, such as fever, chills, nausea, or vomiting?

R = Region and radiation of pain
- Where is the pain?
- Where does it radiate?

S = Severity of pain
- Would you describe your pain as none, mild, moderate, severe, or excruciating?
- Rate your pain on a scale from 0 to 10, with 0 representing "no pain" and 10 being "the worst imaginable pain."
- What is the pain intensity at its worst, best, and now?

T = Temporal aspects of pain
- Is the pain better or worse at any particular time of the day or night?
- When does it start or when does it stop?
- Is it intermittent or constant, or does it occur only when you're moving?

Additional pain assessment elements

Include the following additional elements in your initial assessment plan and treatment:
- detailed history consisting of:
  – medication usage
  – treatment history
  – previous surgeries and injuries
  – impact on quality of life and activities of daily living.
- physical examination, emphasizing the body system involved in the pain complaint (for example, the musculoskeletal or neurologic system)
- psychosocial assessment, including family history of depression or chronic pain
- appropriate diagnostic workup to determine the cause of pain and to rule out any contributing, treatable causes.

A thorough pain assessment enables the clinician to develop an effective pain treatment regimen and evaluate its effectiveness.

Two assessment guides include pain as part of pressure ulcer assessment. The AHCPR[14] treatment guidelines include an example of a sample pressure ulcer pain assessment guide in Attachment A. There's a place to check either yes or no regarding pain. Ayello's[24,25] ASSESSMENT mnemonic asks the clinician to quantify the patient's pain experience including the presence of pain, when the pain occurs (for example, is it episodic or constant), and if the patient is receiving measures for pain relief. The caregiver completes the following boxes under t = tenderness to touch or pain: Tenderness

to touch—no pain, pain present on touch, anytime, or only when performing ulcer care.[24,25] The mnemonic PQRST, which outlines the specific questions to ask the patient, is another useful tool for assessing a patient's pain.

A complete and thorough pain assessment enables the clinician to develop an effective pain treatment regimen and evaluate its effectiveness. (See *Additional pain assessment elements*.)

PRACTICE POINT

Pain is the fifth vital sign.

Pain intensity scales

Pain intensity scales are used to determine how much pain the patient is having by utilizing a simple verbal, visual, or numeric measure. The gold standard for assessing pain intensity is self-report and the utilization of standard pain intensity instruments.[26,27] Standard pain intensity instruments consist of a range of choices indicating the severity of pain as experienced from the patient's perspective. Pain intensity scales are unidimensional, quantitative measures designed to measure the sensory aspect of a patient's pain and to obtain a more objective approximation of his pain by minimizing inaccuracies.[27]

The use of pain intensity scales to quantify pain levels and determine patients' responses to pain treatments has been mandated in all hospitals by JCAHO.[4] Two of the most widely accepted and utilized pain assessment scales are the Numeric Pain Intensity Scale and the FACES Pain Rating Scale.[28] Another scale that is sometimes used is the Visual Analog Scale (VAS). The VAS is a 10-cm line that has no numbers on it. At one end is the term "no pain," and at the

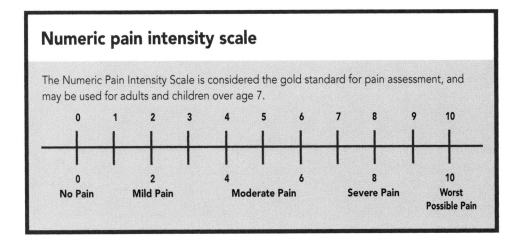

Numeric pain intensity scale

The Numeric Pain Intensity Scale is considered the gold standard for pain assessment, and may be used for adults and children over age 7.

| 0 | 1 | 2 | 3 | 4 | 5 | 6 | 7 | 8 | 9 | 10 |

| 0 | 2 | 4 | 6 | 8 | 10 |
| No Pain | Mild Pain | Moderate Pain | Severe Pain | Worst Possible Pain |

other end is the phrase "pain as bad as it could possibly be."[2]

Numeric pain intensity scale

The Numeric Pain Intensity Scale is commonly known as the gold standard for pain assessment for adults and children over age 7.[2,28] The scale is a 10-cm line with the words "no pain" at one end, "worst possible pain" at the other end, and the numbers zero to ten (0 to 10) running from one end of the scale to the other. (See *Numeric pain intensity scale.*) The patient is asked to select a number on the scale, which represents the level of pain he's experiencing. Zero indicates no pain, 5 indicates moderate pain, and 10 indicates the worst possible pain.[2] The Numeric Pain Intensity Scale is sometimes presented verbally;[2,28] however, visual presentation may help to standardize the process of pain assessment and assist hearing impaired patients. The scale has been translated into many languages.[6]

The pain intensity rating scale aids in the adequate assessment and treatment of pain. It also helps clinicians choose the appropriate classification of pain medication recommendations based on any given patient response.[12,28,29] Whether the patient has a response to the interventions can also be determined by using the scale if the numbers show a downward trend on repeated assessments.

FACES Pain Rating Scale

The FACES Pain Rating Scale (FPRS)[30] consists of six faces that range from a happy, smiling face (no pain) to a crying, frowning face (worst pain). Face 0 indicates an absence of pain, face 1 indicates minor pain, face 2 indicates more pain, and so forth. face 5, the last face on the scale, indicates extreme pain. The patient is asked to choose the face that most closely reflects his own pain at that point in time. (See *FACES Pain Rating Scale,* page 228.) The FPRS is preferred for use with children when compared with other pain intensity scales.[28] The validity and reliability in adult patients hasn't been established, although the FPRS has been used in studies with a geriatric population and a high degree of agreement was found between the FPRS and the VAS ($r = 92$, $p < 0.5$).[31] It has been used with cognitively impaired patients and those for whom English is the second language. A high consistency between the two scales was noted when utilized on any population.

After the initial pain assessment has been completed, reassessment should be

FACES Pain Rating Scale

The FACES Pain Rating Scale may be used for children ages 3 and older, for cognitively impaired patients, and for non-native speakers of English.

Do you have:

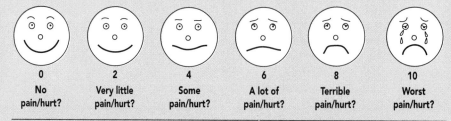

0	2	4	6	8	10
No pain/hurt?	**Very little pain/hurt?**	**Some pain/hurt?**	**A lot of pain/hurt?**	**Terrible pain/hurt?**	**Worst pain/hurt?**

From Wong, D.L.; Hockenberry-Eaton, M.; Wilson, D.; Winkelstein, M.L.; and Schwartz, P. *Wong's Essentials of Pediatric Nursing*, 6th ed. St. Louis: 2001. © Mosby, Inc. Reprinted with permission.

performed at regular intervals. Reassess the patient after administration of pain medication or nondrug pain-relieving interventions to ensure that optimal pain relief has been achieved.

Pain management

Accurate and continuous pain assessment is the foundation of successful pain management.[6,26] However, evidence demonstrates that pain is poorly assessed. Seventy-six percent of physicians with patient care responsibilities in oncology rated poor pain assessment as the number one barrier to adequate pain management.[7] Donovan et al.[32] found that of the 58% of hospitalized patients reporting excruciating pain, fewer than half had a member of the health care team ask them about their pain or note the pain in their records. The use of pain assessment measures has been shown to improve pain management for patients.[31,33] However, problems in using pain assessment scales persist. One problem is that clinicians aren't always comfortable or knowledgeable in the use of pain rating scales. Knowledge and confidence by the clinician is needed as the use of pain scales typically requires that the clinician explain to the patient how the scales work.

After pain has been identified, its cause should be determined and treated. "The goal of pain management in the pressure ulcer patient is to eliminate the cause of pain, to provide analgesia, or both."[13]

Dressing changes, debridement, wound edema, infection, turning, and positioning are some of the factors that can cause wound pain. An appropriate plan of action can be implemented after the specific cause has been identified. For example, if the pain results from dressing changes, medication prior to dressing changes or switching to a different dressing may be indicated. "Besides medications, pain may be treated with physical and occupational therapy to decrease muscle spasms, decrease contractures, and aid in wound debridement and cleaning. Proper seating, positioning, and adaptive equipment may also help to decrease pain."[14] The optimal way to treat the pain of pressure ulcers has yet to be determined.

PRACTICE POINT

Pain management should include interventions that:
- educate the patient
- improve activities of daily living (ADLs) and quality of life
- provide palliation to the dying patient
- decrease or eliminate pain with minimal adverse effects
- minimize patient's dependency on health care workers and family members.

Pain medication

The World Health Organization[34] (WHO) developed a three-step analgesic ladder for the treatment of cancer pain that has been accepted for use in patients with nonmalignant pain.[7] (See *WHO analgesic ladder*.) The WHO approach advises clinicians to match the patient's reported pain intensity of 0 to 10 with the potency of the analgesic to be prescribed, starting with non-opioid analgesics and progressing to stronger medications if pain isn't relieved.[7] For example, a patient who reports a pain score of 1 to 3 (mild pain) should receive a non-opioid with or without an adjuvant. If he reports a score of 4 to 6 (moderate pain), a weak opioid with or without an adjuvant should be administered. If the patient's pain score is from 7 to 10 (severe pain), he should be given a strong opioid with or without an adjuvant.

An adjuvant medication is a drug that has a primary indication other than pain but is analgesic for some painful conditions.[6] Examples of adjuvant medications are anticonvulsants or tricyclic antidepressants. (See *Adjuvant agents,* page 230.) Adding an adjuvant medication is

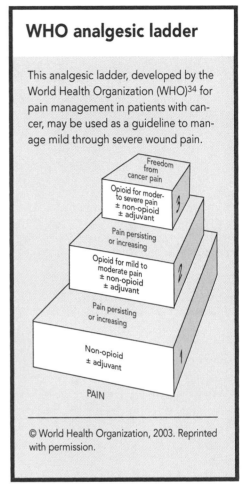

WHO analgesic ladder

This analgesic ladder, developed by the World Health Organization (WHO)[34] for pain management in patients with cancer, may be used as a guideline to manage mild through severe wound pain.

Freedom from cancer pain

Opioid for moderate to severe pain ± non-opioid ± adjuvant — 3

Pain persisting or increasing

Opioid for mild to moderate pain ± non-opioid ± adjuvant — 2

Pain persisting or increasing

Non-opioid ± adjuvant — 1

PAIN

© World Health Organization, 2003. Reprinted with permission.

most useful in addressing the burning or stabbing symptoms of neuropathic pain. Using a combination of drugs such as an opioid and a non-opioid can enhance pain relief because the two drugs work synergistically. The opioid works on the CNS to alter the perception of pain and the non-opioid works on the periphery to block painful impulses. Using a combination method may decrease the need for higher doses of opioids.

Step 1: Non-opioid analgesics

Acetaminophen or nonsteroidal anti-inflammatory drugs (NSAIDs) should be initiated first. These agents should be administered on a regular rather than an

Adjuvant agents

Drug class	Name	Indications
Tricyclic antidepressants	Amitriptyline Desipramine Nortriptyline	• Multi-purpose • Any chronic pain • Neuropathic pain
Anticonvulsants	Carbamazepine Clonazepam Gabapentin Valproic acid	• Burning, neuropathic, lancinating pain
Systemic local anesthetics	Lidocaine Mexiletine	• Burning pain
Topical anesthetics	Capsaicin EMLA cream Lidocaine gel Lidocaine 1% Lidocaine 4%	• Analgesic for intact skin (use on wound periphery prior to dressing changes) • Before changing vacuum-assisted-closure (VAC) dressing (instill solution through the VAC tubing, with the VAC at 50 mmHg and clamp tubing for 15 to 20 minutes)* • Saturate gauze 15 to 20 minutes prior to dressing change

* Systemic absorption and toxicity can occur in large wounds.

as-needed basis to increase their effectiveness and maintain a constant level of the medication in the blood. When using NSAIDS, if one group doesn't work, try another group. (See *Non-opioid analgesics.*)

NSAID groups include:
• salicylates: aspirin, diflunisal, choline magnesium trisalicylate, salsalate
• propionic acids: naproxen, ibuprofen, fenoprofen, ketoprofen, flurbiprofen, suprofen
• acetic acids: indomethacin, tolmetin, sulindac, diclofenac, ketorolac
• oxicams: piroxicam.

Ketorolac tromethamine may provide increased analgesia in comparison to oral NSAIDs and is available for administration both I.V. and I.M. but is limited to a five-day period of utilization and may not be useful in the management of persistent (chronic) pain. Although studies are limited, some researchers are exploring the effects of topical opioids in the treatment of painful skin ulcers. Twillman and colleagues [35] used nine case studies to report decreased pain at the site of an open ulcer when a morphine infused gel dressing was utilized in persons with painful skin ulcers due to a variety of medical conditions. The researchers report remarkable efficacy in eight out of the nine patients studied and felt there should be further research in this area as so many patients stand to gain pain relief from such a modality.

Tricyclic antidepressants, such as amitriptyline, imipramine, nortriptyline, and despiramine have been shown to relieve neuropathy and post-hepatic neuralgia, but are contraindicated in patients with coronary disease.[7]

Hydroxyzine (Vistaril, Atarax) has analgesic, antiemetic, and mild sedative activity as well as antihistamine effects. These drugs may provide analgesic properties and cause sedation that may help to induce sleep in patients with chronic pain. Some analgesics have caffeine as an additional ingredient to increase their potency and are useful in the management of headaches, uterine cramping, episiotomy and dental pain. Diabetic patients with neuropathic pain or other patients with conditions arising from peripheral nerve syndromes may benefit from the use of certain anticonvulsants, such as gabapentin, phenytoin, carbamazepine, sodium valproate, clonazepam[7].

Opioids vary in strength from mild to very strong and are available in different forms such as oral, oral-transmucosal, rectal, transdermal, subcutaneous, I.V., and I.M. forms. The oral form is preferred for long-term use. However, in the case of preprocedural or postprocedural pain, such as debridement, it might be better to use an I.V. route to allow for better pain control and faster ability to increase the dosage as needed. Whether an oral or I.V. route is used, doses should be scheduled on a regular basis to avoid breakthrough pain. If breakthrough pain occurs when the patient is on a long acting (sustained-release) opioid regimen, a short acting (immediate-release) opioid can be added and utilized together with the long-acting opioid to provide pain relief in between. Breakthrough pain is most likely to occur when the patient is moved, or if a dressing change is required, if tubes are being manipulated, or if the patient has an increase in activity.

Constipation can be one of the most common adverse reactions with the use of opioid analgesics. This adverse effect can be easily remedied by taking stool softeners, laxatives, and increasing fiber and fluids (especially water). It's better to anticipate constipation and treat it before it happens. The most common ad-

---

Non-opioid analgesics

- Acetaminophen
- Aspirin
- Tramadol
- Non-steroidal anti-inflammatory drugs
    - Celecoxib
    - Ibuprofen
    - Ketorolac
    - Rofecoxib
    - Salsalate

---

verse effects of opioids also include sedation, nausea, vomiting, itching, urinary retention, and sensory or motor deficits.

Many clinicians fear respiratory depression and subsequently undertreat pain. Respiratory depression might occur with the use of opioids. This primarily affects patients with chronic obstructive pulmonary disease or any other pulmonary disease. This side effect can be decreased or eliminated with the use of lower doses at first that are increased gradually while monitoring the patient's respiratory status.

Meperidine (Demerol) is not recommended for the management of persistent (chronic) pain[7]. Disadvantages include the hazards of normeperidine, a metabolite of meperidine. Repeated doses of meperidine can cause an accumulation of normeperidine, which causes central nervous system excitability and toxicity. This toxicity will be manifested in the patient by twitching, numbness, seizures, and hallucinations.[2] Coma and death are also possible. According to the 1999 APS Principles of Analgesic Use in the Treatment of Acute and Cancer Pain [7], "although the oral doses of meperidine have about one quarter of the analgesic effectiveness of similar parenteral doses, they produce just as much of this

Combination or weak opioids

- Acetaminophen with codeine
- Hydrocodone with acetaminophen
- Oxycodone with acetaminophen
- Propoxyphene
- Propoxyphene with acetaminophen

toxic metabolite." The American Pain Society also warns that patients with compromised renal function are particularly at risk for the accumulation of this toxic metabolite.

EVIDENCE-BASED PRACTICE

Caretakers tend to underutilize opioid analgesics because of the fear of addiction. Caretaker education is very important, especially in the home care setting where the caregiver is the one deciding when to give the patient pain medication. Addiction to opioids should be a concern, but the fear of addiction has been greatly exaggerated. Studies have shown that when a patient takes an opioid for pain relief the incidence of addiction is about 1%. The length of time on the analgesic or the amount given is irrelevant for addiction.[16] Although the incidence of addiction is low, the potential for abuse does exist. Clinicians should remain diligent and responsible for monitoring the patient who is on opioids. An indication that abuse is developing is if the patient begins to use the drug for reasons other than pain relief.

Step 2: Opioid for mild to moderate pain

Weak opioids, or opioids combined with NSAIDs, may be used if step 1 is ineffec-

tive. (See *Combination or weak opioids.*) Propoxyphene and combined propoxyphene drugs are step 2 drugs, but these agents should be avoided in elderly patients because the drug metabolite may cause CNS and cardiac toxicity. Codeine may cause excessive constipation, nausea, and vomiting.[36]

Step 3: Opioid for moderate to severe pain

Use opioids, such as morphine and morphine-like agents, when steps 1 and 2 are ineffective. (See *Opioids: Morphine and morphine-like agents.*)

Morphine is the drug of choice for chronic pain. Morphine is more cost-effective than meperidine, available for many different routes, and is easily titratable. It has fewer, easily treatable adverse effects. The adverse effects of constipation and nausea are usually treated with antiemetic drugs and laxatives. Other adverse effects are usually dose-related and can be resolved with adjustments in the dosage.[6]

PRACTICE POINT

Helpful hints for using opioids:
- Oral-transmucosal fentanyl citrate works in 10 minutes (good for dressing changes).
- Fentanyl patches should be used only on patients who have been taking other opioids. It will take 2 to 3 days for the first patch to reach maximum effect. If immediate pain relief is required, a short-acting opioid can be used along with the patch and then discontinued when the patch begins to work.
- Use short-acting agents (at 10% to 15% of total daily dose) for breakthrough pain.
- Titrate up to long-acting agents if patient needs more than two breakthrough doses on a normal day.
- Don't wait for constipation to begin. Start patient on stool softeners and laxatives to avoid this common adverse effect.

- To taper or discontinue opioid analgesics, decrease the dose by 25% every 2 to 3 days. Monitor for pain or withdrawal symptoms, as these would indicate the tapering is too rapid.

PRACTICE POINT

Symptoms of withdrawal or abstinence from opioids include:
- tachycardia
- hypertension
- diaphoresis
- piloerection
- nausea and diarrhea
- abdominal pain
- body aches
- psychosis.

The presence of these symptoms may indicate that the opioid medication is being tapered too quickly, and not that the patient is addicted to it.

Some researchers are exploring the effects of topical opioids in the treatment of painful skin ulcers.[35] One study reported decreased pain at the site of an open ulcer when a morphine-infused gel dressing was used in patients with painful skin ulcers due to a variety of medical conditions. The researchers report remarkable efficacy in eight out of the nine patients studied.

Nonpharmacologic treatment modalities

Management of pain from wounds can require a combination of pharmacologic and nonpharmacologic treatments; the latter may include the use of music, massage, and relaxation techniques. Many nonpharmacologic treatments can be used prior to, and in conjunction with, medications. These include physical and occupational therapy, repositioning the

> ## Opioids: Morphine and morphine-like agents
>
> - Morphine
> - Dolophine
> - Fentanyl patch
> - Levorphanol
> - Oxycodone

patient, support surfaces, and local wound care.

Physical and occupational therapy

Physical and occupational therapy services may be a valuable asset to utilize in conjunction with pharmacologic therapy. Passive and active range-of-motion exercises should be taught to the patient and his caregivers. Additional measures include the following:
- Patients with peripheral vascular disease may benefit from a walking program to facilitate development of collateral circulation in the lower extremities.
- Application of a transcutaneous electrical nerve stimulation unit may help to decrease pain, particularly in patients with chronic or acute wounds. It's believed that the electrical stimulation provided by the unit helps to inhibit pain transmission cells.
- Hot or cold packs can be applied to decrease spasms in the affected area.
- Stretching exercises help to decrease contractures.
- Exercise helps to decrease muscle spasms with massage.

Local pain management

The use of appropriate dressings and dressing techniques can help to relieve pain during and between dressing changes. Findings from the international study by Moffatt et al.[19] reveal the importance of pain-free dressing changes. All respondents agreed that gauze dressings caused the most pain, while pain was noticeably less severe with the use of hydrogels, hydrofiber, alignates, and soft silicone dressings.

Dressing types

Pain at dressing change is typically overlooked when formulating a care plan. Many products are available for wound care; choose products carefully to provide the patient with a pain-free experience. (See chapter 9, Wound treatment options.) Patients who express discomfort despite careful product selection should be given medication prior to dressing changes.

Hydrogel dressings are soothing to the patient and easily removed without pain. These dressings are especially useful for burns or other wounds that evoke a burning sensation.

Calcium alginate dressings help to absorb exudates in heavily draining wounds. Excess exudate in the wound can lead to pressure that increases pain; likewise, exudate on the wound periphery can erode the periwound skin, causing maceration that may increase pain and, possibly, extend the original wound. Calcium alginate dressings help the wound maintain the proper degree of moisture and are painlessly removed.

Hydrocolloid dressings are occlusive dressings that decrease pain by preventing exposure of the wound to air. These dressings absorb moderate amounts of exudate, which helps to decrease maceration to the periwound skin. However, their adhesive properties can cause trauma if not removed properly.

Foam dressings absorb moderate to high amounts of exudates and don't adhere to the wound, which makes dressing changes more comfortable for the patient.

Transparent dressings maintain a moist wound environment that insulates the wound surface; however, they must be removed carefully to avoid trauma to the wound and surrounding skin. Use with caution on patients who have fragile skin.

All of the above moist-wound dressings can be left on wounds for a longer period of time than wet-to-dry dressings. This decreases the frequency of dressing changes, thereby decreasing the opportunities for the patient to experience pain associated with dressing changes.

The following suggestions will ease the dressing change process for your patients:

• Change dressings in a timely manner. Excess exudate on periwound skin or dressings allowed to dry on a wound may increase the patient's pain.
• Protect the periwound skin with skin barrier wipes or ointment to prevent excoriation, trauma, maceration, or dermatitis that can delay wound healing, increase wound size, and increase patient discomfort.
• Use warm normal saline solution or noncytotoxic wound cleaners to clean wounds.
• Don't use cytotoxic solutions such as betadine or hydrogen peroxide to clean wounds. They not only deter wound healing, they may cause burning, adding to the patient's discomfort.
• Provide pressure relief for your patients.
• Keep the patient's heels off the bed at all times.
• Avoid using tape on elderly patients or patients with fragile skin.
• Consider using anti-shear dressings, originally designed for burn patients; they may assist in decreasing pain by increasing the amount of serous drainage associated with weepy limbs. These dressings also prevent shearing of the epidermal layer of fragile skin.

- Give pain medication around the clock if necessary to keep the pain under control.
- Keep in mind that pharmacologic management is the gold standard for moderate to severe pain.
- Explain dressing change procedures to the patient before dressing changes.
- Allow the patient or his family members to participate in dressing changes if they want to be involved.
- Offer the patient distraction techniques, such as conversation, TV, and videos during dressing changes.
- Inform the patient that he may call a "time-out" if pain is present during dressing changes.
- Ensure that the patient has adequate rest and sleep. Lack of rest and sleep will decrease the patient's pain threshold, decrease his mental performance, and increase his emotional response to pain.
- Teach the patient to substitute tapping, rubbing, and gentle slapping for scratching.
- Instruct the patient in relaxation techniques and the use of visual imagery when encountering a potentially pain-provoking situation.
- Fentanyl patches, transparent dressings, tincture of benzoin, and triamcinolone acetonide inhaler puffed onto the skin are helpful for dermatitis associated with adhesive dressings.
- Use moist wound therapy to enhance autolytic debridement as an alternative to surgical or sharp debridement to eliminate pain associated with sharp debridement.
- Assess for pain and medicate the patient before and after dressing changes or debridement.
- Allow the patient to select the time for dressing changes if appropriate.
- Check wound for signs and symptoms of infection and treat them.
- Don't pack the wound aggressively.

- Assess pain when the patient is at rest to provide adequate pain control.
- Control edema to avoid decreased blood flow to the wound, which may lead to additional pain.
- Eliminate or decrease pain from other possible pain sources.
- Instruct the patient and his family regarding pain management to alleviate fear of addiction with the use of opioids.
- Explain the role that pain control plays in improved wound healing.
- Reevaluate the pain management plan when needed. Document the effectiveness of the analgesic or other treatments for pain relief with a pain score. This will help to assess if the pain management program is working.
- Address other factors, such as loss of function, inability to perform ADLs, and possible changes in body image to help the patient deal with ancillary problems that might contribute to his pain.

PRACTICE POINT

Wet-to-dry dressings can desiccate a wound, thus causing pain on removal. Avoid these dressings in favor of moist wound therapy dressings to promote a healing environment and patient comfort.

Summary

Pain assessment scales can be useful in the role of pain management. The scales enable the clinician to accurately assess the patient's pain, thereby facilitating effective treatment modalities to help decrease the pain associated with any wound. Pain is detrimental for patients because it can exhaust them, affect their ability to perform their ADLs, add to feelings of decreased worth as a person, affect their interactions with loved ones and friends, deter wound healing, and overall diminish their quality of life and the quality of death for patients who are in the process of dying. As clinicians, we are obligated to provide adequate pain relief for our patients by using some or all of the many treatment modalities available to us.

Show what you know

1. Which of the following most accurately defines pain? Pain is:

A. an objective finding based on prolonged elevation of the patient's blood pressure and pulse rate.
B. a state of discomfort evidenced by the person being unable to sleep.
C. a physical consequence of wound care.
D. whatever the experiencing person says it is.

ANSWER: D. McCaffery's classic definition of pain is that it's whatever the experiencing person says it is.[6] A is wrong as research has shown that sudden severe pain may elevate vital signs, but this only occurs for a short time.[6] B is wrong as research has shown that patients can sleep even though they have moderate or severe pain.[6] C is incorrect because, although pain may be a consequence of wound care, this isn't a definition of pain.

2. Which of the following statements best describes the Numeric Pain Intensity Scale? It's a:

A. 10-cm line with the words "no pain" at one end and the "worst possible pain" at the other end.
B. series of faces ranging from smiling to frowning.
C. rainbow of colors starting with green and ending with red.

D. a decision tree for determining which medications to give to a person experiencing pain.

ANSWER: A. B refers to the Faces Pain Rating Scale. C doesn't describe a pain scale. D refers to the WHO analgesic ladder.

3. According to the WHO Analgesic Ladder, which medications should you use initially for relief of mild pain?

A. None
B. Non-opioid with or without an adjuvant
C. Opioid with or without an adjuvant
D. Opioid

ANSWER: B. A non-opioid is the drug recommended to use for mild pain. An adjuvant can be added to the non-opioid if there is neuropathic pain, as well as nociceptive pain. A is wrong as drugs are part of the WHO analgesic ladder. C and D are wrong as they are part of step 2 in the ladder.

References

1. "Pain Terms. A List with Definitions and Notes on Usage Recommended by the IASP Subcommittee on Taxonomy," *Pain* 6(3):249-252, June 1979.
2. Acute Pain Management Guideline Panel. *Acute Pain Management: Operative or Medical Procedures and Trauma, Clinical Practice Guideline*, No.3. Rockville, Md.: AHCPR, 1992.
3. McCaffery, M., and Beebe, A. *Pain: A Clinical Manual for Nursing Practice.* St. Louis: Mosby–Year Book, Inc., 1989.
4. Dahl, J.L., and Gordon, D.B. "Joint Commission Pain Standards: A Progress Report," *APS Bulletin* 12(6), 2002.
5. American Pain Society. *Pain: The Fifth Vital Sign.* Available at *www.ampainsoc.org/advocacy/fifth.htm.* November 1995.
6. McCaffery, M., and Passero, C. *Pain: Clinical Manual,* 2nd ed. St. Louis: Mosby–Year Book, Inc.1999.

7. *Principles of Analgesic Use in the Treatment of Acute Pain and Cancer Pain,* 4th ed. Glenview, Ill.: American Pain Society, 1999.

8. American Geriatric Society. "The Management of Persistent Pain in Older Persons," *AGS Panel on Persistent Pain in Older Persons* 50(6 Suppl):S205-S224, June 2002.

9. Krasner, D. "The Chronic Wound Pain Experience: A Conceptual Model," *Ostomy/Wound Management* 41(3):20-29, April 1995.

10. Krasner, D. "Caring for the Person Experiencing Chronic Wound Pain," in *Chronic Wound Care: A Clinical Source Book for Healthcare Professionals*, 3rd ed. Edited by Krasner, D.L. Wayne, Pa.: HMP Communications, 2001.

11. Krasner, D. "Managing Wound Pain in Patients with Vacuum-Assisted Closure Devices," *Ostomy/Wound Management* 48(5):38-43, May 2002.

12. National Pressure Ulcer Advisory Panel, "Pressure Ulcer Prevalence, Cost, and Risk Assessment: Consensus Development Conference Statement," *Decubitus* 2(2):24-28, May 1989.

13. Van Rijswijk, L., and Braden, B.J. "Pressure Ulcer Patient and Wound Assessment: An AHCPR Clinical Practice Guideline Update," *Ostomy/Wound Management* 45(1A Suppl):56S-67S, January 1999.

14. Bergstrom, N., et al. "Pressure Ulcer Treatment," *Clinical Practice Guideline #15.* Rockville, Md.: AHCPR, 1994.

15. Pieper, B. "Mechanical Forces: Pressure, Shear and Friction," in *Acute and Chronic Wounds: Nursing Management,* 2nd ed. Edited by Bryant, R.A. St. Louis: Mosby–Year Book, Inc., 2000.

16. Rook, J.L. "Wound Care Pain Management," *Advances in Wound Care* 9(6):24-31, November-December 1996.

17. Szors, J.K., and Bourguignon, C. "Description of Pressure Ulcer Pain at Rest and Dressing Change," *Journal of Wound, Ostomy, and Continence Nurses* 26(3):115-20, May 1999.

18. Hollinworth, H. "Nurse's Assessment and Management of Pain at Wound Dressing Changes," *Journal of Wound Care* 4(2):77-83, February 1995.

19. Moffatt, C.J., et al. "Understanding Wound Pain and Trauma: An International Perspective," EWMA Position Document: *Pain at Wound Dressing Changes* 2-7, 2002.

20. Krasner, D. "Using a Gentler Hand: Reflections on Patients with Pressure Ulcers Who Experience Pain," *Ostomy/Wound Management* 42(3):20-29, April 1996.

21. Dallam, L., et al. "Pressure Ulcer Pain: Assessment and Quantification," *Journal of Wound, Ostomy, and Continence Nursing* 22(5):211-17, September 1995.

22. Franks, P.J., and Collier, M.E. "Quality of Life: The Cost to the Individual," in *The Prevention of Pressure Ulcers.* Edited by Morrison, M.J. St. Louis: Mosby–Year Book, Inc., 2001.

23. Langemo, D.K., et al. "The Lived Experience of Having a Pressure Ulcer: A Qualitative Analysis," *Advances in Skin & Wound Care* 13(5):225-35, September-October 2000.

24. Ayello, E.A. "Teaching the Assessment of Patients with Pressure Ulcers," *Decubitus* 5(4):53-54, July 1992.

25. Ayello, E.A. "A Pressure Ulcer ASSESS-MENT Tool," *Advances in Skin & Wound Care* 13(5):247, September-October 2000.

26. Fink, R., and Gates, R. "Pain Assessment," in *Textbook of Palliative Nursing.* Edited by Ferrell, B.R., and Coyle, N. Oxford University Press, 2001.

27. Keele, K.D. "The Pain Chart," *Lancet* 48(2):6-8, 1948.

28. Wong, D.L., and Baker, C.M. "Pain in Children: Comparison of Assessment Scales," *Pediatric Nursing* 14(1):9-17, January-February 1988.

29. Flaherty, S.A. "Pain Measurement Tools for Clinical Practice and Research," *Journal of the American Association of Nurse Anesthetists* 64(2):133-140, April 1996.

30. Wong, D.L.; Hockenberry-Eaton, M.; Wilson, D.; Winkelstein, M.L.; and Schwartz, P. *Wong's Essentials of Pediatric Nursing,* 6th ed. St. Louis: Mosby, 2001.

31. Simon, W., and Malabar, R. "Assessing Pain in Elderly Patients Who Can't Respond Verbally," *Journal of Advanced Nursing* 22(4):663-669, October 1995.

32. Donovan, M., et al. "Incidence and Characteristics of Pain in a Sample of Medical-Surgical Patients," *Pain* 30(1):69-78, July 1987.

33. Faires, J.E., et al. "Systematic Pain Records and Their Impact on Pain Control: A Pilot Study," *Cancer Nursing* 12(6):306-13, December 1991.

34. *Cancer Pain Relief,* 2nd ed., Geneva: World Health Organization, 1996.

35. Twillman, R.K., et al. "Treatment of Painful Skin Ulcer with Topical Opioids," *Journal of Pain and Symptom Management* 17(4):288-92, April 1999.

36. Derby, S., and O'Mahony, S. "Elderly Patients," in *Textbook of Palliative Nursing.* Edited by Ferrell, B.R., and Coyle, N. Oxford University Press, 2001.

37. McCaffery, M., and Robinson, E.S. "Your Patient is in Pain, Here's How You Respond," *Nursing* 32(10):36-45, October 2002.

Part Two

Wound classifications and management strategies

CHAPTER 13

Pressure ulcers

Elizabeth A. Ayello, PhD, RN, APRN,BC, CWOCN, FAAN
Sharon Baranoski, MSN, RN, CWOCN, APN, FAAN
Courtney H. Lyder, ND, GNP, FAAN
Janet Cuddigan, PhD, RN, CWCN

OBJECTIVES

After completing this chapter, you'll be able to:

- discuss the significance of the pressure ulcers as a health care problem

- describe the etiology of a pressure ulcer

- define pressure ulcer classification systems

- state how to complete a risk assessment tool

- discuss strategies for pressure ulcer prevention

- discuss strategies for treating a patient with pressure ulcers

- state the prevalence and incidence of pressure ulcers around the world.

Pressure ulcers as a health care problem

Pressure ulcers have been seen as a nursing problem throughout time. The reality is that pressure ulcers are a global health care concern and more than a nursing issue. All health care providers need to be responsible for the prevention and treatment of pressure ulcers.

Over the centuries, pressure ulcers have been referred to as decubitus ulcers, bedsores, and pressure sores. The term pressure ulcer has become the preferred name of choice because it most closely describes the etiology and resultant ulcer. A pressure ulcer is "any lesion caused by unrelieved pressure resulting in damage of underlying tissue. Pressure ulcers are usually located over bony prominences (such as the sacrum, coccyx, hips, heels) and are staged according to the extent of observable tissue damage. Pressure ulcers vary from superficial tissue damage to deep craters exposing muscle and bone."[1]

Treatment interventions have varied along with the terminology. Wax, honey, feathers, leaves, bugs, ointments, and magic potions survived for centuries as

Skin: An essential organ

The Payne-Martin Classification System for Skin Tears divides skin tears into three categories based on whether tissue is lost in the tear.

Category I
Skin tears without tissue loss

Category I linear-type skin tear

In this Category I, linear-type skin tear, note areas of senile purpura.

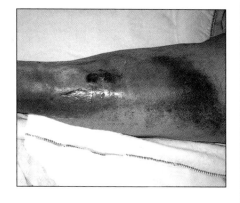

Category I flap-type skin tear

This Category I, flap-type skin tear has an epidermal flap covering the dermis to within 1 mm of the wound margin.

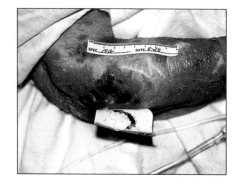

Category II
Skin tears with partial tissue loss

Category II scant tissue loss–type skin tear

Less than 25% of the epidermal flap has been lost in this Category II, scant tissue loss–type skin tear.

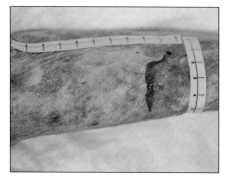

(continued)

Skin: An essential organ *(continued)*

Category II moderate to large tissue loss–type skin tear

More than 25% of the epidermal flap has been lost in this Category II, moderate to large tissue loss–type skin tear.

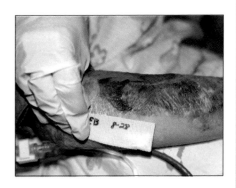

Category III
Skin tears with complete tissue loss

Category III skin tear

The epidermal flap is absent in this Category III skin tear (skin tear with complete tissue loss).

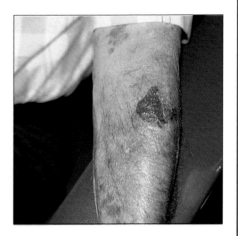

Wound assessment

Maceration

This photograph shows maceration of the surrounding skin caused by an overwhelmed dressing.

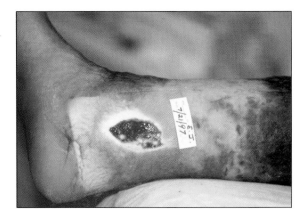

Wound edges with epithelialization

In this photograph, wound edges are attached and epithelialization present.

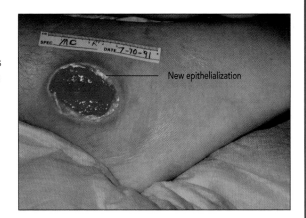

Wound terminology

Using current terminology is imperative for an accurate assessment. The photograph at right labels this wound's characteristics as well as its length and width.

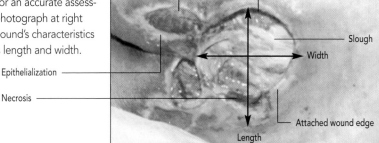

Wound debridement

Slough

Necrotic tissue that's moist, stringy, and yellow (devitalized issue) is referred to as *slough*.

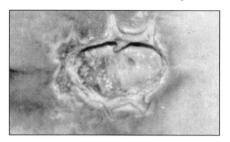

Eschar

In a wound that has become dehydrated, necrotic tissue turns thick, leathery, and black. This tissue is referred to as *eschar*.

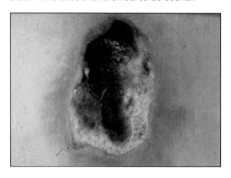

Differentiating tendon from slough

Performing debridement requires knowing where and what to cut. For example, tendon and slough both are yellow, and the clinician must be able to distinguish between them.

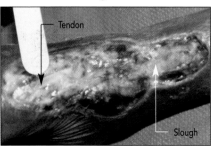

Surgical debridement case series

This pressure ulcer with slough and eschar requires surgical debridement due to advancing cellulitis.

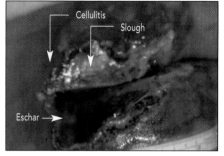

This photograph shows the same pressure ulcer after surgical debridement. Note the absence of eschar. Cellulitis is still present.

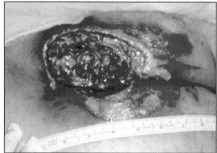

The same pressure ulcer after 7 days of treatment shows minimal necrotic tissue and significant amounts of granulation tissue. Note the change in the cellulitis surrounding the wound.

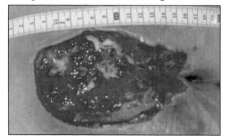

Wound debridement *(continued)*

Sharp debridement at the bedside

Small wounds may be debrided at the bedside, as shown below.

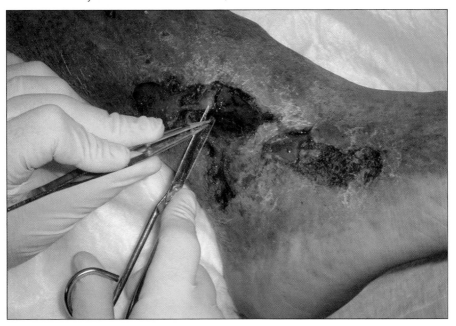

Notice the increased size of this ulcer after debridement.

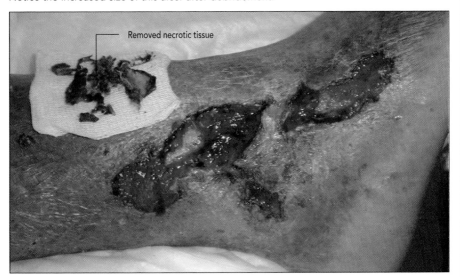

Removed necrotic tissue

Photographs above courtesy of Steven Black, MD.

Seating, positioning, and support surfaces

Multiple sensors integrated into a mat may be used to "map" the entire body area that comes in contact with the support surface. This pressure map of a patient lying face up on a horizontal support surface shows varying degrees of pressure exerted by the patient's heels, calves, thighs, buttocks, shoulders, and head.

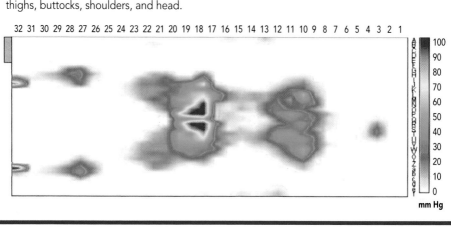

Pressure ulcers

Pressure ulcers are commonly staged using the National Pressure Ulcer Advisory Panel classification system described here.

Stage I

Observable, pressure-related alteration of intact skin whose indicators as compared to an adjacent or opposite area on the body may include changes in one or more of the following parameters: skin temperature (warmth or coolness), tissue consistency (firm or boggy feel), sensation (pain, itching). The ulcer appears as a defined area of persistent redness in lightly pigmented skin; in darker skin tones, the ulcer may appear with persistent red, blue, or purple hues.

STAGE I PRESSURE ULCER

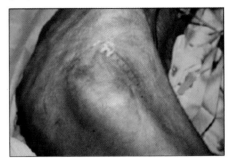

Stage II

Partial-thickness skin loss involving the epidermis or dermis. The ulcer is superficial and presents clinically as an abrasion, blister, or shallow crater.

STAGE II PRESSURE ULCERS

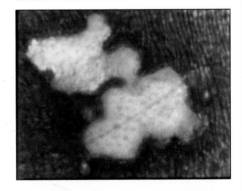

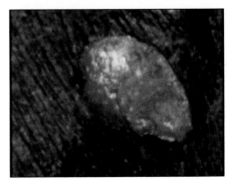

(continued)

Pressure ulcers *(continued)*

Stage III

Full-thickness skin loss involving damage or necrosis of subcutaneous tissue that may extend down to, but not through, underlying fascia. The ulcer presents clinically as a deep crater with or without undermining of adjacent tissue.

STAGE III PRESSURE ULCER

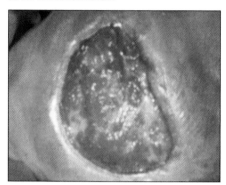

Stage IV

Full-thickness skin loss with extensive destruction, tissue necrosis, or damage to muscle, bone, or supporting structure (such as tendon or joint capsules).

STAGE IV PRESSURE ULCERS

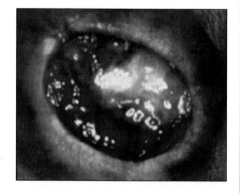

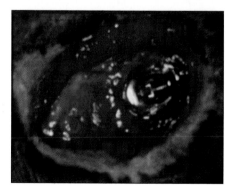

Reprinted with permission from the National Pressure Ulcer Advisory Panel slide series #1. Available: *www.npuap.org.*

Vascular ulcers

Vascular ulcers include wounds resulting from arterial, venous, and lymphatic conditions.

Arterial ulcer

This photograph shows a necrotic great toe with blisters on the toes and foot, representing arterial insufficiency.

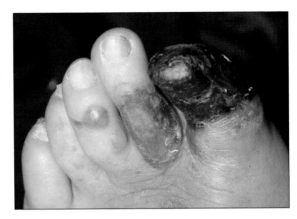

Venous ulcer

This photograph shows a venous ulcer. Venous ulcers are typically moist with irregular edges and firm, fibrotic, and indurated surrounding skin.

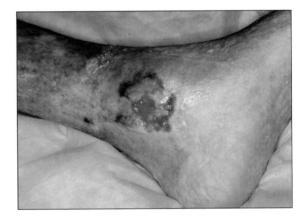

Lymphedema

This photograph shows lymphedema with fibrosis and scarring.

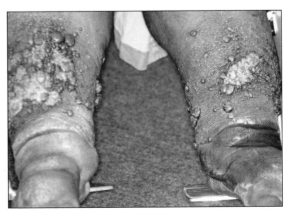

Diabetic foot ulcers

Ulcer on the sole

Repetitive, moderate pressure can cause skin breakdown and ulcers in the neuropathic foot, as shown here.

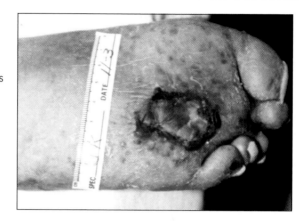

Charcot's foot with infection

This photograph shows Charcot's foot with infection present. Treatment of such wounds may include administration of parenteral antibiotics and surgical debridement of necrotic and infected tissue.

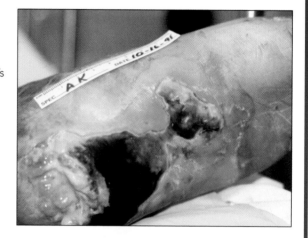

Callus with thick rim of tissue

Diabetic ulcers typically have a thick rim of keratinized tissue surrounding the wound, as shown here.

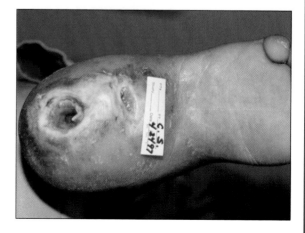

Ulcers in sickle cell disease

This is an example of an ulcer secondary to sickle cell disease. It has all the classic findings of a venous stasis ulcer, but ultrasound demonstrated no venous reflux.

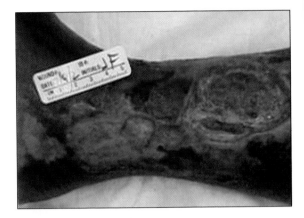

This wound had no infection, but wasn't healing. For this type of wound, the best treatment is surgical debridement.

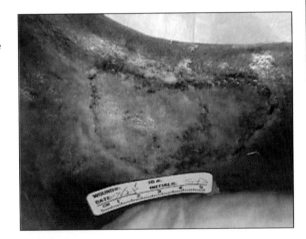

This is the same wound after surgical debridement. Note the healing that has occurred.

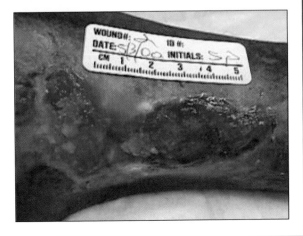

Complex acute wounds

Surgical closure of a pressure ulcer

This photograph shows markings made for gluteal fasciocutaneous flaps for surgical closure of a stage III pressure ulcer.

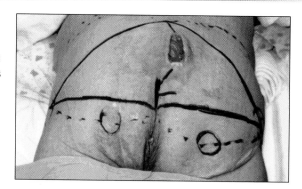

Shown here is surgical closure of the same ulcer.

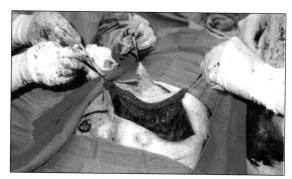

Necrotizing fasciitis

Shown here is necrotizing fasciitis of the abdomen.

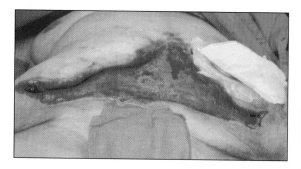

Calciphylaxis

This photograph shows calciphylaxis of both extremities in a patient with end-stage renal failure. Despite aggressive local wound care, the wounds never healed, and the patient died of sepsis.

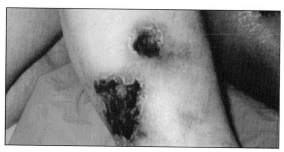

Complex acute wounds *(continued)*

Extravasation

Extravasation can cause tissue loss that may evolve into extensive wounds, as shown in this I.V. site 24 hours after infiltration of calcium chloride.

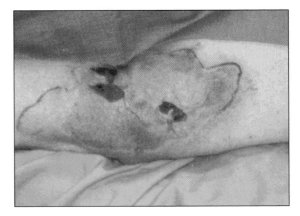

Shown here is the same site 48 hours later after wound debridement.

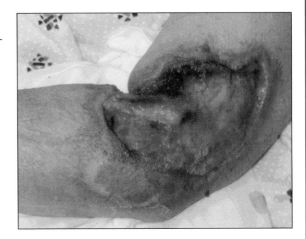

This photograph shows the same site after surgical debridement down to viable tissue.

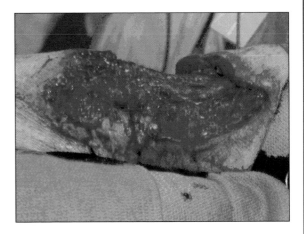

Atypical wounds

Wounds with uncommon etiologies are called *atypical wounds*.

Vasculitis

This photograph shows reticulated erythema and necrotic ulcers on the thighs of a patient with vasculitis.

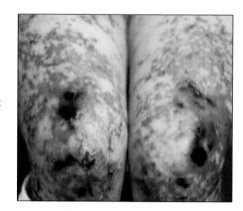

Pyoderma gangrenosum

In a patient with inflammatory bowel disease and pyoderma gangrenosum, this ulcer on the lateral leg shows areas of cribriform scarring.

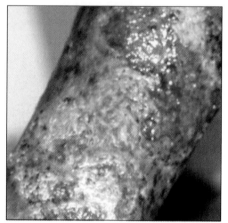

Shown here is peristomal pyoderma gangrenosum in a patient with Crohn's disease.

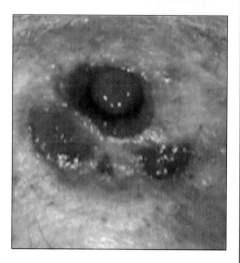

Atypical wounds *(continued)*

Infectious causes

Shown here is the leg and foot of a patient with Hansen's disease due to *Mycobacteria leprae*. In addition to neuropathic changes of the toes and plantar aspect of the foot, this patient has a large lateral leg ulcer as well.

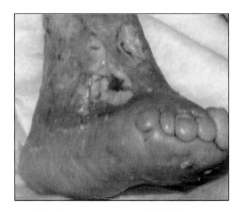

Cryofibrinogenemia

This patient has painful punctate ulcers on the feet and legs secondary to cryofibrinogenemia.

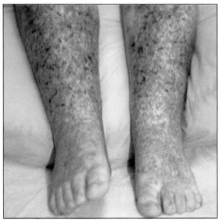

Calciphylaxis

Shown here is necrotic plaque with livedo reticularis in a dialysis patient with end-stage renal disease and calciphylaxis.

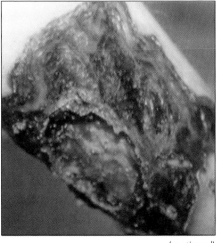

(continued)

Atypical wounds (continued)

Malignancies

Shown here is a right medial leg ulcer in a venous distribution secondary to T cell lymphoma.

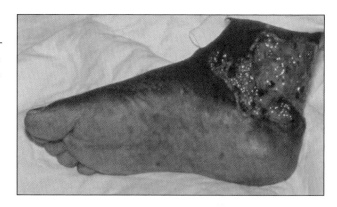

Factitial dermatitis

This photograph shows an angulated factitial ulcer on the breast. The term *factitial dermatitis* denotes a self-imposed injury.

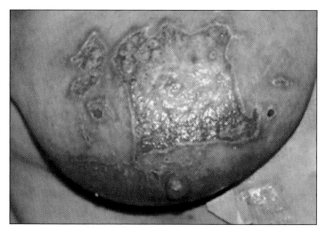

caregivers searched for the right answer. Today, research supports using moist wound therapy to promote a microenvironment conducive to healing. Numerous products and dressing choices are available for clinicians to utilize in their practice. (See chapter 9, Wound treatment options.)

The incidence and prevalence of pressure ulcers is truly an enigma. Pressure ulcers aren't a reportable event in all health care settings, so data is speculative at best. We do know, however, that the numbers are significant enough to warrant a national health care initiative in the United States. As early as 1989, the federal government focused their attention on pressure ulcers with the appointment of a panel charged with the development of the Agency for Health Care Policy and Research (AHCPR) guidelines. Another federal initiative that supports the fact that many peoples get pressure ulcers is Healthy People 2010. The objective is to reduce the incidence of pressure ulcers in the long-term care population by 50%.[2] In addition, the Centers for Medicare and Medicaid Services (CMS, formerly the Health Care Financing Administration) considers a pressure ulcer to be a sentinel event in a resident of a long-term care facility who has been assessed as being at low risk for a pressure ulcer. According to CMS, the only residents who are at high risk are those who have impaired transfer or bed mobility, are comatose, malnourished, or have end-stage disease; other patients are at low risk.[3] Given the attention that regulatory agencies have shown to pressure ulcer occurrence, pressure ulcer risk assessment should be a priority of patient care.

The financial cost to institutions and facilities isn't precisely known. Published estimates of treatment costs vary by hospital, long-term care, and home care settings; the one certainty is that pressure ulcers do create a financial burden for the facility, patient, and family. Pressure ulcers cost institutions valuable staff time, supplies, and reputation.

Pressure ulcer practices should be supported by scientific, evidence-based practice, not anecdotal success stories. This presents a problem. We don't have adequate research-based, randomized clinical studies to support our current practices. Wound care interventions and modalities have often been based on "it works for me." We need to encourage health care providers to participate in research studies so that we'll have the evidence in the future to direct and improve our clinical decision process, thereby improving patient outcomes.

Wound etiology

Pressure ulcers are believed to be localized wounds that develop over bony prominences due to excessive pressure, which leads to ischemia and necrosis, eventually resulting in tissue ulceration. The primary factor causing pressure ulcers is pressure. Maklebust[4] defined pressure as "a perpendicular load or force exerted on a unit of area." The correlation between tissue compression and ischemia is supported in the literature. The amount of pressure and the duration of that pressure are inversely proportional.[5] Low amounts of pressure over long periods of time can be just as detrimental to tissue as high amounts of pressure over short periods of time. The long-held standard of 32 mm Hg as a critical closing pressure is being revisited. Continued research is needed in the areas of capillary pressure, the application of uniform pressure, and the application of localized pressure. (See chapter 11, Seating, positioning, and support surfaces.)

Body tissues differ in their ability to tolerate pressure. The blood supply to the skin originates in the underlying

Pressure gradient

In the illustration to the right, the V-shaped pressure gradient results from the upward force (upward arrows) exerted by the supporting surface against downward force (downward arrows) exerted by the bony prominence. Pressure is greatest on tissues at the apex of the gradient and lessens to the right and left of this point.

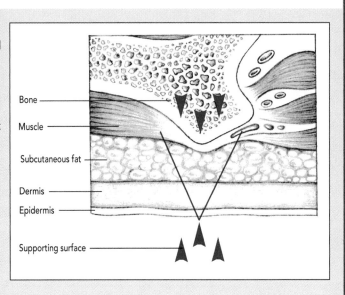

Bone

Muscle

Subcutaneous fat

Dermis

Epidermis

Supporting surface

muscle. Muscle is more sensitive to pressure damage than skin.[6] Tissue tolerance is further compromised by extrinsic and intrinsic factors. Examples of extrinsic factors are moisture, friction, and irritants. Intrinsic factors affecting the ability of the skin and supporting structures to respond to pressure and shear forces are numerous. Age, spinal cord injury, nutrition, and steroid administration are among intrinsic factors believed to affect collagen synthesis and degradation.[7] Other intrinsic factors that affect tissue perfusion are systemic blood pressure, extra corporeal circulation, serum protein, smoking, hemoglobin and hematocrit, vascular disease, diabetes mellitus, vasoactive drugs, and increase in body temperature. [7]

PRACTICE POINT

Muscle tissue dies first from pressure. Look at a variety of extrinsic and intrinsic factors that could put your patient at risk for pressure ulcers.

How do pressure ulcers occur? This is an interesting and challenging question. Literature reviews demonstrate only that the etiology of pressure ulcers continues to remain largely unclear. One theory is that pressure ulcers begin from the bone outward. Deep tissue injury near the bone occurs first, and it isn't until later when the tissue death continues and reaches the outer layer of the skin (the epidermis) that the skin breaks.[8] The pressure gradient model[8] has been used to explain how pressure translates into tissue death. (See *Pressure gradient*.) External pressure is transmitted from the epidermis inward toward the bone as well as counter-pressure from the bone. Pressure is transmitted from the body surface to the underlying bone, compressing all of the tissue in between. The greatest pressure occurs over the bone, gradually decreasing at the skin level. Blood vessels, fascia and muscle, subcutaneous fat, and the skin are compressed between these two counter pressures.

Muscle and subcutaneous fat have a low tolerance for decreased blood flow, making them less resilient than skin to pressure. Destruction of tissue below the skin level isn't seen until surface damage is evident. Unless there's an impairment in the nervous system resulting in loss of sensation, a patient will normally shift their weight by changing their position when pressure is exerted against the skin for a period of time.[4]

PRACTICE POINT

Patients with altered sensation are at risk for the development of pressure ulcers.

The second theory on pressure ulcer formation is that skin destruction occurs at the epidermis and proceeds downward to the deeper tissues. Makelbust and Sieggreen[8] call this theory the "top to bottom model." The injury is seen as intact skin with blanchable erythema. This is the least-favored model of pressure ulcer development, given its limited evidence base.

Friction and shear are also mechanical forces contributing to pressure ulcer formation. The tissue injury resulting from these forces may look like a superficial skin insult. Shear and friction are two separate phenomenon, yet often work together to create tissue ischemia and ulcer development.

Shear is a "mechanical force that acts on an area of skin in a direction parallel to the body's surface. Shear is affected by the amount of pressure exerted, the coefficient of friction between the materials contacting each other, and the extent to which the body makes contact with the support surface."[9] Think of this as pulling the bones of the pelvis in one direction and the skin in the opposite direction. (See *Shearing force.*) The deeper fascia slides downward with the bone

Shearing force

Shear injury is a mechanical force parallel, rather than perpendicular, to an area of tissue. In the illustration below, gravity pulls the body down the incline of the bed. The skeleton and attached deep fascia slide within the skin, while the skin and superficial fascia, attached to the dermis, remain stationary, held in place by friction between the skin and the bed linen. This internal slide compromises blood supply to the area.

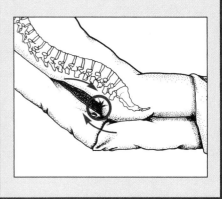

and the superficial fascia remains attached to the dermis. This insult and compromise to the blood supply creates ischemia and leads to cellular death and tissue necrosis. Shear and friction go hand in hand — you'll rarely see one without the other.

PRACTICE POINT

You won't see shear injury at the skin level because it occurs underneath the skin. You will see friction injury. Elevation of the head of the bed increases shear injury in the deep tissue, and may account for the number of sacral ulcers we see in practice.

Pressure ulcer sites

Shown in the illustration to the right are the most common sites where pressure ulcers develop.

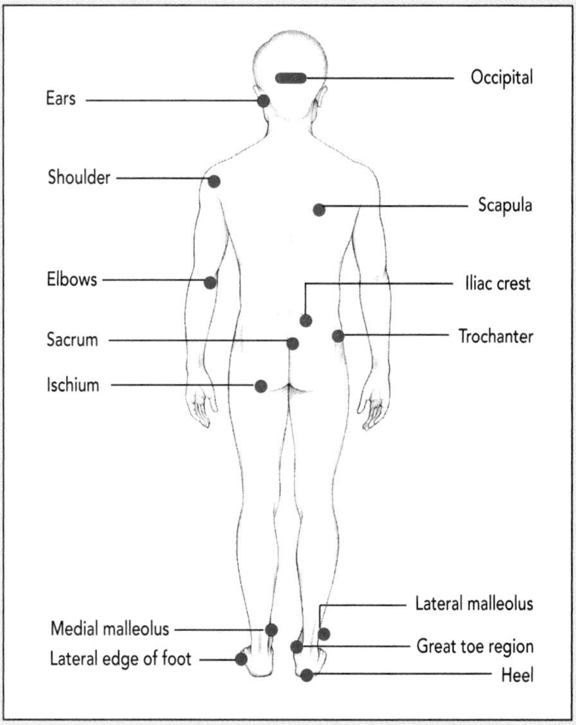

Ears

Shoulder

Elbows

Sacrum

Ischium

Occipital

Scapula

Iliac crest

Trochanter

Medial malleolus

Lateral edge of foot

Lateral malleolus

Great toe region

Heel

Friction is the "mechanical force exerted when skin is dragged across a coarse surface such as bed linens."[9] Simply stated, it's two surfaces moving across one another. A skin insult caused by friction looks like an abrasion or superficial laceration. Friction, however, isn't a primary factor in the development of pressure ulcers. It can contribute to an insult or stripping of the epidermal layer of the skin, creating an environment conducive to further insult. An alteration in the coefficient of friction increases the skin's adherence to the outside surface (the bed). Friction then combines with shearing forces and the ultimate outcome may be a pressure ulcer. Tissues subjected to friction are more susceptible to pressure ulcer damage.[10] The three mechanical forces (pressure, friction, and shear) may act in concert to create tissue damage. Other patients at risk for pressure ulcers from friction are elderly people, those with uncontrollable movements such as spastic movements, and those who use braces or appliances that rub against the skin.[8]

Theories on the etiology of a pressure ulcer need continued research. Those described here may be correct, but additional research and basic science hold the answers to many unanswered questions.

Most pressure ulcers occur in the lower part of the body over bony prominences such as the sacrum, coccyx, ischial tuberosities, greater trochanters, elbows, heels, scapulae, iliac crests, and lateral and medial malleoli.[8] (See *Pressure ulcer sites*.) Other areas, where pressure ulcers may be overlooked, include the occiput (especially in infants and toddlers), ears, and the great toe region. Several national surveys demonstrated that the most common site for pressure ulcers among patients in acute care facilities is the sacrum, with heels being second.[11-13] The incidence of heel ulcers has increased incrementally over the past decade, creating a need for prevention protocols targeting the heels.

 PRACTICE POINT

Careful observation of the sacrum and the heels is warranted because these are the most frequent sites of pressure ulcers.

Clinicians have sought guidance about a particular type of pressure ulcer seen on the heels. Their concerns are being addressed by the National Pressure Ulcer Advisory Panel (NPUAP) Task Force on unstageable deep-tissue injury ulcers. Typically, these wounds appear as dusky, boggy, or discolored areas of purple ecchymosis. Often these areas deteriorate rapidly from intact skin to deep open wounds. The belief is that these ulcers aren't true stage I or II ulcers. The NPUAP Task Force is reviewing the literature, probable etiology, and implications for documentation and classification, as well as prevention and treatment, of these ulcers.

Prevention

Preventing pressure ulcers is of vital importance. Elements of pressure ulcer prevention include identifying individuals at risk for developing pressure ulcers, preserving skin integrity, treating the underlying causes of the ulcer, relieving pressure, paying attention to the total state of the patient to correct any deficiencies, and educating the patient and his family.

Risk factors and risk assessment

Risk assessment is used to identify:
- patients at risk
- the level of risk
- the type of risk.

Identifying individuals at risk for pressure ulcers enables clinicians to make decisions about when to begin using preventive measures. This is important for the most effective use of resources because the level of risk guides the intensity and cost of preventive interventions. We tend to prescribe preventive protocols based on total scores, often ignoring the type of risk — and missing the point of a risk-based protocol. We should custom design protocols according to which pressure ulcer risk assessment subscale scores are low (that is, which risk factors are high). So, for example, if your patient has low subscores on activity, mobility, and moisture, and high scores for nutrition, you should customize interventions to prevent pressure and control moisture, but you don't need a big nutritional intervention, maybe just maintenance.

The clinical practice guidelines on pressure ulcer prevention from the Agency for Health Care Policy and Research (AHCPR; now the Agency for Health Care Research and Quality) are considered an important starting point for identifying at-risk patients and determining the need for prevention interventions. For example, the AHCPR Panel for Prediction and Prevention of Pressure Ulcers[14] suggests that bedridden patients and those with impaired ability to change position are at risk for pressure ulcers because of immobility. The guideline also suggests that these individuals should be assessed for additional factors that increase risk for developing pressure ulcers, which include incontinence, nutritional factors such as inadequate dietary intake or impaired nutritional status, and altered level of consciousness.[14] All risk assessments should be documented using a validated tool.

The many pressure ulcer risk assessment tools include the Norton Scale,[15] the Gosnell Scale,[16] the Braden Scale,[17] the Knoll Scale,[18] and the Waterlow Scale.[19] Deciding which scale to use can be challenging. Reviewing the reliability (consistency) and validity (accuracy) of each validated risk assessment scale should always be the first step in the decision-making process. Reliability for risk assessment scales is usually described by inter-rater reliability. "A common measure of inter-rater reliability for a risk assessment tool is percentage agreement, which looks at the percentage of instances in which different raters assign the same score to the same patients. Validity, or accuracy, is measured by the ability of the tool to correctly predict who will or won't develop a pressure ulcer."[20]

Predictive validity is dependent on the sensitivity and specificity of the tool. Sensitivity "is the percentage of individuals who develop a pressure ulcer who were assessed as being at risk for a pressure ulcer. A tool has good sensitivity if it correctly identifies true positives while minimizing false negatives. Specificity is the percentage of individuals who don't develop a pressure ulcer who were assessed as being not at risk for developing an ulcer. A tool has good specificity if it identifies true negatives and minimizes false positives."[20,21] Because of the amount of clinical research supporting their reliability and validity, the Norton and the Braden Scales are mentioned in the AHCPR guidelines as appropriate to use to determine pressure ulcer risk assessment.

Braden Scale

The Braden Scale is the most commonly used pressure ulcer assessment scale in the United States. Available in many languages and used world wide, this copyrighted tool, created in 1987 by Barbara Braden and Nancy Bergstrom, is available at *http://www.bradenscale.com.braden.pdf.* The Braden Scale has six subscales: sensory perception, moisture, activity, mobility, nutrition, and friction/shear.[17] (See *Braden Scale: Predicting pressure ulcer risk*, pages 248 and 249.) The scale is based on the two primary etiologic factors of pressure ulcer development — intensity and duration of pressure and tissue tolerance for pressure. "Sensory perception, mobility, and activity address clinical situations that predispose a patient to intense and prolonged pressure, while moisture, nutrition, and friction/shear address clinical situations that alter tissue tolerance for pressure."[20]

Each subscale contains a numerical range of scores, with 1 being the lowest score possible. The sensory perception, mobility, activity, moisture and nutrition subscales have scores ranging from 1 to 4. Friction/shear is the only subscale where scores range from 1 to 3. Definitions of each subscale as to patient characteristics to evaluate are given for each numerical ranking. The Braden Scale score is derived from totaling the numerical ratings from each of the six subscales. Six is the lowest possible score and 23 is the highest.

A low numerical score means the patient is at high-risk for developing pressure ulcers. The original risk score was 16.[17] Subsequent research is the basis for the recommendation to use 18 as the risk score for elderly,[22] Black, and Hispanic patients.[23,24] Although Braden and Bergstrom[20,21] suggested the following levels of risk based on total Braden Scale scores: 15 to 18, at risk; 13 to 14, moderate risk; 10 to 12, high risk; and 9 or below, very high risk; in practice, many clinicians just have two categories — patients who are at risk for pressure ulcers and those who aren't. Determining the risk level is helpful in deciding on appropriate prevention strategies. Clinical judgment should play a part in interpreting the total Braden Scale score because not all risk factors are quantified on the scale.

After the total Braden Scale score is computed, a patient's risk and need for preventive protocols can be determined. Because each health care agency may differ in terms of staffing patterns, access to clinicians who specialize in wound care, and the preventive products utilized, it's difficult to prescribe a set of protocols that will fit all circumstances; however, a broad outline of protocol development has been developed. More specific protocols should be written by each agency, and staff education for use of these protocols must be provided prior to their implementation.[20,21] (See *Braden score interventions*, page 250.)

Questions have surfaced regarding when to assess patients and when to do risk reassessment. These two aspects of care are both very important. The AHCPR clinical practice guideline on pressure ulcer prevention recommends that initial pressure ulcer risk assessment be done upon admission as well as reassessments at periodic intervals.[14] The guideline doesn't provide time frames for reassessments, however. Reassessment intervals should be based on the acuity of the individual for whom the pressure ulcer risk is being calculated. Studies by Bergstrom and Braden[22,25] found that in a skilled nursing facility, 80% of pressure ulcers develop within 2 weeks of admission and 96% develop within 3 weeks of admission. The following recommendations for assessment and reassessment are based on this research.[20-22,25]

• Acute care — Initial assessment on admission, reassess at least every 48 hours or whenever the patient's condition changes.

• Long-term care — Initial assessment on admission, then reassess weekly for the first 4 weeks, monthly to quarterly after that, and whenever the resident's condition changes.

• Home health care — On admission, then reassess with every visit.

As far as what time of day a pressure ulcer risk assessment should be done, research demonstrates that no particular time of day is better than another to do a pressure ulcer risk assessment. Outside of home care, patient care activities can vary from shift to shift. Risk assessment can be scheduled on either the day or evening shift, according to when it will best fit with staffing patterns and be performed most consistently.[20,21]

Importance of risk assessment

Some clinicians believe that an informal pressure ulcer risk assessment is sufficient and that a formal risk assessment is unnecessary. On the contrary, an informal risk assessment can't take the place of a formal risk assessment like one conducted using the Braden Scale. Research has shown that in the absence of formal risk assessment, clinicians tended to intervene consistently only at the highest levels of risk. In some studies, for example, turning — considered an important part of pressure ulcer prevention — was prescribed for fewer than 50% of patients at mild or moderate risk for developing pressure ulcers. Pressure reduction was prescribed more than turning, but not with adequate consistency.[26]

In a study that introduced formal risk assessment and linked levels of risk to preventive protocols, the incidence of pressure ulcers dropped by 60%; severity of pressure ulcers and cost of care decreased as well.[26] This could be due to better identification of patients at mild

(Text continues on page 250.)

Braden Scale: Predicting pressure ulcer risk

SENSORY PERCEPTION Ability to respond meaningfully to pressure-related discomfort	**1. Completely limited:** Unresponsive (doesn't moan, flinch, or grasp) to painful stimuli due to diminished level of consciousness or sedation OR limited ability to feel pain over most of body surface.	**2. Very limited:** Responds only to painful stimuli. Can't communicate discomfort except by moaning or restlessness OR has a sensory impairment that limits the ability to feel pain or discomfort over half of body.
MOISTURE Degree to which skin is exposed to moisture	**1. Constantly moist:** Skin is kept moist almost constantly by perspiration or urine. Dampness is detected every time patient is moved or turned.	**2. Often moist:** Skin is often but not always moist. Linen must be changed at least once per shift.
ACTIVITY Degree of physical activity	**1. Bedfast:** Confined to bed.	**2. Confined to chair:** Ability to walk severely limited or nonexistent. Can't bear own weight and must be assisted into chair or wheelchair.
MOBILITY Ability to change and control body position	**1. Completely immobile:** Doesn't make even slight changes in body or extremity position without assistance.	**2. Very limited:** Makes occasional slight changes in body or extremity position but unable to make frequent or significant changes independently.
NUTRITION Usual food intake pattern NPO: Nothing by mouth IV: Intravenously TPN: Total parenteral nutrition	**1. Very poor:** Never eats a complete meal. Rarely eats more than one-third of any food offered. Eats two servings or less of protein (meat or dairy products) per day. Takes fluids poorly. Doesn't take a liquid dietary supplement OR is NPO or maintained on clear liquids or I.V. fluids for more than 5 days.	**2. Probably inadequate:** Rarely eats a complete meal and generally eats only about half of any food offered. Protein intake includes only three servings of meat or dairy products per day. Occasionally will take a dietary supplement OR receives less than optimum amount of liquid diet or tube feeding.
FRICTION AND SHEAR	**1. Problem:** Requires moderate to maximum assistance in moving. Complete lifting without sliding against sheets is impossible. Frequently slides down in bed or chair, requiring frequent repositioning with maximum assistance. Spasticity, contractures, or agitation leads to almost constant friction.	**2. Potential problem:** Moves feebly or requires minimum assistance. During a move, skin probably slides to some extent against sheets, chair, restraints, or other devices. Maintains relatively good position in chair or bed most of the time but occasionally slides down.

Used with permission from Barbara Braden, PhD, RN, FAAN, and Nancy Bergstrom, PhD, RN, FAAN. © 1988.

3. Slightly limited:
Responds to verbal commands but can't always communicate discomfort or need to be turned
OR
has some sensory impairment that limits ability to feel pain or discomfort in one or two extremities.

4. No impairment:
Responds to verbal commands. Has no sensory deficit that would limit ability to feel or voice pain or discomfort.

3. Occasionally moist:
Skin is occasionally moist, requiring an extra linen change approximately once per day.

4. Rarely moist:
Skin is usually dry; linen only requires changing at routine intervals.

3. Walks occasionally:
Walks occasionally during day, but for very short distances, with or without assistance; spends majority of each shift in bed or chair.

4. Walks frequently:
Walks outside the room at least twice per day and inside room at least once every 2 hours during waking hours.

3. Slightly limited:
Makes frequent though slight changes in body or extremity position independently.

4. No limitations:
Makes major and frequent changes in position without assistance.

3. Adequate:
Eats over half of most meals. Eats a total of four servings of protein (meat, dairy products) each day. Occasionally will refuse a meal, but will usually take a supplement if offered
OR
is on a tube feeding or TPN regimen that probably meets most nutritional needs.

4. Excellent:
Eats most of every meal and never refuses a meal. Usually eats a total of four servings of meat and dairy products. Occasionally eats between meals. Doesn't require supplementation.

3. No apparent problem:
Moves in bed and in chair independently and has sufficient muscle strength to lift up completely during move. Maintains good position in bed or chair at all times.

Braden score interventions

- At risk: 15 to 18 — Consider a protocol of frequent turning, facilitating maximal re-mobilization, protecting the patient's heels, providing a pressure-reducing support surface if the patient is bedridden or confined to a chair, and managing moisture, nutrition, and friction and shear. If other major risk factors are present (advanced age, fever, poor dietary intake of protein, diastolic blood pressure below 60 mm Hg, or hemodynamic instability), advance to the next level of risk.

- Moderate risk: 13 to 14 — Consider a protocol of frequent turning, facilitating maximal remobilization, protecting the patient's heels, providing a pressure-reducing support surface, providing foam wedges for 30-degree lateral positioning, and managing moisture, nutrition, and friction and shear. If other major risk factors are present, advance to the next level of risk.

- High risk: 10 to 12 — Consider a protocol that increases the frequency of turning, supplements turning with small shifts in position, facilitates maximal remobilization, protects the patient's heels, provides a pressure-reducing support surface, provides foam wedges for 30-degree lateral positioning, and manages moisture, nutrition, and friction and shear.

- Very high risk: 9 or below — Consider a protocol that incorporates the points for high-risk patients. Add a pressure-relieving surface if the patient has intractable pain, severe pain exacerbated by turning, or additional risk factors such as immobility and malnutrition. A low-air-loss bed is no substitute for a turning schedule.

- Managing moisture — Use a commercial moisture barrier, and use absorbent pads or diapers that wick and hold moisture. Address the cause of the moisture if possible, and offer a bedpan or urinal and a glass of water in conjunction with turning schedules.

- Managing nutrition — Consult a dietitian and act quickly to alleviate nutritional deficits. Increase the patient's protein intake and increase his calorie intake if needed. Provide a multivitamin containing vitamins A, C, and E.

- Managing friction and shear — Elevate the head of the bed no more than 30 degrees and have the patient use a trapeze when indicated. Use a lift sheet to move the patient. Protect the patient's elbows, heels, sacrum, and back of head if he's exposed to friction.

- Other general care issues — Don't massage reddened bony prominences and don't use donut-type devices. Maintain good hydration and avoid drying out the patient's skin.

Adapted with permission from Ayello, E.A., and Braden, B. "How and Why to Do a Pressure Ulcer Risk Assessment," *Advances in Skin & Wound Care* 15(3):125-32, May-June 2002.

and moderate risk and a more consistent use of preventive interventions for patients in all risk categories.

Patient care to prevent pressure ulcers

Preventing pressure ulcers can best be accomplished by using a multidisciplinary approach.[14] Any good prevention program begins with assessing the patient's skin. The skin should be assessed and its condition documented daily in acute and long-term care settings and at each home care visit. Careful attention to preventing skin injury during performance of activities of daily living is paramount. The bathing schedule should be individualized based on the patient's age, skin texture, and dryness or excessive oiliness of the skin. Use of nondrying products to clean the skin is recommended. Avoid excessive friction and hot water when cleaning. Use nonalcoholic moisturizers after bathing. A daily bath may not be needed for all patients; elderly patients, for example, may benefit from "lotion" baths.

For the incontinent patient, moist barriers and ointments should be considered as treatment options. Soiled skin should be cleaned immediately and products to protect the skin applied. If containment products are used, follow the correct methods of application. Reasons for incontinence should always be determined and appropriate measures to address the cause of the incontinence should be implemented.

The skin should be protected from injury. Pad bony prominences using dressings such as films, hydrocolloids, foams, stockinettes, or roller gauze. Don't massage reddened bony prominences because this can lead to further tissue damage. Keep the patient's heels off the bed; use pillows, wedges, and foot elevation devices as indicated. A folded bath blanket under the calves can "float the heels," completely relieving heel pressure in a bedridden patient.

PRACTICE POINT

Keep the patient's heels off the mattress!

Be careful not to drag your patient during transfers or position changes. Use appropriate devices, such as a turn sheet or mechanical lifting device, to prevent friction injuries to the patient's skin. Use the 30-degree lateral position for patients in bed. Keep the head of the bed below 30 degrees to prevent shearing injuries, unless contraindicated due to the patient's clinical condition.

Although no random clinical studies have documented the effects of specific nutritional interventions in preventing pressure ulcers, a large prospective cohort study by Bergstrom and Braden[22] found that nursing home residents who developed pressure ulcers had a significantly lower intake of protein. Clinicians need to ensure that a patient's caloric, protein, and vitamin and minerals needs are met. Recommendations from the dietitian can be an important source of assistance in helping patients to get their required nutrients.

Physical and occupational therapists are important members of the pressure ulcer team, a valuable resource for maximizing the patient's mobility. Their expertise in selecting appropriate size wheelchairs and evaluating seating angles and postural alignment can't be over emphasized. Patients who are confined to a chair should be repositioned every hour, with small shifts in weight made every 15 minutes. Although most clinicians consider turning and repositioning a bedridden patient every 2 hours a standard of care, the appropriate turning interval for all patients has yet to be determined by research. For some, 2 hours may be too long, whereas for others every 2 hours may not be necessary, as for palliative care patients, where frequent repositioning would cause more pain and suffering than benefit.

PRACTICE POINT

Turning schedules should be developed based on the individual patient's needs and care goals.

Appropriate pressure relieving devices and surfaces need to be used. (See chapter 11, Seating, positioning, and support surfaces.) Devices such as "donuts" shouldn't be used.

Ongoing monitoring and documentation is essential. Communication of the prevention plan to all members of the health care team, including the patient and his family, is imperative. Supplement your verbal teaching with one of the many prevention booklets designed for use by the consumer. An example is the NPUAP booklet, "Consumer Education Guide-What are Pressure Ulcers," which can be downloaded from the NPUAP Web site (www.npuap.org). This pamphlet is an easy-to-read guide that can be used for a wide variety of patients. In addition, the AHCPR has a consumer version in Spanish.

Pressure ulcer staging

A comprehensive wound assessment includes many parameters, one of which is staging. (See chapter 6, Wound assessment.) Once the wound etiology is known, the correct classification system to describe the wound can be selected. For example, arterial and venous ulcers are described by their characteristics. Diabetic or neuropathic ulcers are now being classified by the American Diabetes Association, Wagner Grading System for Vascular Wounds, or San Antonio Diabetic Wound Classification System. The NPUAP staging system was designed specifically for pressure ulcers. An outcome of the first NPUAP consensus conference[27] was the NPUAP staging system for pressure ulcers, which was based on Shea's[28] and the International Association of Enterostomal Therapists[29] (now called WOCN) staging systems. Pressure ulcer staging is a system to describe the level of tissue destroyed. It provides practitioners with a common language to communicate with each other what the pressure ulcer looks like clinically. Staging is only part of the total assessment of the ulcer, which includes other factors such as surrounding skin and presence of infection, to name a few. (See chapter 6, Wound assessment.) Among the staging systems used, Shea's[28] is the earliest to be used in the United States, with the NPUAP staging system[27] being the most widely used.

Pressure ulcers should be staged by determining the deepest area of tissue insult. Necrotic wounds can't be staged since visualization of the wound bed is necessary to determine the level of tissue involvement. Staging of necrotic wounds should be done after the necrotic tissue is removed. (See chapter 8, Wound debridement.) The wound should be described and you should note that it's unstageable at this time. Be sure to offload the area and begin other appropriate treatments.

PRACTICE POINT

Even though you can't "stage" an unstageable ulcer, remember that the tissue damage could worsen and still needs to be treated.

NPUAP classification of pressure ulcers staging definitions

The most widely used pressure ulcer staging tool, the NPUAP classification system for staging pressure ulcers is described below.

Stage I

The original definition of a stage I pressure ulcer was "nonblanchable erythema of intact skin, the heralding lesion of skin ulceration."[27] Given the diversity of people with different skin pigmentation, detecting stage I pressure ulcers can be a challenge if clinicians only use color as an indicator. To provide a more cultural-ly sensitive definition, NPUAP revised the definition to include indicators that went beyond color: "An observable pres-sure-related alteration of intact skin whose indicators, as compared with the adjacent or opposite area on the body, may include changes in 1 or more of the following: skin temperature (warmth or coolness), tissue consistency (firm or boggy feel), and/or sensations (pain, itching). The ulcer appears as a defined area of persistent redness in lightly pig-mented skin, whereas, in darker skin tones, the ulcer may appear with persis-tent red, blue, or purple tones."[30] NPUAP continues to refine this stage I definition.

Ayello and Lyder[31] reported that peo-ple with darkly pigmented skin had the lowest prevalence of stage I pressure ul-cers, but the highest prevalence of stage II to IV ulcers. The incidence of pressure ulcers was higher in people with darkly pigmented skin in several studies con-ducted by Lyder and colleagues.[23,24] In unpublished data, Lyder found a higher accuracy of 78% versus 58% when the new revised stage I definition was used.[32] One study[33] provided evidence to support skin temperature (warmth or coolness) as part of the revised stage I definition. Sprigle and colleagues[33] also found that warmth or coolness was present in 85% of patients with stage I pressure ulcers.

Staging concepts

Pressure ulcer staging is only appropriate to use to define the maximum depth of tissue "wounded." Some clinicians have erroneously used it in reverse order to describe improvement in the ulcer. Use of the NPUAP staging system to describe healing is physiologically inaccurate and shouldn't be done. (See *NPUAP position statement on reverse staging*, page 254.) When stage IV pressure ulcers heal to progressively more shallow depth, they

don't replace lost muscle, subcutaneous fat, and dermis before they re-epithelial-ize. Instead, the wound is filled with granulation tissue. Therefore, the ulcer doesn't heal from a stage IV to III, II to I. More information about why clini-cians shouldn't follow this inaccurate practice of "reverse staging" can be found in the NPUAP position statement on reverse staging or on the NPUAP Web site (*www.npuap.org*).

Pressure ulcer staging concepts may not address all forms of pressure ulcers. Clinicians often struggle with the con-cept of deep-tissue injury that presents as a purplish color, most often seen in the heel area. What do we call these ul-cers — stage I, stage III, or stage IV? NPUAP has called together a task force to review these deep-tissue injury wounds. A tentative definition of deep tissue injury is: A pressure-related injury to subcutaneous tissues under intact skin. Initially, these lesions have the ap-pearance of a deep bruise. These lesions may herald the subsequent development of a Stage III or Stage IV pressure ulcer even with optimal management.

Pressure ulcer treatment

The AHCPR developed evidence-based guidelines on the management of pres-sure ulcers and published their results, Treatment of Pressure Ulcers, in December, 1994.[9] The guideline pro-vides the foundation for evidence-based pressure ulcer management.

A pressure ulcer won't heal unless the underlying causes are effectively man-aged. A general assessment should in-clude identifying and effectively manag-ing the medical diseases, health problems (such as urinary incontinence), nutrition-al status, pain level, and psychosocial health that may have placed the patient at risk for pressure ulcer development.

NPUAP position statement on reverse staging

What is staging?

Staging is an assessment system that classifies pressure ulcers based on anatomic depth of soft tissue damage.[88,89] This assessment system only describes the anatomic status of the ulcer at the time of assessment. Staging of pressure ulcers can only occur after necrotic tissue has been removed, allowing complete visualization of the ulcer bed. Pressure ulcer staging is only appropriate for defining the maximum anatomic depth of tissue damage.

What is reverse staging?

In 1989, due to a lack of research-validated tools to measure pressure ulcer healing, clinicians resorted to using pressure ulcer staging systems in reverse order to describe improvement in an ulcer

Why not reverse stage?

Pressure ulcers heal to progressively more shallow depth; they do not replace lost muscle, subcutaneous fat, or dermis before they re-epithelialize.[90] Instead, the ulcer is filled with granulation (scar) tissue composed primarily of endothelial cells, fibroblasts, collagen, and extracellular matrix. A stage IV pressure ulcer cannot become a stage III, stage II, and/or subsequently stage 1 ulcer. When a stage IV ulcer has healed, it should be classified as a healed stage IV pressure ulcer, not a stage 0 pressure ulcer. Therefore, reverse staging does not accurately characterize what is physiologically occurring in the ulcer. The progress of a healing pressure ulcer can only be documented using ulcer characteristics or by improvement in wound characteristics using a validated pressure ulcer healing tool.[90]

How should you document a healing pressure ulcer?

NPUAP does recognize that federal regulations require long-term care facilities to reverse stage at the present time; however, long-term care facilities are encouraged to also document in the medical record appropriate healing using either descriptive characteristics of the wound (such as depth, width, and presence of granulation tissue) or using a validated pressure ulcer healing tool. If a pressure ulcer reopens in the same anatomical site, the ulcer resumes the previous staging diagnosis (once a stage IV, alway a stage IV).

What is NPUAP doing to replace reverse staging?

Since 1996, NPUAP has developed and validated the Pressure Ulcer Scale for Healing (PUSH) tool.[91] This tool documents pressure ulcer healing. Presently, this tool is being pilot tested for adoption by the U.S. Health Care Financing Administration Minimum Data Set Post Acute Care system.

Unless these major areas are effectively addressed, the probability of the pressure ulcer healing is unlikely.

The comprehensive management of pressure ulcers includes cleaning, controlling infections, debridement, dressings that promote a moist wound environment, nutritional support, and redistributory pressure (turning and use of support surfaces). (See chapter 11,

Seating, positioning, and support surfaces.) The use of adjunctive therapies to heal pressure ulcers should be considered for recalcitrant pressure ulcers.

Pressure ulcer assessment

As discussed above, no universal system for pressure ulcer classification exists — and until staging of the pressure ulcer occurs, effective treatment can't commence. Staging alone, however, doesn't determine the seriousness of the ulcer. In the United States, most systems use four stages to classify ulceration and the NPUAP staging system is the most commonly used.

PRACTICE POINT

Unstageable pressure ulcers are those covered with necrotic tissue. Until the eschar is removed, the ulcer can't be accurately visualized and is therefore unstageable.

Cleaning

Cleaning the pressure ulcer to remove devitalized tissue and decrease bacterial burden is often recommended. Pressure ulcers exhibit delayed healing in the presence of high levels of bacteria.[34] Solutions that don't traumatize the ulcer should be used.[35] Normal saline solution (0.9%) is usually recommended because it isn't cytotoxic to healthy tissue.[9] Although the active ingredients in newer wound cleaners may be noncytotoxic (surfactants), the inert carrier may be cytotoxic to healthy granulation tissue. Review of all ingredients is warranted. Hellewell et al.[36] found that antiseptic cleaners were the most cytotoxic to granulation tissue.

The mechanical method used to deliver the cleaning agent must provide enough pressure to remove debris without presenting trauma to the ulcer bed. Optimal pressure to clean an ulcer is between 4 to 15 pounds per square inch (psi).[37] A 35-ml syringe with a 19 gauge needle creates an 8 psi irrigation pressure stream,[9] which was found to be more effective in removing bacteria than other irrigation pressures.[38] It should be noted that irrigation pressures exceeding 15 psi can cause trauma to the ulcer bed and may drive bacteria into the tissue.[39] New technology such as battery-powered, disposable irrigation devices can provide an alternative to loosen wound debris from the syringe and needle system.

Debridement

The presence of necrotic devitalized tissue promotes the growth of pathologic organisms and prevents wounds from healing.[40] Therefore, debridement is a very important step in the management of pressure ulcers. There's no optimal debridement method; therefore, selection of the debridement method should be based on the goals of the patient, absence or presence of infection, amount of necrotic tissue present, and economic considerations for the patient and the facility.

Many types of debridement, including surgical, autolytic, enzymatic, mechanical, and laser, are available. (See chapter 8, Wound debridement.) However, surgical (or sharp laser) debridement is considered by many the most effective type of debridement because it involves the cutting away (with a scalpel) of necrotic tissue.[41] In addition, surgical debridement is relatively quick and can be done at the bedside. Surgical debridement is essential when cellulitis or sepsis is suspected.[42] Autolytic debridement involves the use of a semi-occlusive or occlusive dressing (hydrocolloids, hydrogels). This type of debridement uses the body's own natural enzymes to digest necrotic tissue. It's relatively painless, but takes much longer than sharp debridement. Watch closely for signs and symptoms of infection. Enzymatic debridement uses proteolytic enzymes (such as papain and urea, collagenase, and trypsin) to remove necrotic tissue. This form of debridement is slow and can be expensive.[41] Mechanical debridement uses wet-to-dry gauze to adhere to the necrotic tissue, which is then removed. Upon removal of the gauze dressing, necrotic tissue and wound debris are removed. However, healthy granulation tissue is also removed. This can delay wound healing.[41]

Pressure redistribution

The use of support surfaces is an important consideration in redistributing pressure. (See chapter 11, Seating, positioning, and support surfaces.) The use of dynamic support surfaces in high risk patients has lead to improved outcomes and cost savings. The CMS has divided support surfaces into three categories for reimbursement purposes. Group one devices are those support surfaces that are static; they don't require electricity. Static devices include air, foam (convoluted and solid), gel, and water-overlay mattresses. These devices are ideal when a patient is at low to moderate risk for pressure ulcer development. They redistribute pressure, may decrease shearing, and are relatively inexpensive. If foam is used, it should weigh 1.3 lb per cubic foot and be more than 3″ (7.5 cm) thick.

Group two devices are powered by electricity or a pump and are considered dynamic in nature. These devices include alternating and low-air-loss mattresses. These mattresses are good for patients that are at moderate to high risk for pressure ulcers or have full-thickness pressure ulcers. The advantages of alternating air mattresses include portability, redistribution of pressure, reduced shearing, and moderate cost. The disadvantage of some of these mattresses is their

inability to reduce heat accumulation on the patient's body. The advantages of low-air-loss mattresses are pressure reduction, low moisture retention and reduction of heat accumulation. The disadvantage of low-air-loss beds is that they can be expensive.

Group three devices are also considered dynamic in nature. This classification comprises only air-fluidized beds. These beds are electric and contain silicone-coated beads. They're used for patients at very high risk for pressure ulcers, and after flap or graft surgery. They're often used for patients with nonhealing full-thickness pressure ulcers or those with numerous truncal full-thickness pressure ulcers. The advantages of air-fluidized beds are that they redistribute pressure and reduce heat accumulation, moisture retention, and shearing forces. The patient's ability to move in a fluidized bed is hampered and considered a disadvantage of the product. Few studies demonstrate significant differences within the support surface classifications and preventing or healing pressure ulcers. Therefore, the level and type of risk factors should guide the level and type of support surface selected.

Dressings

The use of moist wound therapy dressings is a major component in managing a pressure ulcer. (See chapter 9, Wound treatment options.) At present, it's conservatively estimated that there are thousands of different dressings available for pressure ulcer management. Dressings can be broken down into several classifications: gauze, nonadherent gauze, transparent films, hydrocolloids, foams, alginates, hydrogels, collagens, antimicrobials, composites, and combinations. Matching the dressing to the wound bed characteristics is essential. A guiding principle is to maintain a moist environment.

Although nongauze dressings are usually more expensive than gauze dressing, less frequent dressing changes, faster healing rates, and decreased rates of infection can make nongauze-based dressing more cost-effective over time.[43-46] It's also important to note that wet-to-dry gauze dressings are a form of debridement and shouldn't be used on ulcers with good granulation tissue. No specific dressing heals all pressure ulcers within an ulcer classification. Consequently, a careful assessment of the pressure ulcer, the patient's needs, and environmental factors (frequency of dressing changes to increase adherence) must be considered. (See chapter 9, Wound treatment options.)

Nutrition

Nutrition is important to maintain the body in positive nitrogen balance, thereby increasing wound healing. It's important to increase protein stores for patients with pressure ulcers who are malnourished. In the absence of deficiency, however, little empirical evidence exist showing that vitamins and mineral supplements aid in pressure ulcer healing or prevention.[47-50] Therefore, providing supplements to patients without protein, vitamin, or mineral deficiencies should be avoided. The use of enteral and parental nutritional support should always be considered when the patient is unable to meet his caloric needs.

Monitoring healing

Since the use of reverse staging of pressure ulcers to monitor healing is inappropriate, several instruments have been developed and validated to assess the healing of pressure ulcers. The two most widely used tools are the Pressure Sore Status Tool (PSST)[51] and the Pressure Ulcer Scale for Healing (PUSH).[52] The PSST is comprised of 13 variables used to provide a numerical indicator of the status of the pressure ulcer (healing or deteriorating).[51] The score ranges from 1, which indicates tissue health (or healed) to 65, which indicates wound degeneration. The variables that comprise the PSST score include: size (length and width), depth, edges, undermining, necrotic tissue type, necrotic tissue amount, exudate type, exudate amount, skin color of surrounding wound, peripheral tissue edema, peripheral tissue induration, granulation tissue, and epithelialization. The PSST provides a comprehensive assessment of the pressure ulcer. This tool is currently being evaluated for use with other wound types.

The PUSH tool[52] is comprised of only three variables: surface area (length and width), exudate amount, and tissue appearance to derive a numerical indicator of the status of the pressure ulcer. (See *NPUAP PUSH tool*, page 258.) A score of 0 would indicate that the pressure ulcer has healed, with the highest score of 17 indicating wound degeneration. The PUSH tool intentionally took a "minimalist approach." Using research databases on its development, PUSH seeks to select the minimal number of assessment parameters needed to monitor healing or deterioration of the ulcer. This makes it ideal for quality assurance monitoring of large groups of patients and identifying patients who are deteriorating and require reassessment and possibly treatment changes. Its brevity, combined with its accuracy in monitoring, makes it ideal for incorporation in the Minimum Data Set-Post Acute Care (MDS-PAC). PUSH isn't intended to provide a comprehensive assessment of pressure ulcers and hasn't yet been validated for other types of wounds, although it's being tested in research studies and clinical use.

The use of high-frequency portable ultrasound to measure wound healing has

NPUAP PUSH tool

PATIENT NAME: _____ PATIENT ID. # _____

ULCER LOCATION: _____ DATE: _____

Directions

Observe and measure the pressure ulcer. Categorize the ulcer with respect to surface area, exudate, and type of wound tissue. Record a subscore for each of the ulcer characteristics. Add the subscores to obtain the total score. A comparison of total scores measured over time provides an indication of the improvement or deterioration in pressure ulcer healing.

LENGTH	0	1	2	3	4	5	Blank
	0 cm²	<0.3 cm²	0.3 – 0.6 cm²	0.7 – 1.0 cm²	1.1 – 2.0 cm²	2.1 – 3.0 cm²	
× WIDTH		6	7	8	9	10	Sub-score
		3.1 – 4.0 cm²	4.1 – 8.0 cm²	8.1 – 12.0 cm²	12.1 – 24.0 cm²	>24.0 cm²	
EXUDATE AMOUNT	0 None	1 Light	2 Moderate	3 Heavy			Sub-score
TISSUE TYPE	0 Closed	1 Epithelial Tissue	2 Granulation Tissue	3 Slough	4 Necrotic Tissue		Sub-score
							Total score

LENGTH × WIDTH
Measure the greatest length (head to toe) and the greatest width (side to side) using a centimeter ruler. Multiply these two measurements (length × width) to obtain an estimate of surface area in square centimeters (cm²). Do not guess! Always use a centimeter ruler and always use the same method each time the ulcer is measured.

EXUDATE AMOUNT
Estimate the amount of exudate (drainage) present after removal of the dressing and before applying any topical agent to the ulcer. Estimate the exudate as none, light, moderate, or heavy.

TISSUE TYPE
This refers to the types of tissue that are present in the wound (ulcer) bed. Score as a "4" if any necrotic tissue is present. Score as a "3" if any amount of slough is present and necrotic tissue is absent. Score as a "2" if the wound is clean and contains granulation tissue. Score as a "1" if the wound is superficial and reepithelializing. Score as a "0" if the wound is closed.
   4–Necrotic tissue (eschar): Black, brown, or tan tissue that adheres firmly to the wound bed or ulcer edges and may be either firmer or softer than surrounding tissue.
   3–Slough: Yellow or white tissue that adheres to the ulcer bed in strings or thick clumps or is mucinous.
   2–Granulation tissue: Pink or beefy-red tissue with a shiny, moist, granular appearance.
   1–Epithelial tissue: For superficial ulcers, new pink or shiny tissue (skin) that grows in from the edges or as islands on the ulcer surface.
   0–Closed/resurfaced: The wound is completely covered with epithelium (new skin).

PUSH Tool version 3.0, ©1998 National Pressure Ulcer Advisory Panel, Reston Va. Used with permission.

also been introduced. The use of this technology, which can capture three-dimensional measurements, has been shown to be quite beneficial in objectively monitoring healing. Ultrasound is "color blind"; that is, it can detect stage I pressure ulcers in darkly pigmented skin.[7]

Control of infections

All pressure ulcers will become colonized with both aerobic and anaerobic bacteria; therefore, pressure ulcers aren't sterile wounds. (See chapter 7, Wound bioburden.) Because all pressure ulcers will be colonized, avoid swab-culturing the surface of a pressure ulcer. Clean technique is customarily used when treating pressure ulcers. If an ulcer may be infected (independent of a puncture biopsy), most experts assess for the amount of drainage and odor and examine the surrounding tissue for cellulitis. It should be noted that some infected ulcers may not demonstrate the typical signs and symptoms associated with infection; rather, they may appear as nonhealing ulcers.

Until the pressure ulcer infection is controlled, the ulcer won't heal. The use of topical agents such as sulfa silvadene and oral antibiotics for a 1- or 2-week period may be useful. A few studies have noted that cleaning an infected wound with 1% povidone-iodine has been demonstrated to reduce the bacterial load and increase healing. Clearly, additional research is needed to examine the role of topical antibiotics in decreasing bacterial loads in pressure ulcers. Systemic antibiotics should only be used when a systemic infection is suspected.

Adjunctive therapies

The use of adjunctive therapies is the fastest growing area in pressure ulcer management. Adjunctive therapies include electrical stimulation, hyperbaric oxygen, radiant heat, growth factors, and skin equivalents. Except for electrical stimulation, published research substantiating the effectiveness of adjunctive therapies in healing pressure ulcers is scarce.

Electrical stimulation is the use of electrical current to stimulate a number of cellular processes, such as increasing fibroblasts, neutrophil macrophage collagen, DNA synthesis, and increasing the number of receptor sites for specific growth factors.[53] Electrical stimulation appears to be most effective on stage III and IV pressure ulcers that were unresponsive to traditional methods of healing. Although there's much data to suggest that electrical stimulation is effective in healing pressure ulcers, the optimal electrical charge needed to stimulate pressure ulcer healing remains unclear. The literature suggests an optimal electrical charge of 300 to 500 uA/sec produces positive effects on the pressure ulcer.[54] However, additional research is needed to determine the optimal electrical charge based on the characteristics of pressure ulcers (for example, stage, depth, and amount of drainage).

Hyperbaric oxygen is believed to promote wound healing by stimulating fibroblast, collagen synthesis, epithelialization, and control of infection.[55] However, controlled clinical studies couldn't be found regarding the association of hyperbaric oxygen and the healing of pressure ulcers. The limited literature that does exist suggests that topical hyperbaric oxygen doesn't increase tissue oxygenation beyond the superficial dermis.[56]

Research into radiant heat (normothermia) as an adjunctive therapy to heal pressure ulcers is being conducted. It's believed that increasing the thermal wound environment not only increases blood flow, but promotes fibroblasts and

Incidence and prevalence, 1999 to 2000

The chart below shows pressure ulcer incidence and prevalence data collected by the National Pressure Ulcer Advisory Panel (NPUAP) for 1999 and 2000.

PRESSURE ULCER INCIDENCE

	1999 to 2000	Pre -1990
Acute care	0.4% to 38% Best estimate: 7%	5% to 11%
Long-term care	2.2% to 23.9%	No data
Home care	0% to 17%	No data

PRESSURE ULCER PREVALENCE

	1999 to 2000	Pre -1990
Acute care	10% to 17% Best estimate: 15%	3% to 14%
Long-term care	2.3% to 28%	15% to 25%
Home care	0% to 29%	7% to 12%

Adapted with permission from the National Pressure Ulcer Advisory Panel (NPUAP), Cuddigan, J., et al., eds. *Pressure Ulcers in America: Prevalence, Incidence, and Implications for the Future.* Reston, Va.: NPUAP, 2001.

other factors associated with pressure ulcer healing as well.[57] Mustoe et al.[58] investigated the role of radiant heat in healing pressure ulcers; their findings suggest that radiant heat is beneficial to pressure ulcer healing. Additional research is needed to increase knowledge about the benefits of radiant heat in pressure ulcer healing.

The use of growth factors and skin equivalents in healing pressure ulcers is emerging. The use of cytokine growth factors (for example, recombinant platelet-derived growth factor-BB [rhPDGF-BB]) and fibroblast growth factors (bFGF) and skin equivalents are currently being studied. Only one multicenter, randomized double-blind study was found.[58] This study enrolled 45 patients with stage III or IV pressure ulcers who were randomized to either treatment group 1 (300ug/ml of rhPDGF), treatment group 2 (100 ug/ml rhPDGF) or treatment group 3 (placebo). After 4 weeks of treatment, patients in group 1 had a 40% reduction in ulcer area, group 2 had a 71% reduction in ulcer area and group 3 had a 17% reduction in pressure ulcer area. Clearly, the use of growth factors may have a crucial impact on the future of wound healing. However, additional research is needed to evaluate the efficacy of specific growth factors in healing pressure ulcers.

Prevalence and incidence

It has been said, "what can be measured can be managed." To improve pressure ulcer care, the number of patients with pressure ulcers must be accurately determined. Doing so will require careful attention to prevalence and incidence data. The data represent the percentage of patients with pressure ulcers among all those surveyed in a setting (prevalence) and the percentage of patients who developed pressure ulcers after admission to the setting (incidence).

In 1989, at its first consensus conference, NPUAP brought attention to the pressure ulcer problem in the United States by reporting prevalence and incidence data.[27] (See *Incidence and prevalence, 1999 to 2000*.) They set a national goal to reduce the incidence of pressure ulcers by 50% by the year 2000.[27] During the next decade, NPUAP engaged in an active program to improve pressure ulcer practice through education, research, and public policy.

At the close of the 20th century, NPUAP assessed the progress toward this goal through its Pressure Ulcers Challenge 2000 project. This 2-year project included a Medline database search for all articles on pressure ulcer incidence and prevalence published and indexed between January 1, 1990 and December 31, 2000. More than 300 studies on pressure ulcer incidence and prevalence were found. Pressure ulcer incidence and prevalence data were analyzed across care settings and in specific populations such as people with spinal cord injuries, elderly patients, infants and children, patients with hip fractures, people of color, and those at the end of life receiving palliative or hospice care.[59]

Study data presented in the NPUAP monograph detailing the results of the project indicate a wide variation in the range of incidence rates (acute care, 0.4% to 38%; long-term care, 2.2% to 23.9%; and home care, 0% to 17%).[59] Inconsistencies in methodology used and the populations studied contribute to these differences and make comparisons and analyses of trends problematic. However, many positive developments in the prevention and treatment of pressure ulcers have occurred over the past decade, including development of evidence-based practice guidelines, standardization of risk assessment, and improved technologies for prevention and treatment.[59] NPUAP estimates that pressure ulcer prevalence in acute care is 15%, with incidence of 7%.[59] Although methodological issues require caution in interpreting the data, the estimates are based on several large studies conducted from 1990 to 2000. (See *Incidence and prevalence, 1990 to 2000*, page 262.)

Prevalence

Due to the variations in the range of prevalence rates, sample characteristics, and study methodologies, these results should be interpreted cautiously. Prevalence rates over the last decade ranged from 10% to 18% in general acute care,[60] 2.3% to 28% in long-term care,[61,62] and 0% to 29% in home care.[62,63] Because of population and methodological differences, valid comparisons can't be made among these studies or to pre-1990 prevalence ranges (for example, 3% to 14% in acute care, 15% to 25% in long-term care, and 7% to 12% in home care).[59] Reported prevalence rates in other countries are:

- Netherlands: 10.1%,[64] 20.4%[65]
- United Kingdom: 1.9%,[66] 7.32%,[67] 9.5%,[68] 14%[69]
- Canada: 29.7%[70]
- Australia: 11.1%[71]
- Iceland: 8.9%[72]
- Sweden: 63.6%[73]

Incidence and prevalence, 1990 to 2000

These tables summarize pressure ulcer incidence and prevalence data* collected by the National Pressure Ulcer Advisory Panel (NPUAP) from 1990 to 2000.

INCIDENCE

CLINICAL SETTING	STAGES I TO IV		STAGES II TO IV	
	Database	**Clinical**	**Database**	**Clinical**
Acute care	17.6% to 19.1%	7% to 38%	0.4%	12.9%
Critical care	—	8% to 40%	—	—
Operating room	—	4% to 21.5%	—	—
Long-term care	—	7% to 23.9%	2.2% to 12.9%	—
Rehabilitation	4% to 6%	0%	—	—
Home care	0% to 6.3%	16.5% to 17%	3.2%	—

SPECIAL POPULATIONS

Hip fracture	19.1%	—	—	—
End of life	0% to 85%			
Spinal cord injury	7.5% to 23.7%	—	—	31%
Infants and children	8% to 19%			

PREVALENCE

CLINICAL SETTING	STAGES I TO IV		STAGES II TO IV	
	Database	**Clinical**	**Database**	**Clinical**
Acute care		10% to18%	—	—
Critical care	—	—	—	—
Operating room	—	8.5%	—	—
Long-term care	2.3% to 12%	23% to 28%	11.2%	—
Rehabilitation	12% to 27%	0% to 25%	—	—
Home care	—	0% to 29%	—	—

SPECIAL POPULATIONS:

Hip fracture	—	—		—
End of life	14% to 28%		—	
Spinal cord injury	15.2% to 30%	10.2%	7.4%	32%
Infants and children	—			

* Incidence and prevalence data are reported according to the methodology used. Data were obtained from existing databases (for example, MDS, medical records) or through clinical observations of the investigator(s). Some investigators considered stages I to IV pressure ulcers, whereas others excluded stage I ulcers from study. Due to differences in methodologies and sample characteristics among studies, valid comparisons between pre-1990 and post-1990 rates can't be made. The reader should be cautioned against using these incidence and prevalence rates to benchmark or determine an "acceptable" pressure ulcer rate for a given setting, facility, agency, or population.

Used with permission from National Pressure Ulcer Advisory Panel (NPUAP). Cuddigan, J., et al., eds. *Pressure Ulcers in America: Prevalence, Incidence, and Implications for the Future.* Reston, Va.: NPUAP, 2001.

- Japan: 5.1%[74]
- France: 5.2%[75]
- Germany: 28.3%.[76]

Three large multisite clinical studies in acute care reported prevalence rates of 14.8%, 15%, and 15% at the end of the 1990s; these studies provide the most accurate and current estimate of prevalence rates in acute care.[77-79] Most pressure ulcers, regardless of setting, are partial-thickness (stages I and II) and are located on the sacrum or coccyx. Heels are the second most frequently occurring location.

Incidence

Use caution when analyzing the reported NPUAP incidence rates of 0.4% to 38% in general acute care,[23,80] 2.2% to 23.9% in long-term care,[25,81] and 0% to 17% in home care.[62,82] Because there was no data from long-term care or home care reported at the original NPUAP 1989 consensus conference, no comparison to the 2001 incidence data can be made. Although the reported range in acute care prior to 1990 was 5% to 11%,[27] NPUAP believes that the difference in the reported ranges doesn't reflect a change in incidence rates over time. This may be due to several factors including differences in incidence rates among studies, staging definitions, incidence rate formulas, populations, and various data sources. Reported incidence rates around the world are as follows:

- United Kingdom: 4.03%[83]
- Canada: 9.7 %[84]
- Sweden: 55%[73]
- Japan: 4.4%.[74]

Prevalence and incidence definitions and formulas

Lack of clarity and consistency in definitions and calculation formulas impedes our understanding of pressure ulcer prevalence and incidence. Standardization of definitions and formulas will enhance comparability of data among future studies. NPUAP recommends the adoption of consistent definitions and formulas for determining pressure ulcer prevalence and incidence.[85] Similarly, the European Pressure Ulcer Advisory Panel (EPUAP) has published a draft statement on prevalence and incidence monitoring.[86]

NPUAP suggests that prevalence should be defined as a "cross-sectional count of the number of cases at a specific point in time, or the number of people with pressure ulcers who exist in a patient population at a given point in time. In assessing prevalence, it doesn't matter in what setting the pressure ulcer was acquired."[85] Suggested standard formulas for obtaining prevalence are:

- Pressure ulcer point prevalence

$$\frac{\text{Number of people with a pressure ulcer} \times 100}{\text{Number of people in a population at a particular point in time}}$$

- Pressure ulcer period prevalence

$$\frac{\text{Number of people with a pressure ulcer} \times 100}{\text{Number of people in a population at a particular period in time}}$$

NPUAP recommends using the following definition of incidence: "the number of new cases appearing in a population indicates the rate at which new disease occurs in a population previously without disease."[14,87] Several approaches to measuring incidence have been used. NPUAP defines "cumulative incidence" as "the rate of new pressure ulcers in a group of patients of fixed size, all of whom are observed over a period of time."[85] The formula is as follows:

- Pressure ulcer cumulative incidence

Pitfalls to calculating prevalence and incidence

Be sure to avoid the following pitfalls when calculating pressure ulcer prevalence and incidence for your facility.

- Define the population and apply the definition consistently throughout the study.
- Count the number of patients with pressure ulcers — not the number of pressure ulcers.
- Count only pressure ulcers, not other wounds.
- Define the stages of the pressure ulcers you count to include and assess them accurately.

Adapted with permission from Ayello, E.A., et al. "Methods for Determining Pressure Ulcer Prevalence and Incidence," in *Pressure Ulcers in America: Prevalence, Incidence, and Implications for the Future*, edited by Cuddigan, J., et al. Reston, Va.: National Pressure Ulcer Advisory Panel, 2001.

$$\frac{\text{Number of people developing a}}{\text{new pressure ulcer} \times 100}$$
$$\overline{\text{Total number of people in a population}}$$
$$\text{at beginning of time period}$$

A problem with using this approach is that it doesn't count pressure ulcers that occur in people admitted to the setting after the study population has been defined. Therefore, it may not be the true incidence of new ulcers in that setting.

Another way is to measure the number of new cases of pressure ulcers that occur in a changing population. In this case, the people who are being studied have varying lengths of stay. Incidence is calculated as the number of people de-

veloping pressure ulcers per 1,000 patient-days, and is called incidence density. Calculate this by using the following suggested formula:

- Pressure ulcer incidence density

$$\frac{\text{Number of people developing a}}{\text{new pressure ulcer} \times 1000}$$
$$\overline{\text{Total patient days free of pressure ulcers}}$$
$$=$$
$$\frac{\text{Number of people developing a pressure ulcer}}{1000 \text{ patient-days}}$$

Using the NPUAP recommended standard formulas alone may not be enough to avoid errors in prevalence and incidence calculations. (See *Pitfalls to calculating prevalence and incidence*.)

Competencies and curriculum

Accurate and current knowledge is essential for clinicians to prevent and treat pressure ulcers. NPUAP has approved a competency based curriculum on pressure ulcer prevention and treatment for registered nurses. Curriculum components include competencies, content outline, a case study with answers, and references. Twelve essential pressure ulcer prevention competencies and eight essential pressure ulcer treatment competencies are recommended. The entire copyrighted registered nurse curriculum document is available free of charge on the NPUAP Web site. The NPUAP competency-based curriculum is an important contribution to nursing practice. The NPUAP Education Committee is also considering developing additional curricula for physicians, dietitians, physical therapists and other health caregivers.

Summary

Pressure ulcers are a common health care problem throughout the world. Intensity and duration of pressure as well as tissue tolerance are the etiologic factors that lead to pressure ulcer development. Results of a pressure ulcer risk assessment using a validated tool can serve as the foundation for developing a pressure ulcer prevention protocol based on the level and type of risk the individual demonstrates. After determining the pressure ulcer stage and other wound factors, a comprehensive plan to treat the pressure ulcer which uses a combination of local wound care, debridement, moist wound healing, cleaning, and pressure relief needs to be implemented. A multidisciplinary approach to patient care that includes patient and family education is essential. Use of the standardized formulas as proposed by NPUAP will provide a basis for universal comparison of prevalence and incidence data.

Show what you know

1. *A pressure ulcer is any lesion caused by:*

   A. incontinence.
   B. unrelieved pressure.
   C. heat.
   D. diabetes mellitus.

ANSWER: B. Pressure is the cause of tissue death in pressure ulcers. Incontinence and diabetes mellitus may be other patient characteristics that may put a patient at risk for pressure ulcers, but in and of themselves don't cause the pressure ulcer. Heat causes burns not pressure ulcers.

2. *A patient is dragged across the bed when transferring to a stretcher. Which one of the following forces that con-tribute to pressure ulcer developed has occurred?*

   A. Electrical stimulation
   B. Shear
   C. Friction
   D. Masceration

ANSWER: C. Shear is the mechanical force that's parallel to the body's surfaces. Electrical stimulation is an adjunct therapy used to heal pressure ulcers. Wetness of the skin isn't a mechanical force

3. *A patient has a 2 by 3 cm sacral pressure ulcer that has some depth and extends into, but not completely through, the subcutaneous tissue. Using the NPUAP staging classification system, this pressure ulcer is:*

   A. Stage I.
   B. Stage II.
   C. Stage III.
   D. Stage IV.

ANSWER: C. The tissue destroyed is into the subcutaneous tissue. It isn't stage I because the epidermis is no longer intact. It isn't stage II because the tissue destroyed is deeper than superficial level and is well into the subcutaneous tissue. It isn't stage IV because this ulcer isn't that extensive and not through the subcutaneous tissue into muscle or bone.

4. *Which of the following Braden Scale scores for an elderly black male would indicate pressure ulcer risk?*

   A. 23
   B. 21
   C. 19
   D. 17

ANSWER: D. The research-based cutscore for onset of pressure ulcer risk for older patients and Blacks is 18. With the Braden Scale, scores at or lower than the cutscore indicate risk for pressure ulcer development. A, B, and C are all wrong answers because they're higher than the cutscore of 18. With the Braden Scale, low numerical scores indicate risk for pressure ulcers.

5. Which one of the following should be included in a care plan to prevent pressure ulcers?

A. Turn and position every 4 hours.
B. Clean skin daily using hot water and soap.
C. Encourage the patient who is confined to a chair to relieve pressure every hour.
D. Limit fluids to 10cc per kg of body weight daily.

ANSWER: C. (See AHCPR 1992 prevention guidelines.) Turn the patient at least every 2 hours. Don't use hot water, but rather warm water, and use lanolin-based soaps to avoid drying the skin. There's no need to limit the patient's fluids.

6. Which one of the following parameters is NOT part of the PUSH tool?

A. Depth
B. Exudate
C. Tissue type
D. Length × width

ANSWER: A. Depth isn't on the NPUAP PUSH tool to measure pressure ulcer healing. Exudate, tissue type, and length × width are the three variables measured on the NPUAP PUSH tool.

7. The best current estimate for pressure ulcer prevalence in acute care in the United States is:

A. 20%
B. 15%
C. 7%
D. 0.8%

ANSWER: B. 7% is the best estimate of incidence, and 0.8% is the target number for Healthy People 2010.

References

1. National Pressure Ulcer Advisory Panel (NPUAP). Cuddigan, J., et al., eds. *Pressure Ulcers in America: Prevalence, Incidence and Implications for the Future.* Reston, VA: NPUAP, 2001.
2. U.S. Department of Health and Human Services. *Healthy People 2010: Understanding and Improving Health,* 2nd ed. Washington, DC: U.S. Government Printing Office, November, 2000.
3. Health Care Financing Administration. *Survey Procedures for Long Term Care Facilities. Investigative Protocol: Pressure Sore/ulcer.* Baltimore, MD: Health Care Financing Administration, 1999.
4. Maklebust, J. "Pressure Ulcers: Etiology and Prevention," *Nursing Clinics of North America* 22(2):359-77, June 1987.
5. Kosiak, M. "Etiology and Pathology of Ischemic Ulcers," *Archives of Physical Medicine and Rehabilitation* 40(2):62, February 1959.
6. Parish, L.C., et al. *The Decubitus Ulcers.* New York: Masson Publishing, 1983.
7. Dyson, M., and Lyder, C. Wound management-physical modalities. In Morison, M., ed., *The Prevention and Treatment of Pressure Ulcers.* Edinburgh: Harcourt Brace/Mosby International, 2001.
8. Maklebust, J., and Sieggreen, M. *Pressure Ulcers: Guidelines for Prevention and Management,* 3rd ed. Philadelphia: Lippincott Williams & Wilkins, 2001.
9. Bergstrom, N., et al. *Treatment of Pressure Ulcers in Adults.* Clinical practice guideline, Number 15. Rockville, MD: Public Health Service, US Dept. of Health and Human Services; Agency for Health Care Policy and Research publication 95-0652, December 1994.
10. Dinsdale, S.M. "Decubitus Ulcers: Role or Pressure and Friction in Causation," *Archives of Physical Medicine and Rehabilitation* 55(4):147-52, April 1974.
11. Barczak, C.A., et al. "Fourth National Pressure Ulcer Prevalence Survey," *Advances in Wound Care* 10(4):18-26, July-August 1997.
12. Meehan, M. "Multisite Pressure Ulcer Prevalence Survey," *Decubitus* 3(4):14-7, November 1990.

13. Meehan, M. "National Pressure Ulcer Prevalence Survey," *Advances in Wound Care* 7(3):27-30,34, May 1994.

14. Panel on the Prediction and Prevention of Pressure Ulcers in Adults. *Pressure Ulcers in Adults: Prediction and Prevention.* Clinical Practice Guideline No. 3. AHCPR Publication No. 92-0047. Rockville, Md.: Agency for Health Care Policy and Research, 1992.

15. Norton, D., et al. *An Investigation of Geriatric Nursing Problems in Hospital.* London: National Corporation for the Care of Old People, 1962.

16. Gosnell, D.J. "An Assessment Tool to Identify Pressure Sores," *Nursing Research* 22(1):55-59, January-February 1973.

17. Bergstrom, N., et al. "The Braden Scale for Predicting Pressure Sore Risk," *Nursing Research* 36(4):205-10, July-August 1987.

18. Abruzzese, R.S. "Early Assessment and Prevention of Pressure Sores," in Lee, B.Y., ed. *Chronic Ulcers of the Skin.* New York: McGraw-Hill Book Co., 1985.

19. Waterlow, J. "Pressure Sores: A Risk Assessment Card,"*Nursing Times* 81(48):49-55, November 27-December 3, 1985.

20. Ayello, E.A., and Braden, B. "How and Why to do Pressure Ulcer Risk Assessment," *Advances in Skin and Wound Care* 15(3):125-32, May-June 2002.

21. Ayello, E.A., and Braden, B. "Why is pressure ulcer risk assessment so important?" *Nursing* 31(11):75-79, November 2001.

22. Bergstrom, N., and Braden, B. "A Prospective Study of Pressure Sore Risk Among Institutionalized Elderly," *Journal of the American Geriatric Society* 40(8):747-58, August 1992.

23. Lyder, C.H., et al. "Validating the Braden Scale for the Prediction of Pressure Ulcer Risk in Blacks and Latino/Hispanic Elders: A Pilot Study," *Ostomy/Wound Management* 44(suppl 3A):42S-49S, March 1998.

24. Lyder, C.H., et al. "The Braden Scale for Pressure Ulcer Risk: Evaluating the Predictive Validity in Black and Latino/Hispanic Elders," *Applied Nursing Research* 12(2):60-68, May 1999.

25. Bergstrom, N., et al. "Predicting Pressure Ulcer Risk: A Multisite Study of the Predictive Validity of the Braden Scale," *Nursing Research* 47(5):261-69, September-October 1998.

26. Braden, B., and Bergstrom, N. "Clinical Utility of the Braden Scale for Predicting Pressure Sore Risk," *Decubitus* 2(3):44, August 1989.

27. National Pressure Ulcer Advisory Panel. "Pressure Ulcers Prevalence, Cost, and Risk Assessment: Consensus Development Conference Statement," *Decubitus* 2(2):24-28, May 1989.

28. Shea, J.D. "Pressure Sores: Classification and Management," *Clinical Orthopaedics and Related Research* 112:89-100, October 1975.

29. International Association of Enterostomal Therapy (IAET). "Dermal Wounds: Pressure Sores. Philosophy of the IAET," *Journal of Enterostomal Therapy* 15(1):9-15, January-February 1988.

30. Henderson, C.T., et al. "Draft Definition of Stage I Pressure Ulcers: Inclusion of Persons with Darkly Pigmented Skin. NPUAP Task Force on Stage I Definition and Darkly Pigmented Skin," *Advances in Skin & Wound Care* 10(5):16-19, September 1997.

31. Ayello, E.A., and Lyder, C.H. "Pressure Ulcers in Persons of Color: Race and Ethnicity," in *Pressure Ulcers in America: Prevalence, Incidence, and Implications for the Future,* edited by Cuddigan, J., et al. Reston, Va.: National Pressure Ulcer Advisory Panel, 2001.

32. Lyder, C.H. *Accuracy of Stage I Pressure Ulcer Definitions in Dark Skinned Individuals.* Unpublished data.

33. Sprigle, S., et al. "Clinical Skin Temperature Measurement to Predict Incipient Pressure Ulcers," *Advances in Skin & Wound Care* 14(3):133-37, May-June 2001.

34. Robson, M.C., and Heggers, J.P. "Bacterial Quantification of Open Wounds," *Military Medicine* 134(1):19-24, February 1969.

35. Barr, J.E. "Principles of Wound Cleansing," *Ostomy/Wound Management* 41(Suppl 7A):15S-22S, August 1995.

36. Hellewell, T.B., et al. "A Cytotoxicity Evaluation of Antimicrobial Wound Cleansers," *Wounds* 9(1):15-20, 1997.

37. Rodeheaver, G.T., et al. "Wound Cleansing by High Pressure Irrigation," *Surgery Gynecology and Obstetrics* 141(3):357-62, September 1975.

38. Stevenson, T.R., et al. "Cleansing the Traumatic Wound by High Pressure Syringe Irrigation," *Journal of the American College of Emergency Physicians* 5(1):17-21, January 1976.

39. Bhaskar, S.N., et al. "Effect of Water Lavage on Infected Wounds in the Rat," *Journal of Periodontology* 40(11):671-72, November 1969.

40. Yarkony, G.M. "Pressure Ulcers: Medical Management," in *Spinal Cord Injury Medical Management and Rehabilitation.* Gaithersburg, MD: Aspen, 1994.

41. Dolychuck, K.N. "Debridement," in Krasner, D., et al., eds. *Chronic Wound Care: A Clinical Source Book for Health Care Professionals*, 3rd ed. Wayne, Pa: HMP Communications, 2001.

42. Galpin, J.E., et al. Sepsis Associated with Decubitus Ulcers," *American Journal of Medicine* 61(3):346-50, September 1976.

43. Kim, Y.C., et al. "Efficacy of Hydrocolloid Occlusive Dressing Technique in Decubitus Ulcer Treatment: A Comparative Study," *Yonsei Medical Journal* 37(3):181-85, June 1996.

44. Bolton, L.L., et al. "Quality Wound Care Equals Cost-effective Wound Care: A Clinical Model," *Advances in Wound Care* 10(4):33-38, July-August 1997.

45. Saydak, S. "A Pilot of Two Methods for the Treatment of Pressure Ulcers," *Journal of Enterostomal Therapy* 7(3):139-42, May-June 1990.

46. Lyder, C.H., et al. "Examining the Cost-effectiveness of Two Methods for Healing Stage II Pressure Ulcers in Long-term Care," Under review.

47. ter Riet, G., et al. "Randomized Clinical Trial of Ascorbic Acid in the Treatment of Pressure Ulcers," *Journal of Clinical Epidemiology* 48(12):1452-60, December 1995.

48. Rackett, S.C., et al. "The Role of Dietary Manipulation in the Prevention and Treatment of Cutaneous Disorders," *Journal of the American Academy of Dermatology* 29(3):447-53, September 1993.

49. Waldorf, H., and Fewkes, J. "Wound Healing," *Advances in Dermatology* 10:77-81, 1995.

50. Erlich, H.P., and Hunt, T.K. "Effects of Cortisone and Vitamin A on Wound Healing," *Annals of Surgery* 167(3):324-28, March 1968.

51. Bates-Jensen, B.M. "The Pressure Sore Status Tool a Few Thousand Assessments Later," *Advances in Wound Care* 10(5):65-73, September-October 1997.

52. NPUAP PUSH Task Force. "Pressure Ulcer Scale for Healing: Derivation and Validation of the PUSH Tool," *Advances in Wound Care* 10(5):96, September-October 1997.

53. Kloth, L.C., and McCulloch, J. "Promotion of Wound Healing with Electrical Stimulation," *Advances in Wound Care* 9(5):42-45, September-October 1996.

54. Gardner, S.E., et al. "Effect of Electrical Stimulation on Chronic Wound Healing: A Meta-analysis," *Wound Repair Regeneration* 7(6):495-503, November-December 1999.

55. Courville, S. "Hyperbaric Oxygen Therapy: Its Role in Healing Problem Wounds," *Caet Journal* 17(4):7-11, 1998.

56. Gruber, R. P., et al. "Skin Permeability of Oxygen and Hyperbaric Oxygen," *Archives of Surgery* 101(1):69-70, July 1970.

57. Xia, Z., et al. "Stimulation of Fibroblast Growth In Vitro by Intermittent Radiant Warming," *Wound Repair Regeneration* 8(2):138-44, March-April 2000.

58. Mustoe, T.A., et al. "A Phase II Study to Evaluate Recombinant Platelet-derived Growth Factor-BB in the Treatment of Stage 3 and 4 Pressure Ulcers," *Archives of Surgery* 129(2):213-19, February 1994.

59. Ayello, E.A., et al. "Methods for Determining Pressure Ulcer Prevalence and Incidence," in Cuddigan, J., et al., eds. *Pressure Ulcers in America: Prevalence, Incidence, and Implications for the Future.* Reston, VA: NPUAP, 2001.

60. O'Brien, S.P., et al. "Sequential Biannual Prevalence Studies of Pressure Ulcers at Allegheny-Hahnemann University Hospital," *Ostomy/Wound Management* 44(suppl 3A):78s-88s, March 1998.

61. Baker, J. "Medicaid Claims History of Florida Long-term Care Facility Residents Hospitalized for Pressure Ulcers," *Journal of Wound, Ostomy, and Continence Nursing* 23(1):23-25, January 1996.

62. Langemo, D.K., et al. "Incidence and Prediction of Pressure Ulcers in Five Patient Care Settings," *Decubitus* 4(3):25-30, August 1991.

63. Oot Giromini, B.A. "Pressure Ulcer Prevalence, Incidence and Associated Risk Factors in the Community," *Decubitus* 6(5):24-32, September 1993.

64. Bours, G.J., et al. "The Development of a National Registration Form to Measure the Prevalence of Pressure Ulcers in the Netherlands," *Ostomy/Wound Management* 45(11):28-40, November 1999.

65. Wendte, J.F. "Monitoring the Prevalence of Pressure Ulcers: Does it Support Implementation Projects?" *European Pressure Ulcer Advisory Panel Review* 4(1):22, 2002.

66. Healey, F. "Wound Care. Waterlow Revisited," *Nursing Times* 92(11):80-84, March 13-19, 1996.

67. Dealey, C. "The Size of the Pressure-sore Problem in a Teaching Hospital," *Journal of Advanced Nursing* 16(6):663-70, June 1991.

68. Hanson, R. "Sore Points Sorted," *Nursing Times* 93(7):66-72, February 12-18, 1997.

69. O'Dea, K. "Pressure Sores. Damage Limitation," *Nursing Times* 92(15):46-47, April 10-16, 1996.

70. Harrison, M.B., et al. "Practice Guidelines for the Prediction and Prevention of Pressure Ulcers: Evaluating the Evidence," *Applied Nursing Research* 9(1):9-17, February 1996.

71. Gruen, R.L., et al. "The Point Prevalence of Wounds in a Teaching Hospital," *Australia and New Zealand Journal of Surgery* 67(10):686-88, 1997.

72. Thoroddsen, A. "Pressure Sore Prevalence: A national Survey," *Journal of Clinical Nursing* 8(2):170-79, March 1999.

73. Gunningberg, L., et al. "The Development of Pressure Ulcers in Patients with Hip Fractures: Inadequate Nursing Documentation is Still a Problem," *Journal of Advanced Nursing* 31(5):1155-64, May 2000.

74. Hagisawa, S., and Barbenel, J. "The Limits of Pressure Sore Prevention," *Journal of the Royal Society of Medicine* 92(11):576-78, November 1999.

75. Barrois, B., et al. "A Survey of Pressure Sore Prevalence in Hospitals in the Greater Paris Region," *Journal of Wound Care* 4(5):234-35, May 1995.

76. Lahmann, N., and Dassen, T. "Prevalence of Pressure Ulcers in Eleven German Hospitals in April 2001," *European Pressure Ulcer Advisory Panel Review* 4(1):17, 2002.

77. Amlung ,S., et al. "National Prevalence Pressure Ulcer Survey: A Benchmarking Approach," in *14th Annual Clinical Symposium on Wound Care. The Quest for Quality Wound Care: Solutions for Clinical Practice*; September 30, 1999 to October 4, 1999. Denver, CO: Sponsored by the Wound Care Communications Network and University of Pennsylvania Medical Center, 1999.

78. CalNOC. A Statewide Nursing Outcomes Database. Linking Patient Outcomes to Hospital Nursing Care: California Nursing Outcomes Coalition: January 18, 2000.

79. Whittington, K., et al. "A National Study of Pressure Ulcer Prevalence and Incidence in Acute Care Hospitals," *Journal of Wound, Ostomy, and Continence Nursing* 27(4):209-15, July 2000.

80. O'Sullivan, K.L, et al. "Pressure Sores in the Acute Trauma Patient: Incidence and Causes," *Journal of Trauma* 42(2):276-78, February 1997.

81. Berlowitz, D.R., et al. "Are We Improving the Quality of Nursing Home Care: The Case of Pressure Ulcers," *Journal of the American Geriatric Society* 48(1):59-62, January 2000.

82. Ramundo, J.M. "Reliability and Validity of the Braden Scale in the Home Care Setting," *Journal of Wound, Ostomy, and Continence Nursing* 22(3):28-34, March 1995.

83. Clark, M., and Watts, S. "The Incidence of Pressure Sores Within a National Health Service Trust Hospital During 1991," *Journal of Advanced Nursing* 20(1):33-36, July 1994.

84. Goodridge, D.M., et al. "Risk Assessment Scores, Prevention Strategies, and the Incidence of Pressure Ulcers Among the Elderly in Four Canadian Health Care Facilities," *Canadian Journal of Nursing Research* 30(2):23-44, Summer 1998.

85. National Pressure Ulcer Advisory Panel (NPUAP) Board of Directors. "An Executive Summary of the NPUAP Monograph Pressure Ulcers in America: Prevalence, Incidence and Implications for the Future," *Advances in Skin & Wound Care* 14(4):208-15, July-August 2001.

86. Defloor, T., et al. "Draft EPUAP Statement on Prevalence and Incidence Monitoring," *European Pressure Ulcer Advisory Panel Review* 4(1):13-15, 2002.

87. Armitage, P., and Berry, G. *Statistical Methods in Medical Research.* Cambridge, Mass.: Blackwell Scientific Pubns., 1987.

88. Maklebust, J. "Policy Implications of Using Reverse Staging to Monitor Pressure Ulcer Status," *Advances in Wound Care* 10(5):32-35, 1997.

89. Maklebust, J. "Perplexing Questions about Pressure Ulcers," *Decubitus* 5(4):15, 1992.

90. Xakellis, G., and Frantz, R.A. "Pressure Ulcer Healing: What Is It? What Influences It? How Is It Measured?" *Advances in Wound Care* 10(5):20-26, 1997.

91. Thomas, D.R., et al. "Pressure Ulcer Scale for Healing:Derivation and Validation of the PUSH Tool. *Advances in Wound Care* 10(5):96-101, 1997.

CHAPTER 14

Vascular ulcers

Mary Y. Sieggreen, MSN, APRN, CS, CVN, APN
Ronald A. Kline, MD, FACS, FAHA

OBJECTIVES

After completing this chapter, you'll be able to:

- identify the arterial and venous vessels in the lower extremities

- describe the anatomy and physiology of the lymphatic system

- describe the pathophysiology of lower extremity ulcers: arterial, venous, lymphatic

- describe systems for classifying venous and lymphatic disease

- state the signs and symptoms that comprise a vascular, arterial, venous, or lymphatic assessment

- discuss vascular laboratory tests done for patients with vascular, arterial, venous, or lymphatic disease

- describe the components of local wound care for a patient with an arterial or venous ulcer

- describe surgical treatment for patients with arterial and venous ulcers

- discuss the treatment of patients with lymphedema

- identify education needs for patients with arterial, venous, or lymphatic disease.

Scope of the problem

"Peripheral vascular disease" is commonly used in reference to an arterial problem, even though the term includes diseases and conditions of the venous and lymphatic systems as well as the arterial system. Patients with leg ulcers may present with a combination of arterial, venous, and lymphatic disease. This chapter describes arterial, venous, and lymphatic anatomy and physiology and examines the causes and treatment of lower extremity vascular ulcers.

Approximately 10% to 35% of the population has some form of venous disease and approximately 8% to 10% of patients have pure arterial insufficiency.[1] It's estimated that between 1% and 22% of the population over age 60 suffers from lower extremity skin ulcers.[2-5] One study found the problem to be underestimated when a self-report survey indicated high numbers of patients cared for their own ulcers without consulting a health care provider.[6] The principal leg ulcer etiology in most patients is peripheral vascular disease. Chronic venous disease is the seventh most common chronic disease. It's the underlying cause in 95% of leg ulcers.[1,7-9] In a U.S. community health survey, 5% of adults had skin changes in the leg and more than 500,000 suffered from venous ulcers. Over 2,000,000 work days are lost in the United States per year due to the associated morbidity of postphlebitic syndrome.[9] Although it's understood that chronic wounds have physical, financial, and psychological affects, it's difficult to measure their effects on a patient's quality of life.[10] It's also difficult to obtain accurate etiological information about leg ulcers and, in about one-third of medical records, no ulcer etiology might be documented.

Vascular anatomy and physiology

Vascular anatomy includes the arterial, venous, and lymphatic systems. Vascular ulcers may develop in any of these systems for a variety of causes.

Arterial system

Lower extremity arterial perfusion begins with adequate cardiac performance. As blood exits the left ventricle, it begins its downward course through the descending thoracic aorta. The intercostal arteries, which arise from the descending thoracic aorta, are the first important collaterals to perfusion in the legs. These become important when they are the sole collaterals in distal aortic occlu-

sions. As the aorta exits the thorax and enters the true abdominal cavity, its caliber begins to decrease after every major arterial branch. Its greatest reduction in size occurs distal to the renal arteries.

Lumbar arteries usually arise as paired vessels at each vertebral level in the abdomen. The lumbar arteries become important collateral pathways to the lower extremities in distal aortic occlusions or severe aorto-iliac occlusive disease. At the level of the umbilicus, the abdominal aorta bifurcates into the common iliac arteries, which branch into internal and external iliac arteries. The internal iliac arteries perfuse the lower sigmoid colon and rectum. They also, by way of the gluteal and pudendal branches, provide another collateral pathway to perfusion of the legs. The external iliac artery becomes the common femoral artery at the level of the inguinal ligament. It's at this level that one can first appreciate the quality of the pulse wave by palpation of the femoral artery.

Aspects of the femoral artery

The common femoral artery bifurcates into the superficial femoral artery and the deep femoral artery. The deep femoral artery is the single most important collateral pathway for perfusion of the lower portion of the leg. Its muscular perforators allow reconstitution of the popliteal artery in superficial femoral artery occlusions. The superficial femoral artery becomes the popliteal artery after it exits the adductor hiatus, also known as Hunter's canal. (See *Arterial system*.)

The superficial femoral artery is the most commonly occluded artery in the legs of patients with peripheral vascular occlusive disease. Its occlusion infrequently results in significant ischemia to the lower leg. Below the knee, the popliteal artery bifurcates into the tibioperoneal trunk and the anterior tibial

Arterial system

This illustration shows the major arteries of the lower extremities.

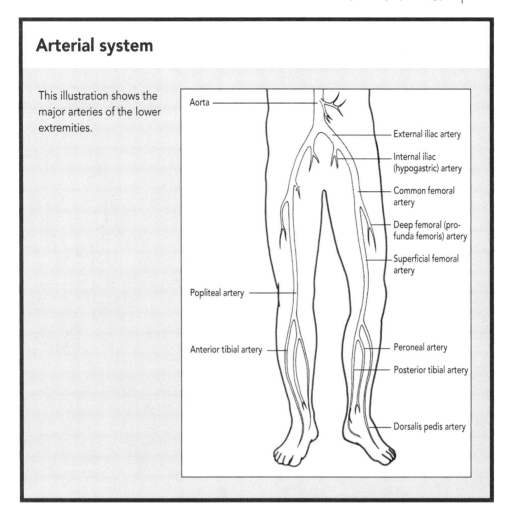

Aorta

External iliac artery

Internal iliac (hypogastric) artery

Common femoral artery

Deep femoral (profunda femoris) artery

Superficial femoral artery

Popliteal artery

Anterior tibial artery

Peroneal artery

Posterior tibial artery

Dorsalis pedis artery

artery. The anterior tibial artery proceeds from the popliteal fossa through the interosseous membrane, which connects the tibia and fibula; it then courses down the anterior muscle compartment into the foot. The tibio-peroneal trunk at a variable distance then bifurcates into the peroneal artery and the posterior tibial artery.

The peroneal artery courses down toward the ankle in the deep muscular compartment whereas the posterior tibial artery descends into the foot in a more superficial fashion. The peroneal artery provides muscular branches, which are important in the proper perfusion of the muscular compartments. The peroneal artery is commonly patent even in the presence of severe lower-extremity peripheral vascular occlusive disease.

Aspects of the tibial arteries

The anterior and posterior tibial arteries proceed into the foot with the anterior tibial artery becoming palpable as it becomes the dorsalis pedis artery. The posterior tibial artery then courses behind the medial malleolus and at this level also becomes palpable. The posterior tibial artery provides both deep and superficial components to the plantar arch. Perforators from the plantar arch pro-

Arterial wall

In the layers of the arterial wall shown here, the plaque formation and thrombus significantly reduce blood flow through the vessel.

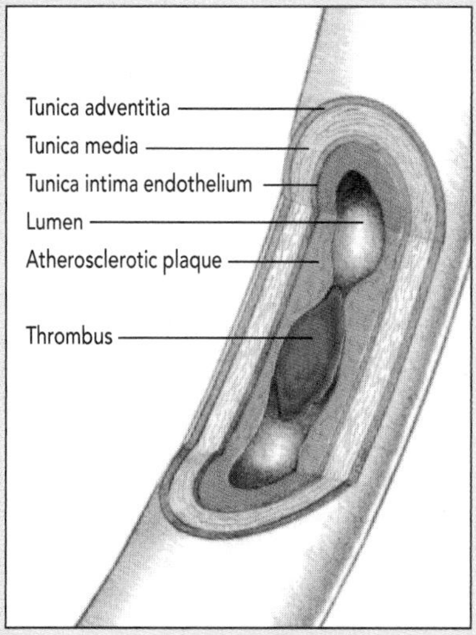

Tunica adventitia
Tunica media
Tunica intima endothelium
Lumen
Atherosclerotic plaque
Thrombus

vide arterial perfusion to the heel, sole, and branches to the digits.

The anterior tibial artery eventually communicates with the plantar arch forming a complete circuit in the foot. The peroneal artery, although it stops above the level of the ankle joint, does provide medial and lateral tarsal branches, which communicate with the distal most portions of the anterior tibial and posterior tibial arteries. This is another important collateral pathway for reconstitution of the plantar arch in patients with occlusive disease. Vascular surgeons can perform bypass operations to any of these named vessels.

Arterial wall architecture

The arterial wall typically consists of three lamina. The outer lamina, the adventitia, is a layer of loose connective tis-

sue that provides moderate strength to the arterial wall. The media, or middle layer, contains both elastic and muscular fibers and is responsible for the arterial strength, elasticity, and contractility. The intima, the innermost layer, is the endothelial lining of an artery and a few cell layers thick. As the arterial tree descends from the center to the periphery, muscular functions become more evident. Vessels below the common femoral artery have a greater propensity for rapid size adjustments in direct relationship to perfusion. The tibioperoneal vessels can quickly accommodate changes in perfusion by relaxation or dilatation.

Arteries are capable of increasing in size to maintain constant shear stress when atherosclerotic accumulation decreases luminal surface area. However, once a stenosis reaches 50% of the vessel diameter, the artery loses its ability to relax any further and any increase in atherosclerotic accumulation impedes arterial perfusion. Further restriction in flow through this stenotic area results in a decrease in the diameter of the artery distal to the stenosis in order to accommodate diminished blood flow. Compliance of an artery decreases as the arterial wall becomes more rigid as seen in calcific atherosclerosis. (See *Arterial wall*.)

Arterial perfusion

As blood descends through successively smaller arterial conduits, it eventually reaches the arteriolar level. Rheologic factors in this precapillary bed play an important role in perfusion. Blood is a non-Newtonian thixotropic fluid; that is, its viscosity is inversely proportional to its shear rate. Shear rate can be equated to the velocity of blood flow. The slower blood is propulsed the more viscous it becomes. The primary determinant of whole blood viscosity at any given shear rate is the hematocrit. As red cell mass increases, blood viscosity markedly increases.

Dehydration or polycythemia, two of many disease states that increase whole blood viscosity, can result in a sludging of blood in the precapillary bed and decrease arterial tissue perfusion. In many elderly patients with arterial occlusive disease, even mild dehydration can result in poor extremity perfusion. Simple rehydration can reduce the red cell mass and allow for better perfusion. In other cases of increased blood viscosity, such as multiple myeloma, plasmapheresis may be necessary to remove the abnormal concentrations of proteins. Nonetheless, in the "normal" atherosclerotic patient, it's the red cell mass, measured by hematocrit, which is the primary determinant of viscosity.

As blood proceeds into the capillary bed, the diameter of the vessel approaches that of the red cell—approximately 8 microns in diameter. Red cells pass through capillaries sequentially. Red cell deformability plays a role in perfusion at this level. In conditions in which the red cell membrane is relatively rigid, tissue perfusion decreases because of increased transit time for a red cell to pass from the precapillary to postcapillary level. Although nutrient and oxygen extraction are increased by this increase in transit time, the per unit perfusion of the tissues is overall decreased. Medications such as pentoxifylline reportedly allow the red cell easier deformability, thereby increasing the per unit perfusion of tissues.[7,8]

In normal states, arterial tissue perfusion is well above minimal requirements. Certain tissues, such as muscle, can change their metabolic requirements. Muscle becomes more efficient under anaerobic conditions—for example, in a person who engages in long-distance running. The process is gradual, but it's useful in patients with claudication. A regular exercise program can increase the distance walked before claudication occurs. Skin doesn't have such a compensatory mechanism.

Venous system

The venous system begins at the postcapillary level. Venules begin to coalesce, forming small veins, which again coalesce into larger veins from the periphery to a more central location. The venous system mimics the arterial system in many respects, but has a greater anatomic variability than the arterial tree. In the leg, the veins that course with the tibial and peroneal arteries are usually paired with numerous cross-linking branches, resulting in a retia appearance in some patients. These branches ascend along the respective arteries to form the popliteal vein, which is the first vein of significant size in the lower leg. The popliteal vein proceeds toward the head and becomes the femoral vein, commonly called the superficial femoral vein—a name that causes confusion because the vein in question is actually a deep vein. The superficial femoral vein joins the deep femoral vein to form the common femoral vein. The deep femoral vein is the deep drainage system of the thigh. (See *Deep and superficial venous systems,* page 276.)

Dual venous system

The leg has a dual venous system—the deep system just described and the superficial system represented by the saphenous veins. The greater saphenous vein courses along the medial aspect of the leg. The dorsal digital veins in the foot coalesce to form the greater saphenous vein. The greater saphenous vein is found medial and anterior to the medial malleolus. It ascends in the leg through a variable course and may be bifurcated or even trifurcated. At knee level, its course becomes deeper in relationship to the skin. As it ascends the leg, it joins the common femoral vein at

Deep and superficial venous systems

This illustration shows deep and superficial veins of the lower extremities.

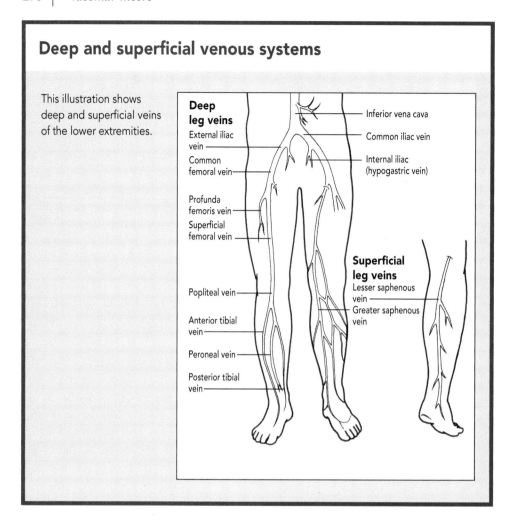

Deep leg veins
External iliac vein
Common femoral vein
Profunda femoris vein
Superficial femoral vein
Popliteal vein
Anterior tibial vein
Peroneal vein
Posterior tibial vein

Inferior vena cava
Common iliac vein
Internal iliac (hypogastric vein)

Superficial leg veins
Lesser saphenous vein
Greater saphenous vein

the fossa ovale. The lesser saphenous vein drains the posterior aspect of the calf. It perforates into the deep compartment of the calf at the level of the popliteal fossa to join the popliteal vein. As the common femoral vein ascends behind the inguinal ligament it becomes the external iliac vein and joins the internal iliac vein to become the common iliac vein. The common iliac veins join at the level of the umbilicus and to the right of the aorta to become the inferior vena cava. The renal veins drain into the vena cava. More cephalad, the hepatic veins join the vena cava, which then empties into the right heart chamber.

The saphenous system is connected to the deep venous system through numerous perforator veins. Perforator veins shunt blood from the subcutaneous tissue and the greater saphenous system into the deep veins of the leg. They cross through the superficial fascia of the leg, hence their name. The location of perforator veins is somewhat variable and some are ascribed proper names. The lowest perforator connecting the saphenous system with the deep venous system is just above the medial malleolus.

Valve anatomy

Unidirectional valves are present in the deep and superficial venous systems and in the perforator veins. These valves are located just before bifurcation points. The greater saphenous vein contains approximately six to eight valves. With rare exception, a valve is always present just below the insertion of the greater saphenous vein into the common femoral vein at the fossa ovale. The orientation of the valves allows venous blood to flow from distal to proximal. Perforator veins' valves are oriented to shunt blood from the lesser saphenous vein and the greater saphenous system into the deep veins of the leg.

Valve anatomy is that of a bileaflet with valve sinuses present on the lateral bases of each valve leaflet. These sinuses represent a dilation in the normal contour of the vein wall. Their function is to assist in valve closure, a passive act caused by the retrograde flow of venous blood into the sinus thereby coapting (fitting together) the two valve leaflets. The valve leaflets are oriented parallel to the surface of the skin. It's the loss of valve function at various levels that results in varying degrees of venous insufficiency. Valve function is lost under a number of disease states. Inability of the valve to coapt can also occur with over-distention of the venous segment. This effectively stretches the valves apart so that they no longer come in direct contact, thereby allowing blood to reflux into the more dependent portion of the vein. Disease states that cause loss of valve function include:

- congenital valve absence
- deep vein thrombosis
- ectasia
- phlebitis
- valve atresia
- venous hypertension
- venous engorgement.

Venous wall architecture

Venous wall anatomy is similar to arterial wall anatomy except that the respective lamina are thinner. The outermost layer of a vein is the adventitia. The media varies most from the arterial media. The media within a vein contains both elastic and muscular fibers, but to a much lesser degree than the arterial media. Nonetheless, a vein can contract and adjust its size to correspond to the degree of venous blood flow. The intima layer is a delicate single layer of endothelial cells.

The relatively thin media accounts for the lack of venous compliance at increased pressures. At low pressures, the venous system is fairly compliant, but once arterial pressure is reached, the venous wall becomes distended and rigid. Venoconstriction occurs in both the superficial and deep veins; the more peripheral the vein, the more readily it contracts. This reactivity is under sympathetic adrenergic control. Peripheral veins are more sensitive to this sympathetic drive than central veins. The ability of veins to relax and dilate enables the venous system to hold 75% of the total blood volume.

PRACTICE POINT

Loss of consciousness can occur from venous pooling in motionless lower extremities—a fate not unknown to young military recruits who must stand at attention for prolonged periods of time.

The upward flow of lower extremity venous blood, although aided by unidirectional valves and arterial pressure, is mostly dependent upon the "muscular pump." Pedal dorsal vein pressure in the supine position should approximate that of central venous pressure. Upon assuming an erect posture, this pressure can approach 100 mm Hg. With active muscle contraction, intra-compartmental pressure markedly increases, thereby causing deep veins of the leg to compress and push venous blood upward. This pressure then approaches 200 mm Hg. This is possible because the muscular compartments of the leg are enclosed by relatively rigid fascial encasement. Back-flush of blood is reduced when valves are competent and reflux into the saphenous system is prevented by the unidirectional perforator valves.

Lymphatic system

The lymphatic system is the least understood of the three vascular systems in the leg. The embryologic development of the lymphatic system is still largely unknown.

Lymphatic vessels are divided into three categories:

• initial or terminal lymphatic capillaries
• collecting vessels
• lymph nodes.

Initial or terminal lymphatic capillaries originate in the superficial dermis. At this level they are valveless—the epidermis doesn't contain lymphatic vessels. From the superficial dermis, the valveless system drains into the deep dermal and subdermal system where valved lymphatic vessels can be identified. Lymphatic valves are similar to venous valves, ascending the leg to drain both the dermis and the muscular beds into lymph nodes, routinely found at the popliteal fossa and the inguinal ligament. The lymphatic chain generally parallels the larger veins in the proximal leg above the knee.

Dissection around the deep femoral artery can disrupt the lymphatic system, resulting in surgically induced lymphedema. Above the level of the inguinal ligament, the lymphatic system drains through series of iliac lymph nodes coalescing into peri-aortic nodes, then into the cisterna chyli and more cephalad into the thoracic duct. The thoracic duct ascends along the thoracic aorta on the right side of the chest and drains into the left jugular vein just above the jugulo-subclavian junction. In addition to the thoracic duct, some patients have an accessory right lymphatic duct, which drains into the right jugular venous system. The thoracic duct traditionally has been considered the main lympho-venous drainage, although other methods of drainage exist, including lympho-venous communications within the various muscle compartments and peripheral lympho-venous communications.

Lymphatic vessel anatomy is similar to, but smaller than, either arterial or venous anatomy. The outer adventitial layer, in particular, is quite minimal. The media contains, in addition to a few elastin fibers, some stria of smooth muscle, which is used to help propel lymphatic flow cephalad via contraction. A single layer of endothelium comprises the intima. The relative size of a lymphatic vessel is between one-seventh and one-tenth the size of a major artery or vein.

Aspects of lymphatic flow

Lymphatic flow occurs as the consequence of four distinct etiologies: capillary blood pressure, osmotic pressure, interstitial fluid pressure (hydrostatic), and oncotic pressure. Intrinsic contractility of the lymphatic vessel wall, as previously stated, aids in cephalad lymphatic flow. The muscular pump aids in flow as it does in the venous system. Positive abdominal pressure, negative thoracic pressure, and pulsatile blood flow aid in cephalic flow of lymph.

The lymphatic system provides a drainage mechanism for acellular interstitial fluid. White blood cells are capable of entering the interstitial space and one of their mechanisms of reentry into the vascular space is by way of the lymphatic channels. Lymph is functionally "filtered" at the node level. The nodes act as a repository for lymphatic cells.

Normal lymphatic circulation requires an intact lymphatic system with essentially normal architecture. Whenever a disruption occurs within the lymphatic drainage system, lymphedema ensues.

Ulcer pathophysiology

The pathophysiology of vascular ulcers varies according to the type of ulcer. Although arterial and lymphatic ulcers are well understood, the pathophysiology of venous ulcers remains less clear.

Arterial ulcers

Arterial ulcers are wounds that won't heal due to inadequate arterial blood flow. Precipitating events for arterial ulcers vary. Limbs with arterial compromise may have minimal but adequate blood flow to maintain tissue viability. Ischemic lower extremity ulcers caused by trauma, although not of arterial etiology, must be treated as arterial ulcers because of deficient arterial blood available for healing.

The location of traumatic ulcers varies depending on the cause, but these wounds are commonly found on the foot or on the anterior tibial area of the lower leg. Traumatic ulcers may be caused by an acute physical injury, such as bumping into a piece of furniture or dropping a heavy object on the foot, or by continual pressure from ill-fitting footwear. Regardless of the cause, when ischemia is present, wound healing is inhibited. Although some wounds heal in the presence of ischemia, arterial inflow must usually be improved for healing to occur. Injury requiring more than baseline oxygen may be caused by blunt trauma, chronic or acute pressure, thermal extremes, chemicals, or decreased cellular nutrition from impaired arterial flow. Increased tissue nutritional need or diminished flow causing tissue hypoxia

Ischemic forefoot

This photograph shows an ischemic forefoot.

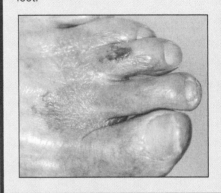

in arterial insufficiency eventually leads to gangrene or tissue necrosis. (See *Ischemic forefoot.*)

Venous ulcers

Venous ulcers are chronic skin and subcutaneous lesions usually found on the lower extremity at the pretibial and the medial supra malleolar areas of the ankle, where the perforator veins are located. Venous ulcers were formerly known as "venous stasis" ulcers because their development was thought to be caused by blood pooled in the veins. More recent literature indicates that venous hypertension rather than venous stasis is both the cause of these ulcers and the reason they don't heal.[11] It's difficult to restore skin integrity in the presence of chronic venous hypertension because the underlying edema must be controlled in addition to healing the ulcer.

Venous ulceration may be precipitated by deep vein thrombosis (DVT), which can remain undiagnosed for years prior to the onset of the ulcer. (See *Venogram*, page 280.) It has long been thought that

Venogram

In this venogram, the patient's left venous valve (B) is intact. On the patient's right (A), collateral veins are present due to venous occlusion, possibly from an undiagnosed deep vein thrombosis.

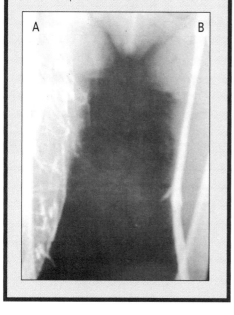

A   B

Hemosiderin deposit

Hemosiderin deposits caused the discoloration seen here in the patient's right leg.

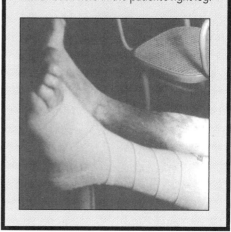

the natural course of lower-extremity DVT is the eventual development of leg ulcers.[12]

Symptomatic and asymptomatic thrombi may cause long-term complications by scarring the intima and creating valvular incompetence. When the valves are rendered incompetent, blood backs into the distal veins during diastole. With loss of perforator valve function, the high intracompartmental venous pressure, which can approach 200 mm Hg during active muscle contraction, results in distention of the saphenous system. This in turn causes a cascading effect with dilation of the greater saphenous vein and worsening of already compromised valvular function. The weight of the column of blood increases the pressure inside the capillaries.

Characteristics of venous ulcers

Venous hypertension distends the superficial veins, resulting in vein wall damage and exudation of fluid into the interstitial space, thereby causing edema of venous insufficiency. Over time, an actual leakage of red cells occurs through these compromised veins. As they break down, the red blood cells deposit hemosiderin into the tissues, causing a form of "internal tattooing" of the skin; the coloration is that of a brownish hue noticeable even in black skin. (See *Hemosiderin deposit*.) The skin loses its normal texture, becomes somewhat shiny and subsequently sclerotic, giving a taut skin appearance in these areas.

Edema and loss of red cells into the subcutaneous tissue occur at the point of greatest gravitational pressure, the ankle. This gives rise to the pathopneumonic features of chronic venous stasis, hyperpigmentation, and stocking distribution induration of the subcutaneous tissues,[13,14] the characteristics of long-standing venous insufficiency called lipodermatosclerosis. These areas are prone to subsequent ulceration or infection; extreme pruritus and excoriation are usually present, potentially aggravating the injured skin. Dermatitis due to endogenous or exogenous sources and severe allergic reactions may complicate the situation. The skin may present as itchy, erythematous, and weeping, or dry and scaly. (See *Venous ulcer with granulating base.*) Chemical or mechanical factors may be responsible for contact dermatitis surrounding a leg ulcer.[15]

Another sequelae of venous hypertension is irritability of the musculature. Many patients with venous insufficiency — even those in whom the condition is mild — report nocturnal leg cramps. Depolarization may occur due to fluid distention of the muscular cells, causing tetanic-like contractions of various muscle groups. Distention of veins in the subdermal plexus results in the varicosities typically seen with venous insufficiency. (See *Varicose veins,* page 282.) The appearance of telangiectasias, more commonly called "spider veins," is the result of distention of the smaller subdermal capillary network. (See *Telangiectasias,* page 282.)

In some circumstances, venous aneurysms can occur due to massive dilation of the greater saphenous vein and its tributaries. Further stagnation of flow in these areas in the presence of an abnormal vessel wall can result in thrombophlebitis, which worsens the venous outflow of the leg and aggravates an already deleterious condition. Thrombosis adheres to the wall of the vein and although recanalization occurs eventually, the valves remain incompetent. In an attempt to compensate for the reduced venous return, the surrounding collateral

Venous ulcer with granulating base

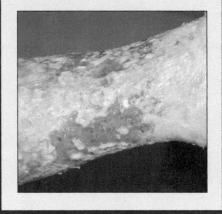

The venous ulcer shown here has irregular borders and a granulating base with surrounding fibrotic tissue.

veins dilate. Chronic edema occurs in the ankle. Increased venous pressure impedes capillary flow, decreasing oxygen available for transport from the capillaries to the tissues, and protein and red blood cells leak into the interstitial tissues. The effect is cumulative, eventually leading to tissue damage, scar formation and, ultimately, ulceration.

Endothelium in the normal saphenous vein facilitates contraction in response to noradrenaline. In varicose veins, the endothelial-enhanced noradrenaline vasoconstriction is decreased. Endothelial damage is thought to be a possible cause of venous dilatation and subsequent varicose veins.[16]

Venous leg ulcers are also correlated with increased ambulatory venous pressures. Nicolaides[17] obtained ambulatory venous pressures on 220 patients admitted with venous problems. The study found that no patients with ambulatory venous pressures (AVP) less than 30 mm Hg had

Varicose veins

Note the presence of varicose veins in the patient's lower extremities, shown here.

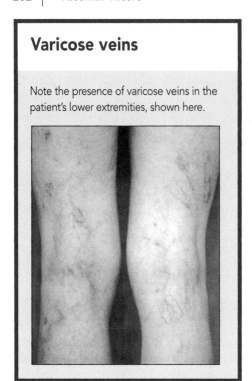

Telangiectasias

Telangiectasias, also known as "spider veins," are shown in the photograph below.

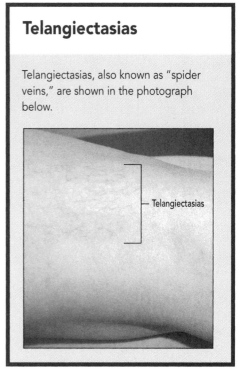

Telangiectasias

---

ulcers while 100% of those with AVP greater than 90 mm Hg had leg ulcers. The incidence of ulceration wasn't preferentially associated with either superficial or deep venous disease.

EVIDENCE-BASED PRACTICE

Nicolaides' study[17] suggests that ambulatory venous pressures should be measured in patients with nonhealing venous ulcers to determine whether they may benefit by a procedure such as a venous valve transplant, which reduces the AVP to less than 30 mm Hg.

Pathogenesis of venous ulcers

Several theories have been proposed to explain the mechanism of venous hypertension leading to ulceration. In 1917, Homans suggested that stasis of blood in dilated veins in the skin may cause anox-

ic cell death, leading to ulcers. Blalock[18] found the blood oxygen content to be higher than normal in varicose veins, suggesting that arteriovenous communications may be responsible for venous hypertension. In 1972, however, a study using radioactive macro aggregates refuted the arteriovenous shunting hypothesis.[19]

Two current hypotheses—the "fibrin cuff" and "white cell trapping" theories—are more recent attempts to explain venous ulcer formation. The fibrin cuff theory states that sustained venous hypertension causes distention of dermal capillary beds, which allow plasma exudate to leak into the surrounding tissue. Fibrin precipitation in the peripapillary space forms fibrin cuffs, which impair oxygen, nutrient, and growth factor transport. The tissues undergo inflammation and fibrosis.[20] A subsequent study suggests that peripapillary fibrin is present, but doesn't influence healing of lower-extremity ulcers.[21]

The white cell trapping theory states that the neutrophil aggregation in the capillaries causes lipodermatosclerosis. Increasing venous pressure is thought to reduce capillary perfusion pressure and flow rate. Low capillary flow rate initiates white blood cell adherence to the cell wall. Endothelial cells and leukocytes interact and release proteolytic enzymes, oxygen-free radicals, and lipid products. The white cells are then activated, damage the vessel walls, increasing capillary permeability and allowing larger molecules such as fibrinogen to exit the capillaries.[22,23]

The trap hypothesis of venous ulceration was proposed by Falanga and Eaglstein.[24] This hypothesis proposes that fibrin and other macromolecules that leak out bind or trap growth factors and other substances necessary for maintaining normal tissues and healing.

Classifying venous disease

Chronic venous insufficiency has been defined as an abnormally functioning venous system caused by venous valvular incompetence with or without associated venous outflow obstruction, which may affect the superficial venous system, the deep venous system, or both.[25] Chronic venous insufficiency can result in postphlebitic syndrome, which manifests as varicose veins and venous ulcers.

In 1994, the American Venous Forum developed a system based on clinical, etiologic, anatomic, and pathophysiologic (CEAP) data to categorize the key elements in chronic venous disease.[26] The CEAP system provides an objective classification method that clarifies relationships among contributing factors and improves communication regarding venous disease. The system is subdivided into seven categories based on objective signs of chronic venous disease.[27] (See *CEAP classification system,* page 284.)

Lymphatic ulcers

Lymphedema pathology is broadly classified under either obstructive or nonobliterative pathology. Obstructive pathology can result from anything that causes perilymphangitis. Nonobliterative pathology can result from endolymphangitis proliferans, primary thoracic duct pathology, lymph node obstruction, congenital defects, or lymphatic thrombosis.

Tumors are the most common form of lymph node obstruction in the United States. Primary thoracic duct pathology is either congenital or surgically acquired. Endolymphangitis can be the result of repeated intraluminal injury due to a host of noxious agents causing repeated injury. Lymphangiectasis is atrophy of the lymphatic channel; this is true atrophy and not a developmental problem. Congenital factors, which cause a nonobliterative pathology, result in either agenesis or hypoplasia. One type of congenital nonobliterative pathology is congenital familial lymphedema, or Milroy's disease, which represents approximately 3% of all cases of lymphedema. Milroy's disease has a female predominance with a variable age of onset, although it typically occurs later in life.[28]

PRACTICE POINT

Unilateral manifestation of edema is unique to Milroy's disease, although the disease can be bilateral.

Lymphatic thrombosis accounts for another form of nonobliterative pathology, for which anticoagulants are ineffective. Recent studies on benzopyrones such as warfarin demonstrated a reduction in lymphedema by stimulating macrophage activity,[29,30] thereby causing increased degradation of protein in lymph fluid with a resulting decrease in the edema.

CEAP classification system

The CEAP classification system for chronic venous disease consists of four elements:
- clinical classification
- etiologic classification
- anatomic classification
- pathophysiology.

Clinical classification (C0-6)

Class	Description
0	No signs of venous disease
1	Telangiectases or reticular veins
2	Varicose veins
3	Edema
4	Skin changes
5	Healed ulcer
6	Active ulcer

Etiologic classification (E_C, E_P, E_S)

- Congenital (E_C)
- Primary (E_P) — with undetermined cause
- Secondary (E_S) — with known cause

Anatomic distribution classification (A_S, A_D, and A_P)

This element consists of classifications A_S, A_D, and A_P, and segments 1 through 18. See table below for a breakdown.

- Superficial veins (A_S)
- Deep veins (A_D)
- Perforating veins (A_P)

Segment	Classification
1	Superficial veins (A_S) Telangiectases/reticular veins Greater (long) saphenous
2	• Above knee
3	• Below knee
4	• Lesser (short) saphenous
5	• Non-saphenous Deep veins (A_D)
6	Inferior vena cava Iliac
7	• Common
8	• Internal
9	• External
10	Pelvic-gonadal, broad ligament, other Femoral
11	• Common
12	• Deep
13	• Superficial
14	• Popliteal
15	Crural: Anterior tibial, posterior tibial, peroneal (all paired)
16	Muscular: Gastrocnemial, soleal, other Perforating veins (A_P)
17	Thigh
18	Calf

Pathophysiologic classification (P_R, P_O)

- Reflux (P_R)
- Obstruction (P_O)
- Reflux and obstruction (P_R, P_O)

Adapted with permission from Kistner, R.L., and Eklof, B. "Clinical Presentation and Classification of Chronic Venous Disease," in Gloviczki, P., and Bergan, J.J., eds., *Atlas of Endoscopic Perforator Vein Surgery*. New York: Springer-Verlag, 1998.

Three classes of lymphedema

Traditional classification divides lymphedema into three categories: congenital, lymphedema precox, and lymphedema tarda. The diagnosis of congenital lymphedema is usually made at or near birth. Lymphedema precox occurs sometime after birth, usually in the peripubital age. However, any lymphedema occurring before age 35 can be grouped under lymphedema precox. Lymphedema tarda merely implies that the age at onset of symptoms is later than age 35. Although this classification has been used for many years, a newer classification of lymphedema more accurately describes the pathology. Under this new classification lymphedema is described as primary or secondary.

Primary lymphedema can either be obstructive or hyperplastic. Obstructive pathologies are usually described according to anatomic location. They are divided into distal obliterative or pelvic obliterative. Primary hyperplastic lymphedema is classified as bilateral hyperplasia or megalymphatics. Bilateral hyperplasia is characterized by capillary angiomata on the sides of the feet. An obstructive process is usually present at the level of the cisterna chyli or thoracic duct and valves can be visualized when examined. Megalymphatics are large valveless lymphatic ducts similar to varicosities. The patient may exhibit little or no leg edema, but chylous reflux is present.

Secondary lymphatic obstructions

Tumor, surgical intervention, or infection may cause secondary lymphatic obstructions. The infectious group can be bacterial or filarial. The most common cause of lymphatic obstruction outside of the United States is from the filarial infection of *Wuchereria bancrofti*. Toxic exposure may also cause a secondary lymphatic obstruction and is typically grouped under the infectious category.

Differentiating a venous disorder from a lymphatic disorder in a swollen extremity with or without tissue loss is a common dilemma. Many disease processes can mimic lymphedema and these need to be excluded in order to make the diagnosis. Arterial venous malformations, lipedema (an abnormal accumulation of fat in the tissues of the leg), erythrocyanosis frigid (bluish discoloration of extremities secondary to cold exposure), factitious edema, and gigantism can also mimic lym-

---

> ## Conditions that mimic lymphedema
>
> These common clinical processes can mimic lymphedema:
> - Allergic disorders
> - Heart failure
> - Hepatic cirrhosis
> - Heredity angioedema
> - Hypoproteinemia
> - Idiopathic cyclic edema
> - Lipidemia
> - Postphlebitic syndrome
> - Renal failure
> - Total body excess free water

---

phedema. (See *Conditions that mimic lymphedema*.)

Diagnosing vascular ulcers

Vascular disease and ulcer etiology can be determined by obtaining a thorough patient history and performing a physical examination. A focused vascular history includes a clear description of the presenting complaint, past medical history for vascular and related conditions, current and previously taken medications, and risk factors. Signs and symptoms of lower extremity vascular disease may include pain, tissue loss, or change in appearance or sensation. Noninvasive vascular laboratory testing is used to identify the location of vascular pathology.

Physical examination

Skin inspection is an important part of the physical examination. Because skin color may indicate arterial perfusion or venous congestion, the color of each toe should be noted and compared to the other foot and toes. Arterial insufficiency causes ischemic tissue to first become pale, progressing to mottled (livedo reticularis) then to dark purple, and finally black. In venous insufficiency the skin appears a dusky ruddy color. Ischemia causes color changes with positioning. Elevating the foot at a 45-degree angle causes the ischemic limb to become pale. Immediately after positioning this foot in a dependent position, it becomes dark red or ruddy. This is the reactive hyperemia of ischemic tissue.

Skin should be palpated for temperature changes. The skin of an ischemic limb is cool or cold, with temperature demarcation that correlates to the diseased artery. Inspection also includes examining the distal extremities for taut or shiny, atrophic skin. Skin in arterial disease becomes thin and atrophied. In chronic venous insufficiency, the skin may become atrophied with scarring from a previous ulcer, or it may have weeping blisters or dry scaly crusts. Skin over lymphedema is firm early in the process but becomes fibrotic as the condition becomes chronic.

Capillary refill, determined by compressing and releasing the toe pad or the ball of the foot is a good indicator of arterial skin perfusion. It should be tested with the foot elevated slightly. Normal capillary refill time takes less than 3 seconds to return from pallor to normal skin color.

Palpating pulses, checking skin temperature, and obtaining arterial pressures are important elements of the arterial assessment. Pulses are palpated for presence, rate, regularity, strength, and equality. The most common objective physical finding is the presence or absence of pulses. Care must be taken when palpating pedal pulses. Examiners commonly mistake a contracting tendon for the presence of a pulse. No universal consensus exists regarding a pulse grading system; conversely, a high degree of observer variability exists in determining the presence or absence of pulses. It can be confusing if clinicians report 2+ or 3+ pulse examinations. Documentation is better facilitated if pulses are recorded as present or absent. However, even this seemingly obvious assessment parameter may not always be accurate. One study found only a 50% chance that two observers would agree with a third observer about the presence or absence of dorsalis pedis or posterior tibial pulses. This same study found the dorsalis pedis congenitally absent in 4% to 12% and the posterior tibial is absent in 0.24% to 12.8% of subjects.[31] Additional descriptors of pulse, such as "weak," or "bounding," can be added to clarify findings.

PRACTICE POINT

The best way to document pulses is to use descriptor terms, such as present or absent, rather than numerical ratings, such as 2+ or 3+. Use modifier words, such as weak or bounding, to further describe and clarify the pulse findings.

Pulses in the foot, present during rest, may disappear with exercise. A patient who presents with claudication but has clearly discernable pulses should have an exercise test done in the vascular laboratory. It's tempting to skip the assessment of the elusive popliteal pulse, particularly when the dorsalis pedis and posterior tibial pulses are strong. While good pedal pulses indicate foot perfusion, finding bounding popliteal pulses may indicate a popliteal aneurysm. Popliteal aneurysms can be a source of emboli to the lower leg with resulting tissue or limb loss.

Patients presenting with foot or leg ulcers should be tested for neuropathy, which is a common finding in the diabetic patient. Neuropathy commonly obscures a traumatic or pressure-induced wound in an ischemic limb. Lack of pain sensation and injury awareness prevents the diabetic patient from seeking care early. Neuropathy is evaluated by testing light touch, reflexes, kinesthesia of the ankle, and vibratory sense. An objective assessment of significant neuropathy is best done by using the 5.07 Semmes-Weinstein monofilament.[32]

Arterial signs and symptoms

Arterial insufficiency is commonly associated with complaints of pain[33] resulting from atherosclerotic arterial changes interrupting blood flow to tissues.[34] Arterial pain is characteristically described as claudication or rest pain — that is, pain that occurs with exercise and is relieved by rest; it occurs in the muscle group distal to the stenosed or occluded artery. While the calf is the most common location for claudication, it can occur in the buttock, thigh, or foot as well and is predictable and reproducible. Claudication is described by patients as a cramping, aching, or muscle weakness.

PRACTICE POINT

When taking a history it's important to ascertain exactly how far the patient can walk before he needs to stop because a shorter distance indicates more severe atherosclerosis. Reported changes in ambulatory distance may indicate progressive atherosclerotic disease.

The patient who presents with leg ulcers and poorly perfused tissue commonly seeks care because of sharp, severe, and possibly, constant pain at the ulcer site and the distal extremity. Pain that occurs at rest represents inadequate perfusion and is a sign of threatened limb viability. He may describe waking up at night with pain across the distal metatarsal area of the foot. In an attempt to relieve the pain he'll get out of bed and may even ambulate. Dependency of the extremity

results in increased blood flow to the foot because of increased hydrostatic pressure. The ischemic pain is relieved by the small contribution of blood flow from collateral vessels. The patient with pain at rest may begin sleeping with his legs dependent and leg edema may develop due to the chronic dependent position.

PRACTICE POINT

Rest pain represents end-stage arterial insufficiency and commonly requires surgical intervention.[35,36]

Patients with extensive sensory neuropathy — for example, diabetics — may not experience pain even with severely ischemic ulcers. On the other hand, these patients may experience such intense hyperesthesia that they cannot bear the light touch of stockings. Ulcers in patients with neuropathy are typically found on the plantar side of the foot and are surrounded by calluses from long-term pressure.

Previous arterial operations for vascular disease, including coronary artery disease and cerebral vascular disease, should be noted when obtaining a history. Vascular disease isn't limited to any one organ but occurs ubiquitously. Medications should be documented, especially vasoconstrictor drugs. Ischemic symptoms are exacerbated by nicotine. Patients with vascular disease shouldn't use tobacco or nicotine gum or patches.

Gangrene in ischemic tissue initially appears pale, then blue gray, followed by purple and, finally, black. Gangrenous tissue eventually becomes black, hard, and mummified. The hardened tissue isn't painful, but significant pain may be present at the line of demarcation between the gangrene and the live but ischemic tissue. Gangrene may be a small skin lesion or extend to an entire limb depending on the location of the arterial lesion. If a small patch of skin is affect-

Blue toe syndrome

This photograph shows "blue toe syndrome" in the second toe caused by tissue ischemia from arteriosclerosis.

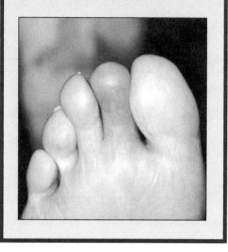

ed, the skin will dry and fall off, producing a skin ulcer. Large areas of gangrene may require debridement, skin graft, or amputation.

Ulcers may appear as small black or dark purple dots or circular areas found on the toes, or around the toe nail beds. (See *Blue toe syndrome*.) Ulcers found in these areas are caused by tissue ischemia from arteriosclerosis or by atheromatous debris embolizing from a proximal artery. Arterial ulcers may also be found between the toes, starting as a small moist macerated spot on the skin surface extending deep into the bony structure of the foot.

Arterial ulcers typically have distinct borders with a pale grey or yellow dry base. The surrounding tissue may appear pale compared to skin elsewhere on the body or it may be reddened if the leg is dependent. Chronic ischemic skin may appear thin and shiny. Foot elevation will produce skin pallor. The red or rud-

dy color of a dependent ischemic limb is called dependent rubor or reactive hyperemia. (See *Dependent rubor*.) Even in a person of color, the difference in hue is discernible when the ischemic limb is compared to the contralateral well-perfused limb.

Arterial pressure is one the most reliable physical findings in peripheral arterial disease.[37] However, lower extremity blood pressures aren't obtained as a part of the routine physical examination. Bilateral brachial pressures should always be obtained on the initial examination to identify whether a discrepancy exists between them. The correct pressure is always the higher of the two pressures. This pressure is used to determine the ankle brachial index when assessing lower extremity perfusion.

Venous signs and symptoms

Patients may report a gradual onset of discomfort associated with venous disease; however, usually no symptoms are present. Most patients describe general nondescript aching rather than specific pain. Some terms used to describe sensations in the legs include: fullness, swelling, tightness, aching, or heavy. These symptoms can be reduced with elevation. Venous insufficiency accompanied by acute DVT may be described as sharp, severe, deep, aching pain.[35] Varicose veins occasionally produce a pulling, prickling, or tingling discomfort localized to the area of the varicose vein.[7] In severe cases of venous insufficiency, a form of claudication can occur. The patient may complain of foot edema that makes it difficult for him to wear shoes.

A venous ulcer is moist and may have a yellow fibrous film covering its surface. This fibrous tissue isn't a sign of infection and doesn't interfere with healing.[38] The ulcer edges are irregular with firm fibrotic and indurated surrounding skin. The surrounding tissue may have brownish rust color, due to the breakdown of the erythrocytes and deposition of hemosiderin. Scar tissue may indicate the site of a previous ulcer. Because of the subcutaneous scarring, there is no allowance for the tissue expansion that occurs with edema in skin of normal elasticity. Scar tissue also prevents blood vessels from transporting oxygen to the skin, further compromising healing.[34,35]

Lymphatic symptoms

In contrast to arterial and venous disease, most patients don't report symptoms other than heaviness due to the weight of the limb. Ambulation is affected because of the limb weight and the inability to wear clothing. However, because of the lower incidence of pedal edema, the patients with lymphedema are less likely to complain of inability to wear shoes. Oozing fluids may cause pruritus.

Tissue loss or ulceration due to lymphatic obstruction with subsequent lymphedema of the extremity is unusual. Tissue loss occurs because of a concurrent secondary pathologic process. Patients with lymphatic obstruction are prone to infectious complications in the affected extremity. These infections can be bacterial but commonly are fungal in origin. Intertriginous folds should be inspected on a frequent basis for the development of ulcers and infections. It isn't uncommon in patients with lymphatic obstruction to acquire cutaneous fungal or bacterial infections. If this isn't controlled by oral agents, then a more aggressive I.V. treatment is required.

Vascular testing

Although an experienced vascular clinician can make a vascular diagnosis on history and physical examination, vascular laboratory studies contribute to the

Dependent rubor

Foot elevation produces skin pallor in patients with ischemic skin. When dependent, the ischemic limb will have a red or ruddy color, as shown here in the patient's right leg. This is called dependent rubor or reactive hyperemia.

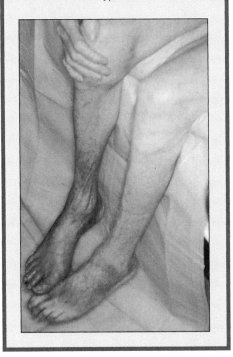

accuracy of the diagnosis. The presence, location, and severity of arterial and venous disease are confirmed by vascular laboratory procedures. Information obtained by vascular studies can predict ulcer healing when the cause is arterial insufficiency.[7] Laboratory tests differentiate among conditions contributing to a nonhealing ulcer.

Noninvasive vascular testing is divided into direct tests that image the vessel itself and indirect tests that demonstrate changes distal to the diseased vessel. These tests include Doppler ultrasound, venous duplex ultrasound, ankle-brachial index

Arteriogram

The arteriogram below shows iliac stenosis.

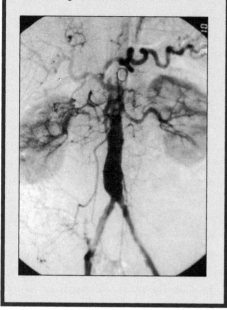

(ABI), transcutaneous pressure of oxygen (TCPO₂), segmental systolic pressures, and plethysmography.

Doppler ultrasound

In a Doppler ultrasound, a transmitting probe sends a signal, which is reflected from an object to the receiving probe. If the signal strikes a moving object such as blood cells, a frequency shift is detected and reflected as sound. The audible signals of venous and arterial flow patterns can be distinguished.

Duplex ultrasound

The venous duplex allows one to evaluate various segments of the venous tree looking for more than 0.5 seconds reflux after either a muscle contraction or manual augmentation of cephalad flow. Another advantage of venous duplex imaging is that it can identify sites of thrombosis with high levels of accuracy. The disadvantage is that it's fairly time-consuming, taking 1 to 2 hours per evaluation for a full leg imaging.

Arteriogram

An arteriogram is an invasive test used to identify an operative lesion in the arterial system by outlining the patent arterial lumen. (See *Arteriogram*.) Indications for a surgical procedure include incapacitating claudication, rest pain, nonhealing ulcers, and gangrene. An arteriogram isn't indicated when the patient is too ill for an operation or won't consider having one.

Arterial testing

Propagation of a pulse wave originating in the heart is easily measured by auscultation of a peripheral artery with a Doppler ultrasound. Recording the Doppler shift demonstrates the normal triphasic signal representing the three phases of the pulsation in a normal peripheral artery. The first wave represents forward flow of blood and arterial distention. The second phase represents the arterial relaxation and subsequent retrograde flow of blood. The third portion of the triphasic Doppler signal is believed to represent the bulging of the aortic valve, which occurs during diastole. The third phase of the triphasic arterial signal is first lost as an artery becomes less compliant and is followed by loss of the second phase of the triphasic Doppler signal. With worsening occlusive disease proximal to the area of auscultation, the normally sharp first wave becomes flattened and broader. In severely diseased arteries, the Doppler signal can be a monophasic, low-amplitude wave. The minimum systolic pressure that can

Arterial waveform changes

The arterial changes corresponding to occluded arteries are illustrated here.

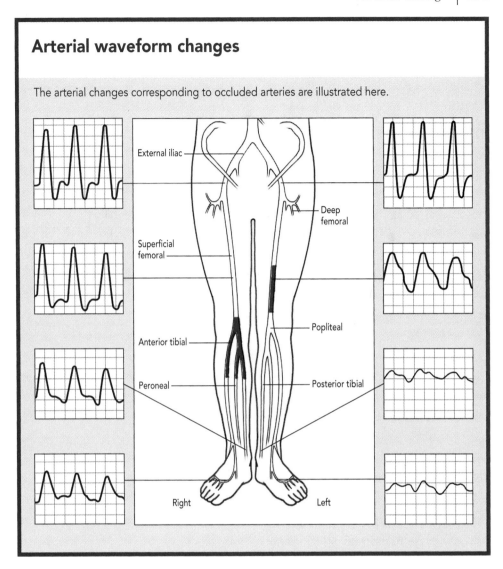

result in forward Doppler flow is used in the calculation of the ABI, a measurement of arterial perfusion in the leg. (See *Arterial waveform changes*.)

Tests for arterial disease include ABI, segmental pressures and waveforms, duplex ultrasound, and exercise treadmill for claudication. Perfusion is indirectly measured in a vascular laboratory by the ABI — the Doppler systolic pressure of the brachial artery divided into the ankle systolic pressure. ABI ratios reflect the degree of perfusion loss in the lower extremity.

In most individuals, the resting ankle pressure in a supine position is equal to the brachial pressure, with an ABI value of one. An individual with claudication may have a normal ABI in this position and have it drop during exercise. Patients with pain even in the resting state will have an abnormally low ABI. With exercise, the ABI in the patient with resting pain usually doesn't fall because

Obtaining an ankle-brachial index

To obtain an ankle-brachial index (ABI), you'll need a sphygmomanometer and a Doppler device. The procedure is performed as follows:

- Take the bilateral brachial blood pressure while the patient is supine. The higher of the two systolic pressures is used as the brachial pressure in the ratio.
- Place the blood pressure cuff on the leg just above the malleoli. Place the Doppler probe at a 45-degree angle to the dorsalis pedis or posterior tibial artery.
- Inflate the cuff until the Doppler signal is obliterated. With the Doppler probe over the artery, slowly deflate the cuff until the

Doppler signal returns. Record the number as the ankle systolic pressure.
- Divide the ankle pressure by the higher of the two systolic pressures. The ratio obtained is the ABI.

ABI Interpretation

ABI	Interpretation
1.0	Normal
0.75 to 0.90	Moderate disease
0.50 to 0.75	Severe disease
Less than 0.5	Rest pain or gangrene
Unreliable	Diabetes

the arteries are already maximally dilated. Inadequate perfusion creates local tissue factors that result in vasodilatation. Collateral pathways can't provide the additional tissue perfusion required resulting in rest pain. A patient with ischemic tissue loss usually has a perfusion picture more consistent with rest pain than claudication.[7] (See *Obtaining an ankle-brachial index*.)

Segmental pressures have been used since the 1950s to determine the location of arterial vascular lesions.[39] Pressures obtained at the level of the thigh, above the knee, calf, and ankle are compared to each other and to pressures in the other leg. An arterial lesion can be isolated with a 20 mm Hg gradient between cuff pressures. If no pressure gradient exists on a limb that claudicates, the patient is asked to exercise and repeat pressures are obtained.

 EVIDENCE-BASED PRACTICE

A falsely high pressure reading is commonly seen in patients with diabetes due to incompressible artery walls caused by medial sclerosis of the arteries.[36] When the vessels are incompressible, toe pressures are obtained as they are reported to be more accurate.

Venous testing

It's possible to perform a crude venous assessment by physical exam using a Doppler ultrasound. By compressing the limb manually, the flow in the veins can be augmented and noted by the audible Doppler signal heard distal to the site of compression. This is a subjective test and reliability is clinician dependent. The introduction of noninvasive vascular testing has provided much anatomic and physiologic information to increase the accuracy of diagnosing venous diseases. Two tests are most commonly used to assess the severity of venous insufficiency. One is the venous photoplethysmography (PPG) and the other is venous duplex imaging.[40]

Plethysmography

Plethysmography records volume changes in the limb. Several types of plethysmography are available:
• air plethysmography, which uses a pneumatic cuff as a segmental volume sensor
• strain-gauge, which uses a fine bore silicone rubber tube filled with mercury wrapped around the limb to be studied
• impedance plethysmography, which measures the relative change in resistive impedance of the passage of an electrical current through a segment of the body
• PPG, which measures the degree of light attenuation, which is proportional to the quantity of blood present and not actual volume change.[7,41]

Air and PPG are the more common tests for chronic venous disease. A photoplethsmograph consists of infrared light emitting diode and a photo sensor mounted on a probe. The probe is applied to the skin over the area to be tested.[7] The advantage of venous PPG is that it's quick and gives assessment of overall venous refill time. On the other hand, it only evaluates the most dependent portion of the leg in the gator area.

Diagnosing lymphedema

The patient history may be helpful in making a diagnosis. Testing modalities have been used for a differential diagnosis. Lymphangiography has recently fallen by the wayside as far as a routine evaluation. Both the radiologic and radionuclide evaluations are becoming less common and harder to obtain even at large medical centers. When in doubt, chemical evaluation of the protein content of the edema fluid within the ex-

tremity will help establish the proper diagnosis. A tissue fluid analysis with a protein content of between 1.0 and 5.5 g/dl is usually indicative of lymphedema, and 0.1 to 0.9 g/dl is more consistent with venous or cardiac edema. The albumin to globulin ratio is usually higher than serum in lymphedema. A complete blood count, plasma protein, albumin, urinalysis and urine protein can help diagnose the source for the edematous limb. Under unusual circumstances, a chromium chloride test can be obtained looking for abnormal losses of protein resulting in extremity edema.[28]

Treating vascular ulcers

Treatment goals for all ulcers include:
• providing an environment conducive to new tissue growth
• protecting the wound
• preventing further tissue destruction.
Topical and systemic treatments should be addressed at the same time. It's imperative to consider etiology when deciding treatment because ulcers aren't all alike and treatment for one type may be inappropriate or harmful to another. A vascular specialist should be consulted for patients with mixed etiology.

Wound infection

Infected leg ulcers, soft-tissue cellulitis, and osteomyelitis are treated by administering I.V. antibiotics. Topical antibiotics aren't indicated for all leg ulcers.[42] Chronic wounds are colonized with normal skin flora and shouldn't be treated with antibiotics.

Biopsy of nonhealing ulcers should be considered if true infection isn't responding to antibiotics or if carcinoma is suspected.

Wound cleaning

A clean wound, free from dead tissue and wound debris, is necessary for healing to occur. Wound cleaning and debridement are the initial steps in wound care. Many commercial wound cleaners and disinfectants are cytotoxic. Povidone iodine, hydrogen peroxide, and 0.25% acetic acid have shown evidence of interfering with fibroblast formation and epithelial growth.[43-46] There may be indications for using cidal agents in a wound; however, their use should be time-limited and each caregiver should have a clear understanding of when the goals have been reached.

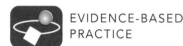

The safest wound cleaner is 0.9% saline solution. Wounds should be cleaned with a force strong enough to dislodge debris but gentle enough to prevent damage to newly growing tissue. The pressure to accomplish this goal ranges from 4 to 15 psi.[48] A 19G needle or 19G angiocatheter distributes approximately 8 psi when used with a 35-cc syringe. A Baxter cap on a saline irrigation bottle is a less expensive method to distribute an adequate amount of pressure. Leg ulcers treated in the home are commonly irrigated with running tap water.

Hydrotherapy or whirlpool has been used to aid in cleaning and debridement of both arterial and venous leg ulcers.[49] A clinical pilot study found that whirlpool followed by vigorous rinsing reduced the bacterial load in venous ulcers more than the whirlpool alone.[50] This may suggest that the vigorous irrigation is the significant factor in cleaning the wound. (See chapter 8, Wound debridement, for more information on wound cleaning.)

Dressings chosen for specific wounds depend on the wound bed condition and the goal for the wound. Many new dressings are designed to support moist wound healing (see chapter 9, Wound treatment options.) Because the skin is fragile in patients with either arterial or venous disease and can be easily injured, tape and adhesive products should be used with extreme caution. Use other methods of securing dressings that won't injury the skin.

Arterial ulcer treatment

Treatment of arterial ulcers must include increasing the blood supply to the area. Positioning the extremity in a dependent position may facilitate blood flow by gravity through collateral vessels. Use caution if devices such as a foot cradle are used for protection because an insensate foot is subject to trauma from the hard wood or metal of the cradle. Debridement of gangrene isn't performed in the presence of ischemia because the blood flow is insufficient to heal the new surgical wound. Ulcers without adequate arterial inflow must be kept dry — a contrast to the principle of moist-wound healing for ulcers with adequate blood supply. Moisture provides a bed for bacterial growth if eschar or gangrenous tissue are present. This tissue, if kept dry, can be left in place until demarcation or debridement is indicated.

Ulcers with adequate blood supply that are expected to heal should be dressed with products that support moist wound healing principles. These dressings include moist saline gauze, hydrocolloids, thin films, and foams. The surrounding intact tissue should be protected from fluid accumulation, which can macerate the healthy skin at the ulcer border. Arterial reconstruction is the treatment of choice to improve the circulation for most patients.[51] Percutaneous intraluminal balloon angioplasty is a consideration for discreet short lesions in the proximal arteries. Treatment for arterial leg ulcers requires reinstating arterial inflow before any other treatment is established. This is usually preceded by a noninvasive vascular test, an arteriogram followed by an angioplasty or an operation. Simultaneously, local ulcer treatment can be determined. Usually the arterial ulcer has a dry ulcer bed. The patient may have several punctate ulcers with regular borders, as well as dry eschar or gangrene distal to the most perfused tissue — usually the tips of the toes or an entire toe. This tissue must be kept dry until adequate arterial perfusion occurs. Moistened gangrenous tissue can provide a medium for bacterial growth. (See *Keeping gangrene dry.*)

Surgical treatment for arterial ulcers

Surgical treatment for arterial ulcers is aimed at restoring tissue perfusion. Bypass grafting may be done using prosthetic grafts or autogenous veins, either reversed or in situ. Percutaneous angioplasty and stent insertions are options, but other than

Keeping gangrene dry

Gangrenous tissue must be kept dry until adequate arterial perfusion is restored to the area. In the photograph below, the necrotic toes are left open to the air with alcohol wipes placed between them to promote drying.

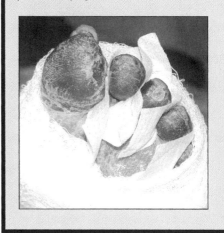

the common iliac arteries, have poor long-term results. Ulcers with large skin loss may need skin grafting to close the defect.

The treatment of ulceration due to arterial insufficiency depends on the level at which the occlusive disease occurs. Operations for arterial insufficiency are generally grouped under three major areas:

- aorto-iliac bypass
- femoral-popliteal bypass
- distal bypasses.

In many patients the occlusive disease is multi-leveled. In these patients, the "rule of thumb" is to improve in-flow first and then, if necessary, perform an outflow procedure. Usually in-flow involves the aorto-iliac segments. The exact operation is tailored to the individual patient's physiologic status and need. An elderly, frail patient with severe aorto-iliac occlusive disease may not be a candidate for an aorto-bifemoral bypass graft. In these patients, an axillo-bifemoral bypass graft is considered. By avoiding an intra-abdominal operation and clamping of the abdominal aorta, the overall morbidity for these operations can be less. However, the trade-off for this is that axillo-bifemoral bypass grafts generally don't have the long-term patency rates that an aorto-bifemoral bypass graft does.

A more recent development in the treatment of aorto-iliac occlusive disease has been percutaneous balloon angioplasty with or without stent placement. Isolated short-segment stenoses can be successfully treated with balloon angioplasty. Short segment stenoses are generally defined as those of less than 10 cm in length, commonly less than 5 cm. With more recent advancement in stent placements, acute occlusions occurring due to atherosclerotic plaque rebound have been decreased. The long-term patency rate for stents approaches that of arterial bypass but only in the aorto-iliac segments. Infra-inguinal balloon angioplasty with or without stent placement is still inferior treatment versus operative intervention. However, this still holds a place in the treatment of high-risk patients.

A femoral-popliteal bypass graft is the standard treatment for femoral popliteal disease. In contrast to aorto-iliac bypasses, where the bypass conduit is that of a synthetic material, the femoral-popliteal segment may have either a prosthetic conduit or an autogenous venous conduit. The patency rate for bypasses of the femoral popliteal segment is dependent upon the choice of conduit and the distal level of the bypass. In above-knee femoral-popliteal operations, the patency rate between autogenous vein and prosthetic material has no significant difference, although long-term patency rates are better when an autogenous venous conduit is used. In the below-knee femoral-popliteal bypasses, prosthetic

material is far inferior to that of autogenous venous conduits.[52] An autogenous venous conduit should be used in the below-knee position whenever possible. (See *Graft patency rates.*)

Below-knee femoral-popliteal bypasses using vein have a higher patency rate than above-knee femoral-popliteal bypasses because a certain amount of atherosclerotic disease at the level of the knee joint can be missed if only anterior-posterior arteriography views are obtained. For this reason, many vascular surgeons require oblique views of the popliteal artery so as to preclude this as a source of decreased long-term patency rates.

Distal bypasses, below the tibial perioneal trunk, require an autogenous venous conduit. This bypass is reserved for patients with tissue loss when pulsatile arterial perfusion to an ischemic area is desired. Although somewhat controversial, either a reversed venous bypass or an in situ bypass can be performed. Patency rates in large series regarding these two techniques is equivalent. The in situ technique is generally reserved for patients with considerable size disparity between the proximal and distal venous conduit, such as the greater saphenous vein. An in situ bypass is technically more demanding and requires more operative time than a reversed venous bypass. Nonetheless, the overall patency between the two techniques is equivalent. Some vascular surgeons advocate the use of prosthetic material for distal bypasses with the creation of a controlled arterial venous fistula in order to promote long-term patency rates of the prosthetic conduit.

A patient who has calf claudication requires improved perfusion to the posterior calf muscles. Claudication can occur in the buttocks, the thigh, or to isolated compartments of the lower leg. The perfusion of the respective symptomatic musculature is what determines the level

Graft patency rates

This chart shows the percentage of grafts that remain patent after 1, 2, 3, and 4 years.

Type of graft	1 year	2 years	3 years	4 years
ABOVE-KNEE FEMOROPOPLITEAL GRAFTS				
Reverse saphenous vein	84%	82%	73%	69%
Polytetrafluoroethylene (PTFE)	79%	74%	66%	60%
BELOW-KNEE FEMOROPOPLITEAL GRAFTS				
Reverse saphenous vein	84%	79%	78%	77%
PTFE	68%	61%	44%	40%
Limb salvage				
Reverse saphenous vein	90%	88%	86%	75%
In-situ vein bypass	94%	84%	83%	
INFRAPOPLITEAL GRAFTS				
Reverse saphenous vein	84%	80%	78%	76%
PTFE	46%	32%	21%	
Limb salvage				
Reverse saphenous vein	85%	83%	82%	82%
PTFE	68%	60%	56%	48%
AT OR BELOW-ANKLE GRAFTS				
Reverse saphenous vein	85%	81%	76%	
In-situ vein bypass	92%	82%	72%	
Foot salvage	93%	87%	84%	

of the outflow portion of the bypass. In patients with combined aorto-iliac superficial femoral popliteal disease, 90% of these patient's claudication can be cured by merely improving the in-flow to the profundal system by some form of aorto-iliac bypass. It's for this reason that routine combined aorto-femoral and femoral-popliteal bypasses should be avoided. In patients with lifestyle-limiting claudication with isolated superficial femoral artery disease, a femoral-popliteal bypass is usually all that's required.

Patients with ischemic tissue loss commonly require pulsatile arterial flow to heal their lesions. If these lesions occur in the foot, then whatever bypass is necessary to restore pulsatile arterial flow to the affected area should be performed. If this requires a femoral distal bypass then this is usually the operation chosen. Combined with the appropriate vascular bypass procedure, an area of ischemic tissue loss with gangrenous edges should be debrided to viable tissue. However, in some patients, if the area of loss is that of dry gangrene, autoamputation can be anticipated once adequate perfusion is restored. Some practitioners allow the gangrenous eschar to autoamputate to enable normal epithelial coverage of the underlying eschar before eschar separation. If, however, the area of tissue loss involves a digit, amputation with primary closure is recommended if no infection is present. This can be done in conjunction with the vascular bypass procedure, or the procedures can be separated by several days if deemed appropriate.

Arterial reconstruction with an in situ graft may be used to revascularize the lower extremity well below the knee. An in situ graft is a vein left in its natural location, anastomosed to the arterial system above and below the arterial stenoses, after the valves are lysed. This procedure allows the surgeon to reconstruct the smaller distal arteries in the lower extremity near the foot. These reconstructed vessels are close to the skin surface. Be careful not to cause injury to underlying vessels when using sharp debridement for these necrotic ulcers. Autolytic debridement is a safer debriding alternative.

Venous ulcers

Venous hypertension and wound care are treated together. Wound care depends on whether the patient can be immobilized. Edema is controlled by conservative means, intermittent elevation, compression bandages, and intermittent pneumatic compression.[53] Studies have demonstrated that moist wound healing combined with compression improves wound-healing rate of venous ulcers.[54] Compression therapy is the mainstay of venous ulcer therapy.[55] Elevating the legs above the heart is recommended whenever the patient can be placed in this position. A compression dressing isn't required when the patient is immobilized with the leg elevated, such as during sleeping hours. Moist gauze dressings with frequent changes can be used instead.

The ambulatory venous patient is best served by semirigid dressings such as the Unna boot, or by multilayered compression wraps. Multilayered compression is

more effective than single layer; both 4-layer and short-stretch bandages have higher healing rates than paste plus an outer support. With the discovery of moist wound healing[56] and the advent of hydrocolloid and foam dressings, occlusive dressings may be used under compression wraps to promote growth of granulation tissue, reduce pain from the dressing rubbing against the ulcer, and promote autolytic debridement. One study found ulcers healed twice as fast with the foam dressing under the Unna boot as those ulcers without the foam.[57]

Compression wraps should be applied starting just below the toes and ending just below the popliteal fossa. A gauze roll or padded gauze dressing is typically used over the wound area. The dressing is covered with an elastic bandage. Stockings reduce ambulatory venous pressure by decreasing venous reflux and improving calf muscle ejection capacity during use.[58] Stockings are graded according to the amount of pressure they exert, from 20 to 60 mm Hg at the ankle. The benefit derived from the stocking is in direct proportion to the fit.

In many cases, patients fail to wear the prescribed compression dressing or stocking because of difficulty donning the stockings or complaints of tightness. The importance of long-term external compression can't be overemphasized. Patients should be taught that the stockings must be replaced every 3 to 6 months. Two pairs should be purchased so that one can be worn while the other is laundered.

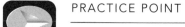

PRACTICE POINT

Long-term compression therapy is an essential part of the treatment of venous leg ulcers.

A pneumatic compression pump may be used to reduce lower extremity edema. One study found improved venous ulcer healing when compression pumps were used; however, third-party payers don't agree with the use of these pumps as a method of treatment.[59-62] One study[63] found 4 hours of compression per day improved ulcer healing when used with compression stockings. In another study,[64] an intermittent pneumatic compression device provided improved healing when used for 1 hour twice weekly in conjunction with conventional dressings.

Surgical treatment for venous ulcers

Surgical treatment for venous ulcers is aimed at correcting the cause of the venous hypertension. Some of these procedures include vein valve transplantation, direct valve repair, and veno-venous bypass. Varicose veins may be treated by excision, ligation, or injection, depending upon the size of the vein.

Surgical treatment for venous insufficiency is still in its infancy compared to the established treatment of arterial occlusive disease. Venous insufficiency can be grouped under two broad categories:
• venous reflux
• venous outflow obstruction.

The net result of both of these disease entities is venous hypertension and the sequelae resulting in venous ulcerations. The mainstay for the treatment of venous insufficiency continues to be good external compression. In many patients, this is all that is required. It acts both as a treatment for various states of venous insufficiency as well as a prophylaxis for the development of the adverse sequelae. In some patients, the use of compression alone is inadequate; for these patients, surgical intervention is usually necessary.

Venous outflow obstruction is usually the result of deep vein thromboses. When it involves isolated segments with normal segments either above or below, the obstruction can result in a cascading event resulting in venous insufficiency. In some patients, the outflow obstruction is the cause of the symptoms. In these patients, bypassing the obstructed segment to relieve the venous outflow obstruction and the corresponding venous hypertension by balloon angioplasty of a sclerotic or stenotic segment with or without stent placement may be necessary.

Other patients require bypass using an autogenous venous conduit. The proximal and distal anastomoses of the venous bypass are dictated by the obstruction site. For example, if a patient has an isolated ilio-femoral thrombosis that has failed to recannulize or has only partially recannulized and the affected leg is symptomatic, a femoral-femoral bypass from the proximal portion of the symptomatic leg to the more distal portion of the contralateral leg can be performed. The saphenous vein is usually used for this but in contrast to arterial bypasses the direction of the valve isn't reversed; rather the valve leaflets are oriented to prevent reflux. Similarly, a bypass from a more proximal vein within a symptomatic leg to the more cephalad iliac vein may be indicated.

In patients with an outflow obstruction, but in whom insufficiency or hypertension is caused by occlusion of the greater saphenous vein, the venous hypertension may be alleviated by isolated partial saphenous vein ligation and stripping. This is usually done at the knee level with stripping of the affected saphenous segment. If, however, the reflux or hypertension is the result of the deep venous system, then stripping the greater saphenous vein wouldn't help and actually may be detrimental due to elimination of one of the venous outflow tracts of the extremity. This information must be known before a surgical procedure is performed to correct venous insufficiency. Three tests are available to evaluate reflux:
• ascending/descending venography
• duplex imaging
• venous PPG.

These tests are all readily available through either a vascular laboratory or a radiology department. Venous PPG can determine whether the deep or superficial system is involved with venous reflux. A better test uses venous duplex, which looks at specific segments of both superficial and deep veins for reflux and can give a more detailed evaluation of the affected extremity. Isolated valve segments of the more proximal venous system can be evaluated using descending venography looking for contrast reflux past the incompetent valve. Venography can also determine sites of stenoses within the venous system as can venous duplex. One of the problems associated with accurate duplex imaging is that it's dependent upon the competence of the technician performing the test. Certain laboratories have more expertise in these areas than do others.

When deep venous insufficiency is due to valvular incompetence, it isn't known how many competent valves are required and in what locations for the deep venous system to become competent again. Research in these areas is ongoing and more attention is now being given to venous insufficiency.

Three techniques are available for surgical correction of venous insufficiency due to valvular incompetence:
• artificial venous valve insertion
• autogenous vein valve transplantation using a segment of vein, usually from the upper extremities or axilla
• direct valvuloplasty.

Autogenous valve transplantation is a procedure in which a segment of vein with a competent valve, usually in the upper extremity or axilla, is identified. This section of vein is rejected and an interposition graft placed at the harvest site. The vein is then transposed into the venous system of the affected extremity maintaining the orientation of the valve to keep the leaflets open in a cephalic di-

rection. Postoperative anticoagulation with heparin and subsequent warfarin is commonly used.

Approximately 75% of the stasis ulcers remain healed at 12-month follow-up after valve transplantation. However, considerable degradation occurs over the course of the second year in these patients, such that only 40% of limbs remain healed.[65] After the second year, results appear to stabilize without further deterioration although the reports on this are limited in both scope and number.

Variations on this procedure using valve segments from other areas or even transposing a deep vein with a competent valve to another deep vein with an incompetent valve can be done. Overall results appeared to be similar to that of transposition of competent vein valve segments.[66]

Direct valvuloplasty is another technique for correcting valvular insufficiency. This is performed by suture approximation of two valve leaflets that don't fully close. It's done either with direct suturing within the areas of the cusps to obtain good apposition, or by external buttressing of an incompetent vein valve sinus. Valve leaflets themselves are brought into apposition by placing the equivalent of a "girdle" around the dilated valve to reduce dilatation and allow the valves to come in apposition in a more normal fashion. This sleeve technique is usually done with prosthetic material. Similarly a transplanted valve that may deteriorate due to dilatation can be made competent again by using this technique.[67]

An external valve repair known as the Psathakis silastic sling procedure has been developed.[68] This involves placing a silastic sling around the popliteal vein then attaching it to the two heads of the biceps femoris muscle. When these muscles contract, the sling is intended to occlude the popliteal vein during ambulation. The problem with this is that the sling becomes intimately adherent to the vein and surrounding tissue and over time no longer functions in this fashion.

In patients where no suitable vein valve segment can be found or it's deemed an inadequate operation, the development of a prosthetic valve with its implantation holds some promise. Currently, a prosthetic venous valve comprised of a complex titanium double leaflet system is being developed and may hold promise.

The appropriate use of adequate compression is necessary in conjunction with all the surgical treatments. The application and management of patients with compression hose is dealt elsewhere within this chapter.

Patients with recurrent leg ulcers due to incompetent perforators in the affected area may benefit from a Linton flap. This procedure requires elevation of the skin and fascia at the site of ulceration and a transection with ligation of the incompetent perforator veins feeding the area. Proper application of compression is required afterward to reduce the local venous hypertension. Results may be very good if compression is used as instructed postoperatively. The morbidity associated with this operation includes tissue slough along the area of incision and the overlying tissue resulting in a prolonged healing period. This may be due to the chronic disease state of the tissue at the ankle.

A new and exciting advancement in technique is the use of an endoscope for subfascial ligation of incompetent perforator veins. Using equipment developed for laparoscopic cholecystectomies, the scope is passed from healthy leg tissue into the subfascial space. The fascia is raised from the underlying musculature, resulting in segments of perforator veins rising so that they can be ligated and transected through the endoscope, thereby avoiding direct incisions in areas of tissue that are tenuous and most likely to have postoperative

Lymphedema

This photograph shows lymphedema of the left leg.

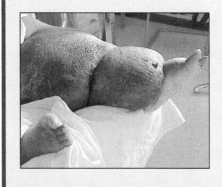

healing problems. The reason for ligating incompetent perforators is to eliminate the venous hypertension associated with reflux of venous blood.[69]

In some patients, the application of a split-thickness skin graft to an otherwise healthy stasis ulcer may be appropriate. This technique shouldn't be used in patients whose underlying venous problems haven't been addressed. The application of a split-thickness skin graft to an ulcer with persistent venous hypertension will fail, even if the patient is compliant with the use of a compression hose.

PRACTICE POINT

Skin grafting of ulcers should only be done after the underlying venous hypertension is corrected.

Lymphedema

Conservative treatment is the treatment of choice for patients with lymphedema. (See *Lymphedema*.) A multimodality approach, including elevation, exercise,

Compression wrapping

This photograph shows a leg being wrapped with a 4-layer compression therapy dressing.

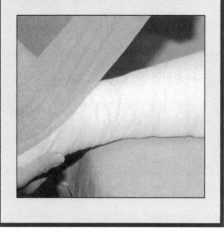

compression garments, manual lymphatic drainage, compression pumps, and preventing infection, is recommended.[29,30,70,71] Patients with lymphedema require a higher degree of compression than those with venous insufficiency. Pressure should be 50 to 60 mm Hg for lymphedema, compared to venous insufficiency, which requires 30 to 40 mm Hg.

A lymph pump is recommended for more rapid reduction of lymphatic fluid to reduce edema in the affected limb. The affected extremity is placed into a long inflatable sleeve that's connected to a pump that inflates the sleeve to a predetermined pressure. Continued elevation of the limb is also necessary. In those who have reducible lymphedema, long-term use of a compression pump is the treatment of choice; however, compliance may be a problem. Once the extremity approaches its smallest obtainable size, a static compression garment is fitted. Between pump uses, the extremity should be wrapped with elastic compression bandages or have temporary compression garments applied to reduce the recurrence of the lymph in the limb. (See *Compression wrapping*.) It may take months to obtain a demonstrable reduction in the size of the extremity in severe cases of lymphedema.

PRACTICE POINT

The effectiveness of lymph pump therapy increases if the patient can be nonambulatory for the initial edema reduction.

Treating lymphedema surgically

Lymphedema has fewer surgical options than the treatment of arterial or venous ulcers. However, patients with severe lymphedema and minimal improvement with compression therapy may benefit from a lymph-reducing surgical procedure. Lymph-reducing operations fall under three broad categories:
- drainage procedures
- excisional therapy
- excisional therapy and skin grafting.

Excisional therapy involves removing a large section of skin and subcutaneous tissue to the muscle fascia and reapproximating the wound edges. The net result is the equivalent of reducing the hem on a waistline. Problems associated with this procedure relate to the undermining of the residual tissue necessary for approximation of wound edges, which can delay healing. In addition, this method doesn't treat the underlying problem of lymphatic outflow obstruction.[71]

Excisional therapy and skin grafting can be performed and may also be used to treat lymphedema. This technique usually involves complete degloving of overlying tissue on the affected extremity and split-thickness skin grafting directly onto the muscular bed. By removing all overlying lymphatic tissue within the dermal and subcutaneous space down to the muscle bed, lymphedema in the area of grafting is no longer a concern. The result is one of marked reduction in the size of the extremity, but any tissue distal to this is left with more exaggerated lymphedema than in the preoperative state. Skin grafts have a 5% to 10% incidence of failure, and when they fail, long-term healing can be a problem.

A drainage procedure for lymphatic obstruction may be considered for patients with lymphatic obstruction at the level of the upper leg or more proximal limb, and those who have short-segment obliteration of lymphatic channels. The procedure is contraindicated for patients with a distal or obliterative disease, and those with combined pelvic and distal obliterative disease.

The drainage procedure currently favored for the treatment of limited lymphatic obstruction is a lymphovenous shunt.[72] In this procedure, a lymph channel, usually at the level of the inguinal region, is anastomosed in an end-to-side fashion to the deep venous system of the leg. This requires microvascular anastomoses. The size disparity between the wall of the lymph channel and that of the wall of the vein is great; for this reason, these procedures have a high failure rate. However, when they are successful, the lymphatic outflow is increased from the extremity and good results can be obtained as long as the lymphovenous anastomosis stays patent. Again, compression garments are necessary for life in these patients.

Measuring healing

Calculating healing rates is problematic when no standard measurement for wound healing parameters exists. Following wounds to complete healing is one method, but not satisfactory if changes in therapy are needed. Healing rates can be expressed as percent of ulcer area, measurement of change in ulcer perimeter, or percent of ulcer area healed. However, the perimeter and surface area is much greater in large ulcers. Using these measurements will give erroneously high healing rates for the larger ulcers compared to smaller ulcers. When percent of ulcer healed is used as a measurement, smaller ulcers will appear to heal faster than large ulcers by comparison.

In another method, ulcers are traced on a celluloid screen, then measured. The area and circumference of the tracing are calculated by a computer program.

Patient education

The patient may inadvertently neglect his ulcer or fail to use prevention measures if he doesn't understand the nature of the condition. Be sure to teach your patient ulcer pathology and treatment rationales, and to recognize and report changes that indicate problems with healing. Patient and family education should also include assessment of educational needs and level of understanding. Teaching methods vary and should be chosen to facilitate the most appropriate method for the patient and his family.

Risk factors

Factors that increase risk for arteriosclerosis include smoking, diabetes, hyperlipemia, and hypertension.[73] Smoking is a factor in 73% to 90% of patients with atherosclerotic arterial disease. Up to 30% of patients with arterial disease are reported to have diabetes,[74] and of those patients with diabetes, 16% to 58% have arterial disease.[75-77] Hypertension is present in 29% to 39% of patients with atherosclerosis, and 31% to 57% of patients with atherosclerosis have hyperlipemia.[74] Risk factor modification

Teaching about arterial ulcers

Teach the patient with an arterial ulcer to:
- monitor arterial or graft patency by palpating pulses
- recognize signs and symptoms of graft failure and what to report
- avoid nicotine in any form
- begin or maintain a regular exercise program
- manage blood glucose, if diabetes is present
- control hyperlipidemia
- manage hypertension
- reduce weight, if indicated
- perform meticulous foot care
- manage ulcer care.

Teaching about venous ulcers

Teach the patient with a venous ulcer to:
- monitor the skin for cracking, ulcers, color, and temperature changes
- use prescription compression stockings
- wear clean stockings daily
- ambulate with stockings on
- avoid extreme temperatures to the skin
- avoid constricting clothing around lower extremities
- maintain ideal body weight
- limit salt intake; avoid smoking
- protect lower extremities from trauma
- avoid prolonged standing or sitting
- elevate feet higher than the heart whenever possible during the day.

is part of the treatment for vascular ulcers to reduce the possibility of further breakdown.

Smoking cessation is critical for patients with arterial insufficiency. The direct relationship between tobacco use and ischemia is well-known. Smokers are nine times more likely to develop claudication than nonsmokers.[78] The link between smoking and vascular disease isn't well recognized; in one study, only 37% of smokers with peripheral vascular disease understood the strong association between smoking and vascular disease.[79] Patients must be informed of the negative effects of smoking on the vascular system and be referred to smoking cessation specialists if needed.

Arterial ulcers

Patients can help themselves by positioning and reducing activities that impair blood flow. After a surgical or percutaneous intervention to restore arterial flow, the patient should continue behaviors that promote vascular health and reduce risk factors. (See *Teaching about arterial ulcers.*)

Venous ulcers

Chronic venous insufficiency is a permanent condition. Because of this, patients are given information about the disease process and rationale for intervention. The more information they have, the more likely they are to manage the condition effectively. Activities that promote venous return are encouraged. Extremity elevation should become a daily routine and external compression is needed for life. Patients must understand the importance of this fact. Protection from trauma to the skin is essential. A small lesion may progress quickly to a large ulcer because of the edema. It may take years to heal, if at all. Small cuts or bruises should have immediate medical attention. Leg exercises to increase muscle pump activity are taught to the patient. Patients are encouraged to use these exercises during long periods of standing or sitting. When sitting, the legs should be elevated. (See *Teaching about venous ulcers*.)

Lymphatic ulcers

Lymphedema and lymphatic obstruction are lifelong problems. Like other chronic problems, management falls to the patient who possesses the problem. Education regarding the etiology of lymphedema and principles for management are the first and most important part of patient education. Usually, when patients know what's behind the pathology of their conditions they can devise creative ways to deal with the manifestations of the disease, or at the very least, figure a way to work the treatment into a schedule that maintains function as long as possible. (See *Teaching about lymphatic ulcers*.)

Manual lymphatic drainage is a therapeutic technique used for patients with lymphedema to increase lymph flow. It consists of movement of the therapist's hands over the patient's skin and subcutaneous tissue. Pressure applied is very gentle and the movements are slow to correspond to the slow lymphatic pulsations. The massage sequence begins at the center of the body and moves to the periphery. The rationale for this is that the lymph nodes must be emptied before they can receive any more lymph from the periphery. Each maneuver is performed in a distal to proximal direction.

 PATIENT TEACHING

Teaching about lymphatic ulcers

Teach the patient with a lymphatic ulcer to:
- keep the affected limb elevated higher than the heart whenever possible
- use the pneumatic pump on schedule to maintain reduced edema
- wear compression garments between pneumatic pump treatments.

Typically, the patient with lymphedema doesn't have access to a therapist who's educated and certified to perform manual therapeutic drainage.[80]

Summary

Success in managing vascular ulcers requires a total patient commitment. Risk factors and ulcer management are so dependent upon the patient's activities that the patient must have as much information as possible to participate in the therapy. An understanding of vascular pathophysiology and its contribution to leg ulcers is critical in the management of the ulcers. Arterial reconstruction is the hallmark of treatment for arterial disease. Venous reconstruction is in its infancy but shows promise to reduce the sequela of postphlebitic syndrome. In general, dry arterial ulcers or those with fixed, stable, dry eschar should be kept dry until the tissue is revascularized. Venous ulcers always require external compression, ultimately in the form of compression stockings. Ulcers associated with lymphedema usually respond when the edema is reduced. A variety of wound care products are available for leg ulcers, but no research exists showing one product to be more effective than another. Economic concerns make it imperative to choose the appropriate dressings and treatment, but research demonstrates little increased benefit of the newer treatments over the old.

Show what you know

1. *The cause of venous ulcers is:*

   A. venous stasis.
   B. venous hypertension.
   C. embolic phenomenon.
   D. varicose veins.

ANSWER: B. Venous stasis was thought to cause venous ulcers because of pooled blood in the veins. However, current literature reports venous hypertension is responsible for increased pressure along the vein wall and in the subcutaneous tissue.

2. *CEAP is a classification system for venous disease. A patient with C-6, E_S, A_D, A_P, P_R classification would have:*

   A. an active ulcer with a known cause, and reflux disease in the deep and perforating veins.
   B. varicose veins of congenital etiology in the superficial veins, with reflux.
   C. skin changes with undetermined cause, disease in the deep veins with obstruction.
   D. a healed ulcer with known cause and deep venous involvement and reflux and obstruction.

ANSWER: A. The CEAP classification stands for clinical, etiologic, anatomic, and pathophysiologic components to the system. C-6 refers to an active ulcer. E_S means etiology is secondary with a known cause. A_D and A_P refer to anatomic distribution of the deep and perfo-

rator veins. And P_R means that reflux is the pathophysiology behind the disease.

3. *Patients with arterial ulcers characteristically have:*

   A. lipodermatosclerosis.
   B. reduced blood flow.
   C. edema.
   D. systemic hypertension.

ANSWER: B. An arterial ulcer by definition is associated with arterial insufficiency. Lipodermatosclerosis and edema are associated with venous ulcers, and systemic hypertension is unrelated to arterial ulcers.

4. *The ankle-brachial index (ABI) is an indicator of loss of perfusion in the lower extremity.*

   A. True
   B. False

ANSWER: A. Perfusion of the lower extremity is indirectly measured by the ABI.

5. *The most important treatment component for venous and lymphatic ulcers is:*

   A. moist wound healing.
   B. antibiotics.
   C. compression.
   D. revascularization.

ANSWER: C. Compression is the most important component — the edema must be managed in order for venous and lymphatic ulcers to heal.

6. *Surgical treatment for arterial ulcers most commonly includes:*

   A. graft.
   B. valvoplasty.
   C. bypass graft.
   D. phlebectomy.

ANSWER: C. Arterial ulcers are associated with arterial insufficiency and a bypass graft is meant to restore the arterial circulation to the ischemic tissues.

7. Lymphedema treatment includes:

A. leg elevation.

B. skin grafting.

C. deep massage.

D. diuretics.

ANSWER: A. Leg elevation is part of the treatment for edema reduction for lymphedema. Skin grafting isn't usually effective. The massage techniques used for manual lymphatic drainage are light massage.

8. The most detrimental activity a patient with any vascular disease can do is:

A. walk into the pain.

B. sleep with legs dependent.

C. use nicotine.

D. fail to monitor pulses.

ANSWER: C. Nicotine shouldn't be used in any form. It constricts vessels and contributes to atherosclerosis and venous disease.

References

1. Young, J.R. "Differential Diagnosis of Leg Ulcers," *Cardiovascular Clinics* 13(2):171-93, 1983.
2. Cornwall, J.V., et al. "Leg Ulcers: Epidemiology and Aetiology," *British Journal of Surgery* 73(9):693, September 1986.
3. Coon, W.W., et al. "Venous Thromboembolism and Other Venous Disease in the Tecumseh Community Health Study," *Circulation* 48(4): 839-46, October 1973.
4. Dewolfe V.G. "The Prevention and Management of Chronic Venous Insufficiency," *Practical Cardiology* 6:197-202, 1980.
5. Callam, M.J., et al. "Chronic Ulcers of the Leg: Clinical History," *British Medical Journal* (Clinical Research Edition) 294(6584):1389-91, May 30, 1987.
6. Nelzen, O., et al. "The Prevalence of Chronic Lower-limb Ulceration has been Underestimated: Results of a Validated Population Questionnaire," *British Journal of Surgery* 83(2):255-58, February 1996.
7. Rutherford, R.B. "The Vascular Consultation" in *Vascular Surgery,* Vol. 1, 4th ed. Philadelphia: W.B. Saunders Co., 1995.
8. Moore, W.S. (ed). *Vascular Surgery: A Comprehensive Review*, Philadelphia: W.B. Saunders Co., 1991.
9. Browse, N.L., et al. *Diseases of the Veins: Pathology, Diagnosis, and Treatment.* London: Edward Arnold, 1988.
10. Phillips, T.J., and Dover, J.S. "Leg Ulcers," *Journal of the American Academy of Dermatology* 25(6 Pt 1):965-89, December 1991.
11. Browse, N.L., and Burnand, K.G. "The Cause of Venous Ulceration," *Lancet* 2(8292):243-45, July 31, 1982.
12. Dodd, H., and Cockett, F. "The Postthrombotic Syndrome and Venous Ulceration" in *The Pathology and Surgery of the Veins of the Lower Limbs.* Edited by Dodd, H., and Cockett, F. New York: Churchill Livingstone, 1976.
13. Burnand, K., et al. "Venous Lipodermatosclerosis: Treatment with Fibrinolytic Enhancement and Elastic Compression," *British Medical Journal* 280(6206):7-11, January 5, 1980.
14. Nicolaides, A., et al. "Chronic Deep Venous Insufficiency in *Haimovici's Vascular Surgery,* 4th ed. Edited by Haimovici, H., et al. Oxford: Blackwell Science, 1996.
15. Powell, S. "Contact Dermatitis in Patients with Chronic Leg Ulcers," *Journal of Tissue Viability* 6(4):103-106, October 1996.
16. Owens, J.C. "Management of Postphlebitic Syndrome," *VD&T*, February-March, 1981.
17. Nicolaides, A.N., et al. "The Relation of Venous Ulceration with Ambulatory Venous Pressure Measurements," *Journal of Vascular Surgery* 17(2):414-19, February 1993.
18. Blalock, A. "Oxygen Content of Blood in Patients with Varicose Veins," *Archives of Surgery* 19:898-905, 1929.
19. Lindemayr, W., et al. "Arteriovenous Shunts in Primary Varicosis? A Critical Essay," *Vascular Surgery* 6(1):9-13, January-February 1972
20. Burnand, K.G., et al. "Peripapillary Fibrin in the Ulcer-bearing Skin of the Leg: The Cause of Lipodermatosclerosis and Venous Ulceration," *British Medical Journal* (Clinical Research Edition) 285(6):1071-72, November-December 1982.

21. Falanga, V., et al. "Pericapillary Fibrin Cuffs in Venous Ulceration: Persistence with Treatment and During Ulcer Healing," *Journal of Dermatology, Surgery, & Oncology* 18(5):409-14, May 1992.

22. Coleridge Smith, P.D., et al. "Causes of Venous Ulceration," *British Journal of Hospital Medicine* (Clinical Research Edition) 296(6638):1726-27, June 18, 1988.

23. Sarin, S., et al. "Disease Mechanisms in Venous Ulceration," *British Journal of Hospital Medicine* 45(5):303-05, May 1991.

24. Falanga, V., and Eaglstein, W.H. "The 'Trap' Hypothesis of Venous Ulceration," *Lancet* 341(8851):1006-08, April 17, 1993.

25. Porter, J.M., et al. "Reporting Standards in Venous Disease," *Journal of Vascular Surgery* 8(2):172-81, August 1988.

26. Ad Hoc Committee of the American Venous Forum. "Classification and Grading of Chronic Venous Disease in the Lower Limbs: A Consensus Statement" in *Handbook of Venous Disorders: Guidelines of the American Venous Forum*. Edited by Gloviczki, P. and Yao, J.S.T. London: Chapman & Hall, 1996.

27. Kistner, R.L., et al. "Diagnosis of Chronic Venous Disease of the Lower Extremities: The CEAP Classification," *Mayo Clinic Proceedings* 71(4):338-45, April 1996.

28. Ernst, C.B., and Stanley, J.C. *Current Therapy in Vascular Surgery,* 3rd ed. St. Louis: Mosby, 1995.

29. Casley-Smith, J.R., et al. "Treatment of Lymphedema of the Arms and Legs with 5,6-benzo-a-pyrone," *NEJM* 329(16):1158-63, October 14, 1993.

30. Miller, L.T. "Lymphedema: Unlocking the Doors to Successful Treatment," *Innovations in Oncologic Nursing* 10(3):53, 58-62, 1994.

31. Lubdbrook, J., et al. "Significance of Absent Ankle Pulse," *British Medical Journal* 1:1724, 1962.

32. Mayfield, J.A., and Sugarman, J.R. "The Use of the Semmes-Weinstein Monofilament and Other Threshold Tests for Preventing Foot Ulceration and Amputation in Persons with Diabetes," *Journal of Family Practice* 49(11 Suppl):S17-S29, November 2000.

33. Taylor, L.M., and Porter, J.M. "Natural History and Nonoperative Treatment of Chronic Lower Extremity Ischemia" in *Vascular Surgery: A Comprehensive Review*. Edited by Moore, W.S. Philadelphia: W.B. Saunders Co., 1993.

34. Blank, C.A., and Irwin, G.H. "Peripheral Vascular Disorders: Assessment and Intervention," *Nursing Clinics of North America* 25(4):777-94, December 1990.

35. Fahey, V.A., and White, S.A. "Physical Assessment of the Vascular System" in *Vascular Nursing*. Edited by Fahey, V.A. Philadelphia: W.B. Saunders Co., 1994.

36. Baker, J.D. "Assessment of Peripheral Arterial Occlusive Disease," *Critical Care Nursing Clinics of North America* 3(3):493-98, September 1991.

37. Brantigan, C.O. "Peripheral Vascular Disease: A Comparison between the Vascular Laboratory and the Arteriogram in Diagnosis and Management," *Colorado Medicine* 77(9):320-27, September 1980.

38. Douglas, W.S., and Simpson, N.B. "Guidelines for the Management of Chronic Venous Leg Ulceration: Report of a Multidisciplinary Workshop," *British Journal of Dermatology* 132(3):446-52, March 1995.

39. Winsor, T. "Influence of Arterial Disease on the Systolic Blood Pressure Gradients of the Extremity," *American Journal of Medical Science* 220, 1950.

40. Belcaro, G., et al. "Noninvasive Tests in Venous Insufficiency," *Journal of Cardiovascular Surgery* 34(1):3-11, February 1993.

41. Nicolaides, A.N., and Miles, C. "Photo-plethysmography in the Assessment of Venous Insufficiency," *Journal of Vascular Surgery* 5(3):405-12, March 1987.

42. Burton, C., "Venous Ulcers," *American Journal of Surgery* 167(1A Suppl):S37-S41, January 1994.

43. Lineaweaver, W., et al. "Topical Antimicrobial Toxicity," *Archives of Surgery* 120(3):267-70, March 1985.

44. Lineaweaver, W., et al. "Cellular and Bacteriologic Toxicities of Topical Antimicrobials," *Plastic & Reconstructive Surgery* 75(3): 94-96, March 1985.

45. Cooper, M., et al. "The Cytotoxic Effects of Commonly Used Topical Antimicrobial Agents on Human Fibroblasts and Keratinocytes," *Journal of Trauma* 31(6):775-84, June 991.

46. McCauley, R.L., et al: "In Vitro Toxicity of Topical Antimicrobial Agents to Human Fibroblasts," *Journal of Surgical Research* 46(3):267-74, March 1989.

47. Maklebust, J. "Using Wound Care Products to Promote a Healing Environment," *Critical Care Nursing Clinics of North America* 8(2):141-158, June 1996.

48. Maklebust, J., and Sieggreen, M. *Pressure Ulcers: Guidelines for Prevention and Management*, 3rd ed., Springhouse, Pa.: Springhouse Corp., 2001.

49. Niederhuber, S.S., et al. "Reduction of Skin Bacterial Load with Use of Therapeutic Whirlpool," *Physical Therapy* 55(5):482-86, May 1975.

50. Bohannon, R.W. "Whirlpool versus Whirlpool and Rinse for Removal of Bacteria from a Venous Stasis Ulcer," *Physical Therapy* 62(3):304-08, March 1982.

51. Husni, E.A. "Skin Ulcers Secondary to Arterial and Venous Disease," in *Chronic Ulcers of the Skin*. Edited by Lee, B.Y. New York: McGraw Hill, 1985.

52. Dalman, R.L. "Long-term Results of Bypass Procedures in *Basic Data Underlying Clinical Decision Making in Vascular Surgery*. Edited by Porter, J.M. and Taylor, L.M. *Annals of Vascular Surgery* 141-43, 1995.

53. Goldman, M.P., et al. "Diagnosis and Treatment of Varicose Veins: A Review," *Journal of the American Academy of Dermatology* 31(3 PH):393-416, September 1994.

54. Cordts, P.R., et al. "A Prospective, Randomized Trial of Unna's Boot versus Duoderm CGF Hydroactive Dressing plus Compression in the Management of Venous Leg Ulcers," *Journal of Vascular Surgery* 15(3):480-86, March 1992.

55. Mayberry, J.C. et al. "Nonoperative Treatment of Venous Stasis Ulcer" in *Venous Disorders*. Edited by Bergan, J.J., and Yao, J.S.T. Philadelphia: W.B. Saunders Co., 1991.

56. Winter, G.D. "Formation of a Scab and the Rate of Epithelialization of Superficial Wounds in the Skin of a Pig," *Nature* 193:293-94, 1962.

57. Loiterman, D.A., and Byers, P.H. "Effect of a Hydrocellular Polyurethane Dressing on Chronic Venous Ulcer Healing," *Wounds* 3(5):178-81, September-October 1991.

58. Noyes, L.D., et al. "Hemodynamic Assessment of High Compression Hosiery in Chronic Venous Disease," *Surgery* 102(5):813-15, November 1987.

59. Pekanmaki, K., et al. "Intermittent Pneumatic Compression Treatment for Postthrombotic Leg Ulcers," *Clinical &*

Experimental Dermatology 12(5):350-53, September 1987.

60. Scurr, J.H., et al. "Regimen for Improved Effectiveness of Intermittent Pneumatic Compression in Deep Venous Thrombosis Prophylaxis," *Surgery* 102(5):816-20, November 1987.

61. Mulder, G., et al. "Study of Sequential Compression Therapy in the Treatment of Nonhealing Chronic Venous Ulcers," *Wounds* 2:111-15, 1990.

62. Allsup, D.J. "Use of the Intermittent Pneumatic Compression Device in Venous Ulcer Disease," *Journal of Vascular Nursing* 12(4):106-11, December 1994.

63. Smith, P.C., et al. "Sequential Gradient Pneumatic Compression Enhances Venous Ulcer Healing: A Randomized Trial," *Surgery* 108(5):871-75, November 1990.

64. McCulloch, J.M., et al. "Intermittent Pneumatic Compression Improves Venous Ulcer Healing," *Advances in Wound Care* 7(4):22-26, July 1994.

65. Raju, S. "Axillary Vein Transfer for Postphlebitic Syndrome." In *Atlas of Venous Surgery*. Edited by Bergan, J.J., and Kistner, R.L. Philadelphia: W.B. Saunders Co., 1992.

66. Kistner, R.L. "Transposition Techniques," in *Atlas of Venous Surgery*. Edited by Bergan, J.J., and Kistner, R.L. Philadelphia: W.B. Saunders Co., 1992.

67. Kistner, R.L. "Valve Reconstruction for Primary Valve Insufficiancy," in *Atlas of Venous Surgery*. Edited by Bergan, J.J., and Kistner, R.L. Philadelphia: W.B. Saunders Co., 1992.

68. Scurr, J.H. "Alternative Procedures in Deep Venous Insufficiency," in *Atlas of Venous Surgery*. Edited by Bergan, J.J., and Kistner, R.L. Philadelphia: W.B. Saunders Co., 1992.

69. Gloviczki, P., and Bergan, J.J. *Atlas of Endoscopic Perforator Vein Surgery*. London: Springer-Verlag, 1998.

70. Pappas, C. and O'Donnell, T. "Long-term Results of Compression Treatment for Lymphedema," *Journal of Vascular Surgery* 16(4):555-63, October 1992.

71. Browse, N. "Reducing Operations for Lymphedema of Lower Limb," Year Book Medical Publishers, Inc., 1986.

72. Felty, C.L., and Rooke, T.W. "Secondary Lymphedema," in *Current Therapy in Vascular Surgery*. Edited by Ernst, C.B., and Stanley, J.C. St. Louis: Mosby, 2001.

73. Barnes, R.W. "The Arterial System" In *Essentials of Surgery*. Edited by Sabiston,

D.C. Philadelphia: W.B. Saunders Co., 1987.

74. Coffman, J.D. "Principles of Conservative Treatment of Occlusive Arterial Disease" in *Clinical Vascular Disease*. Edited by Spittell, J.A. Philadelphia: F.A. Davis, 1983.

75. Kilo, C. "Vascular Complications of Diabetes," *Cardiovascular Reviews &Reports* 8(6):18-23, June 1987.

76. Levin, M.E. and Sicard, G.A. "Evaluating and Treating Diabetic Peripheral Vascular Disease: Part 1," *Clinical Diabetes* 62-70, May-June 1987.

77. Dowdell, H.R. "Diabetes and Vascular Disease: A Common Association," *AACN Clinical Issues* 6(4):526-35, November 1995.

78. Hughson, W.G., et al. "Intermittent Claudication: Prevalence and Risk Factors," *British Medical Journal* 1(6124):1377-79, May 27, 1978.

79. Clyne, CA., et al. "Smoking, Ignorance, and Peripheral Vascular Disease," *Archives of Surgery* 117(8):1062, August 1982.

80. Cavezzi-Marconi, P. "Manual Lymphatic Drainage," in *Phlebolymphoedema: From Diagnosis to Therapy*. Edited by Cavezzi, A., and Michelini, S. Bologna: Edizioni PR, PR Communications, 1998.

CHAPTER 15

Diabetic foot ulcers

Lawrence A. Lavery, DPM, MPh
Sharon Baranoski, MSN, RN, CWOCN, APN, FAAN
Elizabeth A. Ayello, PhD, RN, APRN,BC, CWOCN, FAAN

OBJECTIVES

After completing this chapter, you'll be able to:

* state the significance of foot ulcers in patients with diabetes as a health care problem

* list strategies for preventing foot ulcers in patients with diabetes mellitus

* describe wound characteristics and assessment parameters for a patient with diabetes mellitus

* list options for off-loading for a patient with diabetes mellitus with a foot ulcer.

Diabetes: A growing problem

The American Diabetes Association (ADA) defines diabetes as "a disease in which the body doesn't produce or properly use insulin." Of the 17 million Americans (6.2% of the population) who have diabetes, only 11 million are diagnosed, leaving over one-third, or 5.9 million, people unaware that they have diabetes.[1]

Between 5% and 10% of people with diabetes have type 1 diabetes, an autoimmune disorder that causes destruction of pancreatic β-cells and requires insulin therapy to prevent complications. Type 1 diabetes is characterized by an abrupt onset of clinical signs and symptoms associated with hyperglycemia and strong propensity for the development of ketoacidosis. The clinical onset may be abrupt but the pathophysiologic insult is a slow, progressive phenomenon.[2]

Between 90% and 95% (or 16 million Americans) have type 2 diabetes, making it the most common form of diabetes mellitus.[1] Patients with type 2 diabetes have a relative insulin deficiency because their bodies either fail to make enough insulin or are unable to use insulin properly. Type 2 diabetes is a heterogeneous disorder for which specific secondary genetic causes of the metabolic syndrome are being rapidly identified. Almost 30%

ADA contact information

The American Diabetes Association (ADA) offers much information for the diabetic patient and his family, as well as for health care professionals. General information about diabetes is available, along with advice on exercise, nutrition, and daily meal planning. To contact the ADA:

1701 N. Beauregard Street
Alexandria, VA 22311
1-800-DIABETES
www.diabetes.org

of patients with type 2 diabetes remain undiagnosed.[3] This failure to identify individuals with type 2 diabetes results in progressive morbidity and mortality. Severe insulin resistance can exist for years before the onset of hyperglycemia.

Blacks, Hispanics, Native Americans, and Asian-Americans have the highest prevalence of diabetes mellitus.[2] Type 2 diabetes, which is usually seen in adults, is now being seen in a much younger population.[2] Diabetes incidence has increased 48% in the last 10 years, with a 70% increase in patients in their 30s.

Diabetes is the single most common underlying cause of lower-extremity amputation in the United States. Foot problems are one of the most common complications in diabetics leading to hospitalization.[4-7] Admissions for foot complications account for 20% to 25% of all hospital days for patients with diabetes.[4,8,9] In the United States there are approximately 120,000 nontraumatic lower-extremity amputations performed each year, with 45% to 83% of these amputations involving patients with diabetes.[7,10,11] The risk of lower-extremity amputation in diabetics is 15 to 46 times higher than in nondi-

abetic patients.[4,5,7,10] After the initial amputation, the risk of reamputation or amputation of the contralateral extremity is high — 9% to 17% of patients will experience a second amputation within the same year[4,12] and 25% to 68% will have an amputation of the contralateral extremity within 3 to 5 years.[4,13,14] The 5-year survival rate after a lower-extremity amputation ranges from 41% to 70%.[10,14]

Diabetes is a contributing factor in 75% to 83% of all amputations among Blacks, Hispanics, and Native Americans.[4,7,15] The incidence of lower-extremity amputation is 1.5 times higher in Hispanics and 2.1 times higher in Blacks compared to non-Hispanic whites. (See *ADA contact information*.)

Etiology and risk factors

A number of local and systemic risk factors for foot ulceration and amputations should be considered in the prevention and treatment of the diabetic foot. (See *Ulceration and amputation risk factors in diabetic patients*.) Perhaps the strongest and easiest risk factor to identify is the presence of a previous ulceration or amputation, which indicates the potential for recurrence due to scar formation or biomechanical abnormalities resulting from the previous event. The underlying pathology usually isn't reversible, and most disease processes affecting the diabetic foot will continue to worsen over time.

Neuropathy

Usually, patients with diabetes present with sensory, motor, and autonomic neuropathy, all of which have a devastating impact on multiple systems in the foot. Sensory neuropathy contributes to an inability to perceive injury to the foot due to what's commonly referred to as loss

Ulceration and amputation risk factors in diabetic patients

Risk factor	Relative risk or odds ratio
LOCAL RISK FACTORS	
History of foot ulcer or amputation	1.6 to 18
Sensory neuropathy	2.2 to 18.4
Structural foot deformity (hallux valgus, claw toes) or limited joint mobility (hallux rigidus, equinus)	3.3 to 3.5
Peripheral vascular disease	2.4 to 3.0
Abnormal foot pressures	2.0 to 5.9
SYSTEMIC RISK FACTORS	
Hypertension	1.02 to 2.13
Hyperlipidemia	1.02 to 6.4
Hyperglycemia	1.3 to 3.2
Male gender	2.6 to 5.2
Duration of diabetes	1.06 to 3.0
Age over 65	2.0
Retinopathy	1.07 to 3.7
Poor vision	1.9
Proteinuria	2.4
Obesity	1.2

Adapted with permission from Lavery, L.A., and Gazewood, J.D. "Assessing the Feet of Patients with Diabetes," *Journal of Family Practice* 49(11 Suppl):S9-S16, November 2000.

of protective sensation.[16] Motor neuropathy alters the biomechanics of the foot, which causes increased shear and pressure on the sole. Motor neuropathy contributes to wasting of the intrinsic muscles of the foot, muscle imbalance, structural foot deformity, such as claw toes and subluxated metatarsophalangeal joints, and limited joint mobility. Autonomic neuropathy causes shunting of blood,[17] and loss of sweat and oil gland function, which leads to dry, scaly skin that can easily develop cracks and fissures. The combined effect of these neuropathies is a foot that can't respond to pain, a foot with severe biomechanical impairment, and skin that's poorly nourished and hydrated. Neuropathy provides a permissive environment that limits the body's ability to respond appropriately to injury.

Neuropathy is the most prominent risk factor of lower extremity complications.[7,16] Many lower extremity complications involve sensory neuropathy as a pivotal component of the critical pathway for the development of ulcers and amputations. In patients with neuropathy, pain and loss of function, two of the primary natural warning systems that alert the body to take action and seek medical care, are defective. Patients with diabetes sustain repetitive injuries to their feet that aren't recognized until the

PRACTICE POINT

Assessing protective sensation with a monofilament

A Semmes-Weinstein 10-g (5.07 log) monofilament is commonly used to assess protective sensation in the feet of patients with diabetes. You can order the Semmes-Weinstein monofilament from the following companies:

- Center for Specialized Diabetic Foot Care: 1-800-543-9055
- North Coast Medical, Inc.: 408-283-1900
- Sensory Testing Systems: 1-888-289-9293
- Smith & Nephew Rehabilitation Division: 1-800-558-8633.

Use the 10-g (5.07 log) monofilament wire on each foot at the following 10 sites:

- plantar aspect of the first, third, and fifth digits
- plantar aspect of the first, third, and fifth metatarsal heads
- plantar midfoot medially and laterally
- plantar heel
- dorsal aspect of the midfoot.

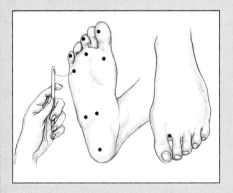

Performing the test

Place the patient in a supine or sitting position. Remove his socks and shoes and provide support for his legs. Touch the monofilament to the patient's arm or hand to demonstrate what it feels like. Then ask him to respond "yes" each time he feels the monofilament on his foot.

Place the patient's foot in a neutral position with his toes pointing straight up, and tell him to close his eyes. Remind him to say "yes" when he feels the monofilament on his foot. Hold the monofilament perpendicular to the patient's foot and press it against the first site, increasing the pressure until the monofilament wire bends into a C shape. Make sure it doesn't slide over the skin. Hold the monofilament in place for about 1 second. Record the patient's response on a foot-screening form. Use a "+" for a positive response and a "-" for a negative response. Then move to the next site.

Test all 10 sites at random and vary the time between applications so that the patient won't be able to guess the correct response. If he has a scar, callus, or necrotic tissue at a test site, apply the monofilament along the perimeter of the abnormality, not directly on it.

Loss of protective sensation is indicated if the patient can't feel the monofilament at any site on his foot. It's essential to teach a patient who has lost protective sensation to inspect and protect his feet.

Adapted with permission from Sloan, H.L., and Abel, R.J. "Getting in Touch with Impaired Foot Sensitivity," *Nursing* 28(11):50-51, November 1998, and from Armstrong, D.G., et al. "Choosing a Practical Screening Instrument to Identify Patients at Risk for Diabetic Foot Ulceration," *Archives of Internal Medicine* 158(3):289-92, February 9, 1998.

damage is so severe that full-thickness ulcerations result. Three primary pathways or mechanisms of injury have been identified in the development of foot ulcers. They include wounds that result from ill-fitting shoes (low-pressure injuries that are associated with prolonged or constant pressure from shoes that are too narrow or too short), repetitive moderate forces on the sole resulting in pressure ulcers on weight-bearing areas, and penetrating injuries from puncture wounds or other traumatic events (high-pressure injuries with a single exposure of direct pressure).

Several screening methods can be used to identify sensory neuropathy, including vibration perception threshold (VPT) testing and pressure assessment with the 10-gram Semmes-Weinstein monofilament (SWM).[16,18,19] These methods are noninvasive and have good sensitivity and specificity to identify patients with loss of protective sensation.[20] Wunderlich[20] and Armstrong and colleagues[16] suggested using a combination of modalities — the SWM, a VPT test, and the University of Texas Subjective Peripheral Neuropathy Verbal Questionnaire, a simple four-question evaluation — to optimize screening for neuropathy.

PRACTICE POINT

The University of Texas Subjective Peripheral Neuropathy Verbal Questionnaire
- Do your feet ever feel numb?
- Do your feet ever tingle, as if electricity were traveling into your foot?
- Do your feet ever feel as if insects were crawling on them?
- Do your feet ever burn?[20]

The SWM presents several potential problems that should be considered before using it. Semmes-Weinstein monofilaments should be purchased from a vendor that sells calibrated instruments because considerable variability exists among different brands of monofilament.[21] Booth and Young found that some brands of monofilaments buckle at greater than 8 g of force rather than the 10 g for which they're designated.[21] In addition, the material properties of the monofilament wear out after repetitive testing. Young and colleagues[22] found that after 500 cycles of testing (or the equivalent of testing 10 sites on each foot for 25 patients) there was an average reduction of 1.2 g of testing force. A worn-out monofilament may result in patients being diagnosed as having neuropathy when they aren't at risk. (See *Assessing protective sensation with a monofilament.*)

For more consistent testing, a VPT testing instrument or VPT meter is useful. The VPT is a quantitative device that measures large nerve function. It's less prone to inter-operator variation than the 10-g monofilament device and doesn't need to be replaced frequently to continue providing accurate results. The VPT meter (XILAS Medical, San Antonio, Texas) is a handheld device with a rubber head that's applied to a bony prominence, such as the medial aspect of the first metatarsal head or the tip of the great toe. The unit contains a linear scale that displays the applied voltage, ranging from 0 to 100 volts. The amplitude is then slowly increased until the patient can feel the vibration. The inability to feel greater than 25 volts is indicative of loss of protective sensation and puts the patient at risk of ulceration and amputation.

Peripheral vascular disease

Peripheral vascular disease (PVD) in patients with diabetes is characterized by multiple occlusive plaques of small- and medium-sized arteries of the infrapopliteal vessels.[17] PVD puts the patient with diabetes at greater risk for foot ulcers and infections secondary to ischemic changes.[7,23] Several theories attempt to explain the microvascular changes that occur in diabetes mellitus. One theory proposes that increased microvascular pressure and flow results in injury to the

Skin examination of a diabetic patient

When providing care for diabetic patients, skin examination is critical to identify signs of impending injury, high-pressure areas, and cracks, maceration, or fissures in the skin.

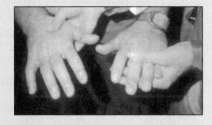

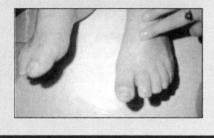

vascular endothelium. This injury causes the release of extravascular matrix proteins, which in turn causes microvascular sclerosis and thickening of the capillary basement membrane. Capillary fragility also leads to micro-hemorrhage, which could be the reason that infection spreads through the tissue planes in patients with diabetes.[17,24] LoGerfo and colleagues[25,26] believe that there's no microcirculatory occlusive process; instead they suggest that some other physiologic abnormality occurs.

Evaluating vascular status should include a history of intermittent claudication, ischemic rest pain, peripheral vascular surgery, and an assessment of bilateral lower-extremity pulses and clinical

signs of ischemia such as dependent rubor, pallor, hair loss, and shiny skin.[27]

Skin and nails

Evaluation of the integument is critical to identify the subtle signs of impending injury; high-pressure areas; and cracks, maceration, or fissures in the skin. (See *Skin examination of a diabetic patient* and *Skin-care teaching tips*.)

Discolored callus or bleeding under a callus is a sign of a preulcerative lesion. Likewise, deformed and thickened nails are commonly the source of abnormal pressure on the nail bed or ingrown toenails. In patients with neuropathy, ulcerations typically form from repetitive pressure from the shoe and nail over the nail bed. Common nail disorders seen in patients with diabetes mellitus include onychomycosis (tinea unguium) and onychocryptosis (ingrown toenail).[27] While these are apparent minor problems in nondiabetic adults, they can result in cellulitis and osteomyelitis in patients with diabetes, neuropathy, and vascular impairment.

Musculoskeletal examination

Ulcers on the sole are a result of excessive, repetitive pressure. Repetitive moderate stress of 30 to 50 psi can cause skin breakdown and ulcers in the neuropathic foot.[7,28-30] Structural and functional foot deformities in patients with diabetes alter the biomechanics of the lower extremities and contribute to developing high-pressure areas that are predisposed to ulceration.

The "tip-top-toe syndrome" is commonly seen in patients with diabetes. Ulcers occur when deformed toes (cocked-up toes, hammer toes, or claw toes) have pressure on them from the top of the shoes, the insole, or both. The lesser digits contract, resulting in a claw toe deformity and subluxation of the metatarsophalangeal joint.[17,28,31] In many instances,

PATIENT TEACHING
Skin-care teaching tips

Teach your diabetic patient the following self-care points:

- Keep your diabetes well controlled. People with high sugar levels tend to have dry skin and less ability to fend off harmful bacteria. Both conditions increase the risk of infection.
- Keep skin clean and dry. Use talcum powder in areas where skin touches skin, such as armpits and groin.
- Avoid very hot baths and showers. If your skin is dry, don't use bubble baths. Moisturizing soaps, such as Dove or Basis, may help. Afterward, use an oil-in-water skin cream, such as Lubriderm or Alpha-Keri. Don't put lotions between your toes — the extra moisture there can encourage fungus to grow. .
- Prevent dry skin. Moisturize your skin to prevent chapping.
- Don't scratch dry or itchy skin because doing so can tear the skin, allowing infection to occur.

- Treat cuts right away. Wash minor cuts with soap and water. Don't use mercurochrome antiseptic, alcohol, or iodine to clean skin because these agents are too harsh. Use an antibiotic cream or ointment only if your doctor says it's okay. Cover minor cuts with sterile gauze. See a doctor right away if you get a major cut, burn, or infection.
- During cold, dry months, keep your home more humid. Bathe less during this weather if possible.
- Use mild shampoos and unscented soaps. Don't use feminine hygiene sprays.
- See a dermatologist about skin problems if you aren't able to solve them yourself.
- Take good care of your feet. Check them every day for sores and cuts. Wear broad, flat shoes that fit well. Check your shoes for foreign objects before putting them on.

this combination of deformities literally pushes the head of the metatarsal through the bottom of the foot. The tips of the toes, dorsum of the toes, and the area beneath the metatarsophalangeal joints are subjected to increased pressure and friction, which can lead to ulceration.[17] Limited joint mobility of the ankle and metatarsophalangeal joints also increases pressure on the plantar part of the foot as the foot can't adequately redistribute pressure.[28,32]

Prevention parameters

Many factors are involved in preventing foot complications. Because the specific elements of a multispecialty approach to prevention haven't been studied individually, it's difficult to prioritize the role of each aspect of care. Both systemic disease factors and local treatment are pivotal elements of long-term prevention.

Treatment of systemic disease processes, such as heart failure, renal insufficiency, and diabetes is essential. Glucose control is critical to slow the multiple disease processes involved in diabetes-related foot complications. Hyperglycemia has been associated with higher risk of ulceration and poor healing response in patients with diabetes.[7] Effective glycemic control can be achieved through a comprehensive team effort that addresses dietary management, self glucose monitoring, proper ex-

Wide-toe shoe

Shoes with a deep toe-box and that are "extra depth" throughout the shoe are the mainstay of diabetic wound preventive care. The deep toe-box is designed to provide enough room to accommodate claw toes or hallux valgus deformity. The shoes typically come with laces, as shown here, or with Velcro closures.

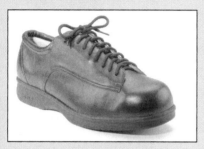

Photograph courtesy of Royce Medical Co.

inforcement for the rest of a high-risk patient's life. Preventing these wounds also requires patience — on the part of health care providers as well as patients.

PRACTICE POINT

The 5 Ps of diabetic ulcer prevention:
- podiatric care
- protective shoes
- pressure reduction
- prophylactic surgery
- preventive education

Additional Ps that should be added are:
- persistence
- patience.

ercise, appropriate medication, and early recognition and treatment of hyperglycemia.[17]

Several clinical studies report reduced amputations of 48% to 78%[33,34] as well as reduced hospitalizations of 47% to 49%,[35,36] when high-risk patients are treated in diabetic foot specialty clinics. Foot care points based on the recommendations of the American Orthopaedic Foot and Ankle Society[37] and the American College of Foot and Ankle Surgery by Frykberg and colleagues[38] have been published with prevention recommendations. Frykberg[30] lists the 5 Ps of prevention as podiatric care, protective shoes, pressure reduction, prophylactic surgery, and preventive education.

Two more Ps should be added to Frykberg's[30] 5 Ps: persistence and patience. Diabetic foot prevention is a chronic disease process requiring persistent attention, patient education, and re-

Podiatric care

Regular foot evaluation should identify any new risk factors such as impending complications, provide debridement of callus and nails, and include evaluation of therapeutic shoes and insoles. These routine encounters with the podiatrist offer an additional opportunity to reinforce key educational elements, such as the need to avoid going barefoot, hydrate the skin, and inspect the feet daily.

Protective shoes and pressure reduction

The primary role of protective shoes is to eliminate the shoe as a source of pathology. Shoes should be evaluated by a podiatrist or pedorthist to make sure they fit correctly. Shoes with a deep toe-box and extra depth throughout the shoe are the mainstay of diabetic prevention care. (See *Wide toe shoe.*) Such shoes allow an accommodative insole to fit without irritating the top or sides of the foot. (See *Wide toe shoe with insert.*) The deep toe-box is designed to provide enough room to accommodate claw toes or hallux valgus deformity. The combination of a correctively sized shoe and accommodative insole can reduce pressure on the sole, top, and sides of the foot by 20%.[39,40] Custom-made shoes are only necessary in a small percentage of high-risk patients with foot deformities that can't be accommodated in off-the-shelf shoes. A number of athletic shoes and comfort shoes have the extra depth and come sized to accommodate wide feet or prominent deformities.

Prophylactic surgery

Prophylactic surgery may be beneficial for some patients to improve joint motion or correct structural deformities. For example, percutaneous lengthening of the Achilles tendon[41] has been shown to reduce foot pressures on the sole in subjects with prior ulceration. Surgical correction of claw toes and resection of dislocated metatarsophalangeal joints have been used frequently to reduce the likelihood of recurrent ulceration.

Preventive education

Education for the patient and his family is a critical aspect of chronic disease management. In a study of ulcer risk factors, a large proportion of patients both with and without foot ulcers lacked the visual acuity, manual dexterity, or joint flexibility to perform simple self-examination checks of their feet. Among ulcer patients, 49% couldn't position or visualize their feet, and 15% were legally blind in at least one eye. When patients are obese or have limited joint mobility or impaired vision, education and self-assessment skills should be addressed to the spouse or caregiver.[7] Repetition and positive reinforcement should be practiced by every member of the health care team to help the patient and his family

Wide-toe shoe with insert

The combination of a correctly sized shoe and an accommodative insole can reduce pressure on the sole, top, and sides of the foot. The insert can be customized to relieve pressure according to the patient's needs, as shown in the top photograph. The insert is then placed inside the shoe, as shown in the bottom photograph.

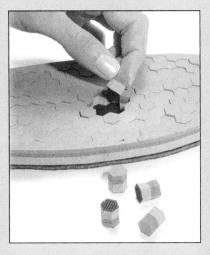

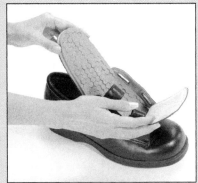

Photographs courtesy of Royce Medical Co.

understand the disease process and protection practices.

International consensus on the diabetic foot: Risk categorization

Category	Risk factors	Ulcer incidence	Amputation incidence	Prevention and treatment
0	No sensory neuropathy	2% to 6%	0	• Reevaluation once a year
1	Sensory neuropathy	6% to 9%	0	• Podiatry every 6 months • Over-the-counter shoes and insoles; evaluate appropriate fit
2	Sensory neuropathy and foot deformity or peripheral vascular disease	8% to 17%	1% to 3%	• Podiatry every 2 to 3 months • Professionally fit therapeutic shoes and insoles • Patient education
3	Previous ulcer or amputations	26% to 78%	10% to 18%	• Podiatry every 1 to 2 months • Professionally fit therapeutic shoes and insoles • Patient education

Adapted with permission from Peters, E.J., and Lavery, L.A. "Effectiveness of the Diabetic Foot Risk Classification System of the International Working Group on the Diabetic Foot," *Diabetes Care* 24(8): 1442-47, August 2001, and from Rith-Najarian, S.J., et al. "Identifying Diabetic Patients at High-Risk for Lower-Extremity Amputation in a Primary Health Care Setting. A Prospective Evaluation of Simple Screening Criteria," *Diabetes Care* 15(10):1386-950, October 1992.

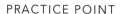

PRACTICE POINT

If a patient can't examine his own feet, be sure to teach his caregivers how to perform the assessment and provide any care the patient can't do unassisted.

Risk stratification

It's important to thoroughly evaluate the lower extremities to identify risk factors and prioritize the patient's treatment according to his needs.[42] A risk classification system endorsed by the International Working Group on the Diabetic Foot provides a validated scheme to stratify subjects based on their risk of ulceration and amputation. Key elements of the lower extremity examination should help to risk stratify subjects and identify the frequency and level of preventive care. (See *International consensus on the diabetic foot: Risk categorization.*)

Wound assessment and classification

Several classification systems can be used to classify diabetic ulcers. The University of Texas ulcer classification system is a validated system that includes a mecha-

University of Texas diabetic wound classification system

	Grade 0	Grade I	Grade II	Grade III
A	Preulcerative or postulcerative lesion, completely epithelialized	Superficial wound, not involving tendon, capsule, or bone	Wound penetrating to tendon or capsule	Wound penetrating to bone or joint
B	Preulcerative or postulcerative lesion, completely epithelialized with infection	Superficial wound, not involving tendon, capsule, or bone with infection	Wound penetrating to tendon or capsule with infection	Wound penetrating to bone or joint with infection
C	Preulcerative or postulcerative lesion, completely epithelialized with ischemia	Superficial wound, not involving tendon, capsule, or bone with ischemia	Wound penetrating to tendon or capsule with ischemia	Wound penetrating to bone or joint with ischemia
D	Preulcerative or postulcerative lesion, completely epithelialized with infection and ischemia	Superficial wound, not involving tendon, capsule, or bone with infection and ischemia	Wound penetrating to tendon or capsule with infection and ischemia	Wound penetrating to bone or joint with infection and ischemia

Reprinted with permission from Armstrong, D.G., et al. "Validation of a Diabetic Wound Classification System: The Contribution of Depth, Infection, and Ischemia to Risk of Amputation," *Diabetes Care* 21(5):855-69, May 1998.

nism to document depth and the presence of infection and vascular impairment—two pivotal factors in predicting clinical outcomes.[6,43] (See *University of Texas diabetic wound classification system.*) The risk of amputation has been shown to be predictive of amputation as wounds increase in depth (grade A to D) and progress from no infection (Grade 0), to infection (Grade I), to PVD (Grade II), and to infection and PVD (Grade III) using the University of Texas system.

A classification scheme first described by Meggit[44] and popularized by Wagner[45] has also been used extensively, but has the disadvantage of not consistently including depth throughout the system. In addition, osteomyelitis is the type of infection included and the only vascular parameters are end-stage disease events of gangrene. Furthermore, the system is difficult to use for more subtle disease processes that are critical for clinical decision-making. (See *Meggit-Wagner ulcer classification,* page 322.)

The ADA Consensus report[1] recommends that wound assessment include a systematic evaluation that includes the following questions:
• Has the patient experienced trauma? Is the ulcer a result of penetrating trauma, blunt trauma, or burn?
• What is the duration of the wound? Is the ulcer acute or chronic?
• What is the progression of local or systemic signs and symptoms? Is the wound getting better, is it stable, or is it deteriorating?
• Has the patient had any prior treatment of the wound or previous wounds? What treatments worked? What failed?

In addition, blood glucose control and comorbidities should be evaluated. Clinical assessment should identify:

Meggit-Wagner ulcer classification

Grade	Wound characteristics
0	Preulceration lesions, healed ulcers, presence of bony deformity
1	Superficial ulcer without subcutaneous tissue involvement
2	Penetration through the subcutaneous tissue; may expose bone, tendon, ligament, or joint capsule
3	Osteitis, abscess, or osteomyelitis
4	Gangrene of digit
5	Gangrene of foot

Reprinted with permission from Wagner, F.W. "The Dysvascular Foot: A System for Diagnosis and Treatment," *Foot & Ankle* 2(2):64-122, September 1981, and from Meggitt, B. "Surgical Management of the Diabetic Foot," *British Journal of Hospital Medicine* 227-32, 1976.

• signs of ischemia — adequate blood flow to heal the wound
• signs of soft tissue or bone infection — unpleasant odor, cellulitis, abscess, or osteomyelitis
• wound depth — undermining or exposed tendon, joint capsule, or bone
• appearance — surrounding callus, devitalized tissue, granulation tissue, drainage, eschar, or necrosis.

Diabetes control, optimized perfusion, infection control, local wound management, and off-loading are central tenets of wound healing.[28] For healing to occur, the ulcer must have adequate perfusion and not be infected. Confirmed vascular occlusion in patients with diabetes mellitus requires revascularization of the ischemic limb when possible. Aggressive debridement of necrotic and infected tissue is imperative for healing.[46,47] Aggressive, sharp debridement is preferred to enzymatic debriding agents for the patient with adequate perfusion. Appropriate wound dressings are needed to maintain a balanced moist-wound environment and promote wound healing.[17] When selecting a dressing, consider its ability to absorb exudate, debride nonviable tissue and reduce microbial contaminants, and promote wound rehydration, as well as its potential to deliver antibiotics to the wound bed.[17] (See chapter 9, Wound treatment options.)

 PRACTICE POINT

Six essentials of the American Diabetes Association's treatment algorithm:[48]
• off-loading therapy
• debridement, early and often
• moist-wound healing
• treating infection
• correcting ischemia (below the knee disease)
• preventing amputation.

Off-loading therapy

Reduction of pressure and shear forces on the foot may be the single most important — and most neglected — aspect of neuropathic ulceration treatment. Off-loading therapy is a key part of the treatment plan for diabetic foot ulcers. The goal is to off-load (reduce) the pressure at the ulcer while keeping the patient ambulatory.[17,39,49] Calhoun and colleagues[17] have defined off-loading as "any measure

Off-loading modalities and wound healing

Off-loading modality	Mean healing time	Percent healed	Source
Total contact cast	• Forefoot ulcers: 30 days • Midfoot and hindfoot ulcers: 63 days	90%	Myerson, M., et al.[50]
Total contact cast	• 38 days	73%	Helm, P.A., et al.[51]
Total contact cast	• 44 days	82%	Sinacore, D.R., et al.[52]
Total contact cast	• Forefoot ulcers: 31 days • Nonforefoot ulcers: 42.1 days	Not reported	Walker, S.C., et al.[53]
Total contact cast	• Midfoot ulcers: 28 days	100%	Lavery, L.A., et al.[54]
Total contact cast Cast boot Half-shoe	• 34 days • 50 days • 61 days	90% 65% 58%	Armstrong, D.G., et al.[55]
Total contact cast Shoe-insole	• 42 days • 65 days	90% 32%	Mueller, M.J., et al. [56]
Scotch cast boot	• 112 days • 181 days	80%	Knowles, E.A., et al.[57]
Half-shoe	• 70 days	96%	Chantelau, E., et al.[58]
Custom splint	• 300 days	Not reported	Boninger, M.L., and Leonard, J.A.[59]

to eliminate abnormal pressure points to promote healing or prevent recurrence of diabetic foot ulcers." Several methods are available to protect the foot from abnormal pressures. (See *Off-loading modalities and wound healing.*) Off-loading strategies must be tailored to the age, strength, activity, and home environment of the patient. In general, however, more restrictive off-loading approaches will result in less activity and better wound healing. Education is critical to improve off-loading compliance. The patient must understand that the wound is a result of repetitive pressure, and that every unprotected step is literally tearing the wound apart.

PRACTICE POINT

Methods to off-load the diabetic foot include:
- bed rest
- wheelchair
- crutches
- foams
- half-shoes
- therapeutic shoes
- custom shoes
- custom splints
- prefabricated walkers and total contact casting.

Applying a total contact cast

The photographs below highlight the major steps in applying a total contact cast.

Foam layer covers toes for protection. Padding is applied over bony prominences before the first layer of casting material is applied.

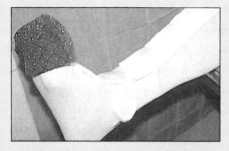

Completed total contact cast.

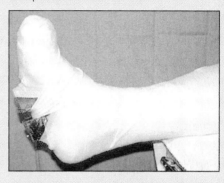

Cast boot covers the total contact cast.

Application of the total contact cast.

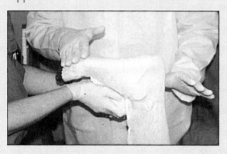

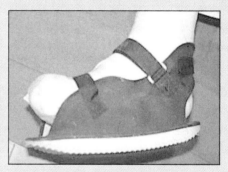

Total contact cast

Total contact casting (TCC) is considered the ideal, gold standard for off-loading the foot. Use of TCC reduces pressure at the ulcer site while still allowing the patient to be ambulatory.[17,49] A skilled clinician is required to apply the molded plaster cast to ensure a proper fit. A TCC is a modification of a traditional fracture cast with minimum cast padding and a covering to protect the toes. The cast is molded to the contour of the foot and leg so that there's no movement within the cast. TCCs are generally changed every 1 to 2 weeks, but in patients with edema or other concerns, the cast may need to be replaced more frequently. (See *Applying a total contact cast.*)

TCC is one of the most effective ways of treating plantar neuropathic foot ulcers described in the medical literature.[49,53,60] Studies[50,52,53,55,56,60-62] have shown that TCC can heal these ulcers in six to eight weeks. The proportion of wounds that heal in descriptive and randomized clinical trials with TCC is consistently much higher than those using topical growth factors, bioengineered tissue, or special dressings.[63-66]

One of the main advantages of using a TCC is that it forces patient compliance with off-loading. The ulcer is protected with every step the patient takes, around the clock. Using TCC to facilitate wound healing is analogous to using a fracture cast to heal a fracture—in both cases, healing is facilitated by rest and immobilization. TCC reduces the patient's activity level,[55] decreases his stride length and cadence, and significantly reduces pressure at the ulcer site.[49,60] The main disadvantages for patients are the same as their complaints with a fracture cast—a cast is heavy and hot, and makes bathing, walking, and sleeping difficult. It would be considered inappropriate to let a patient with an ankle fracture leave the clinic in shoes or a sandal. We shouldn't compromise when treating weight-bearing ulcers.

> **PRACTICE POINT**
>
> TCC shouldn't be used if wound infection is suspected or present.

Removable walkers

There are a number of removable walking boots that have been designed to help protect and heal foot wounds in diabetics, including the DH Pressure Relief Walker, the Conformer Boot, and the AirCast Pneumatic Walker. (See *Removable walking boots*.) Removable walking boots offer several advantages compared to total contact casts. Removable walking boots are relatively inexpensive, and the protective inner sole can be easily replaced if it shows signs of wear. No special training is required to correctly and safely apply these devices, and they can be easily removed to assess and debride the wound.[55,60] The DH Pressure Relief Walker has been shown to be identical to total contact casts in pressure reduction at the site of ulcerations on the sole.[60] The disadvantage to these boots is that patients can remove the walker, so the element of forced compliance that makes the total contact cast attractive is lost.

Removable walking boots

These photographs show examples of prefabricated, removable walking boots, which are used as off-loading devices.

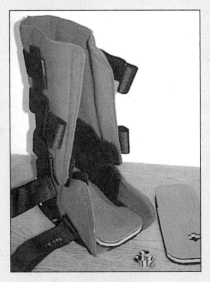

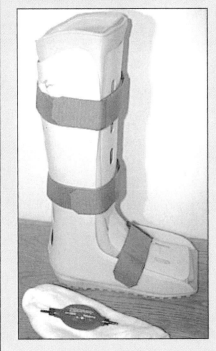

Wedged shoe

This photograph shows an example of a wedged forefront-relief shoe.

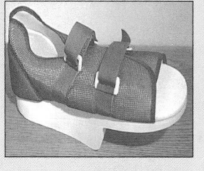

Healing sandals and half-shoes

A number of healing sandals and half-shoes or wedged shoes are available to reduce pressure on the forefoot. (See *Wedged shoe.*) These sandals and shoes are useful for patients who can't tolerate a total contact cast or for those who need a transitional device after removal of a TCC while they're awaiting therapeutic shoes and insoles. Royce Medical's DH healing sandal is a convenient product with Velcro closures, a conforming cover for the forefoot, and a patented pressure reducing insole. Other types of "healing sandals" require a pressure reducing insole added in the office.

Half-shoes, such as the OrthoWedge or Darco products, were originally designed to protect the forefoot after elective surgery. The OrthoWedge shoe has a 1½″ (4-cm) heel wedge at a 10-degree dorsiflexion angle, so that weight is removed from the forefoot area. Studies by Needleman[23] and Lair[67] provide support for its role in postoperative patients following surgery on the forefoot. However, these types of shoes aren't well-accepted by patients because they're difficult to walk in. They typically cause pain of the contralateral extremity, and patients with postural instability can't safely use these devices.

In a randomized clinical trial that compared total contact casts to healing sandals and removable cast boots, patients in the healing sandal group used the device during walking significantly less than subjects in the TCC group.[28,55]

Ankle-foot orthoses

Custom-made ankle-foot orthoses can be used for lower-extremity pathology, including Charcot fractures, tendon injuries, and neuropathic ulcers. (See *Ankle-foot orthoses.*) The Charcot Restraint Orthotic Walker (CROW), for example, was initially described to treat patients with neuropathic fractures. It provides protection to the neuropathic foot and aids in controlling lower-extremity edema. This device looks like a ski boot; it has a rigid polypropylene shell with a rocker bottom sole.[28]

The primary drawback to custom-made devices is that they typically cost about $1,000. If the structure of the foot changes or local edema resolves, the device can no longer be used. Since a number of less expensive, off-the-shelf products are now available to treat neuropathic wounds, custom ankle-foot orthoses are used less commonly. Off-the-shelf devices should be replaced at regular intervals since the materials in the insoles will lose their effectiveness over time.[40] Patients at risk for foot disease who have Medicare Part B are eligible for one pair of custom shoes and three pairs of insoles per calendar year.[68]

PATIENT TEACHING

Always remind your patients to wear properly-fitting shoes and insoles to prevent recurrence after a foot ulcer has healed.

Debridement

Sharp debridement of the ulcer removes devitalized tissue, reduces the bacterial load of the wound, eliminates proteases from the wound bed, and provides a bleeding wound bed. A diabetic ulcer typically has a thick rim of keratinized tissue surrounding it. Debridement must occur through the callus so that all the necrotic tissue is removed. Enzymatic debridement or autolytic debridement may be an option if sharp debridement isn't possible.[27] Ongoing debridement may be needed throughout the healing process.[17,47] Higher healing rates were seen in patients with diabetes who had more frequent debridement.[47] Proper debridement requires that all necrotic and infected tissue be removed.[17]

Treating infection

Poor glucose control is believed to predispose the diabetic patient to infection.[17] Hyperglycemia impairs leukocyte functioning including phagocytosis and intracellular killing function.[17] Patients with diabetes commonly demonstrate a diminished inflammatory response, even when severe soft tissue and bone infections are present. However, frequent wound culture and use of superficial swab cultures in wounds without clinical signs of infection aren't helpful. All open wounds will have a normal flora of bacterial contamination. Routine swab culture will routinely generate a laundry list of bacteria colonizing the wound.[69,70]

Identification of foot infections in the patient with diabetes mellitus requires vigilance because the signs of infection may not be present.[1] *Staphylococcus* and *Streptococcus* are the most common bacteria found in non–limb threatening infected diabetic foot ulcers.[17,30] The ADA[1] recommends that patients with

Ankle-foot orthoses

These photographs show examples of custom-made ankle-foot orthoses.

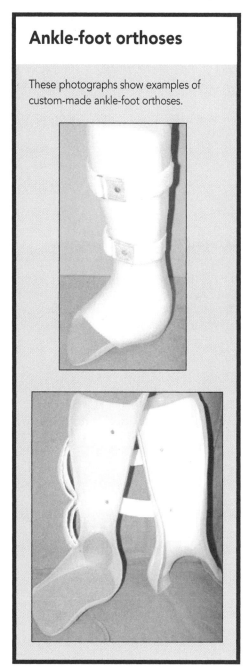

non–limb-threatening infections be treated with oral antibiotics to achieve serum levels and address the usual etiologic organisms (mostly gram-positive). Most of these patients can be treated on an outpatient basis.

Patients with limb-threatening infections should be hospitalized with administration of parenteral antibiotics and surgical debridement of necrotic and infected tissue. Most foot infections that are limb-threatening are polymicrobial with a mixed flora of gram positive and gram negative aerobic and anaerobic pathogens, so broad spectrum antibiotics are indicated. The major pathogens are *S. aureus,* group B streptococci, *Enterococcus,* and facultative Gram-negative bacilli.[1]

Advanced technologies

Many new treatments have been — and are being — developed to improve the outlook for the patient with a diabetic foot ulcer. In 1969, Silver[71] reported on the oxygen gradients in wounds, establishing the need for adequate oxygen in healing tissue. Several authors have suggested hyperbaric oxygen therapy as an adjunct therapy in patients with adequate arterial circulation and a transcutaneous oxygen level below 40 mm Hg.[72,73] Although hyperbaric oxygen has been available for decades, there is little scientific evidence to support its effectiveness.[74] Despite this limited evidence base, the ADA[1] has indicated that adjunctive hyperbaric oxygen may be reasonable to use in treating severe limb- or life-threatening wounds that haven't responded to other treatments.

Several advanced technologies are available for use in treating diabetic ulcers that don't respond to standard therapy. In December 1997, the FDA approved the use of becaplermin (Regranex) in patients with diabetic foot ulcers and adequate circulation. This product, a topical gel that contains recombinant human platelet-derived growth factor, promotes wound healing by stimulating cell migration to the wound. Of the patients treated with Regranex, 50% experienced healing,

compared with 35% of patients in the placebo gel control group;[66] mean time to complete healing was also faster in the patients treated with Regranex.

Engineered skin products are another advanced technology used in wound healing. These products are expected to have an important impact on healing wounds.[75] In 2000, the Food and Drug Administration (FDA) approved the tissue-engineered skin substitute known as Graftskin (Apligraf) for use in noninfected diabetic foot ulcers. This bilayered skin substitute contains cells from human infant foreskins and bovine type I collagen.[63] In a study by Veves and colleagues,[63] more patients treated with Apligraf (56%) had complete wound closure than did those in the control group receiving standard wound care (38%). The median time to healing was 65 days for Apligraf and 90 days for controls.

Interactive wound dressing (Dermagraft) is a fibroblast- derived, manufactured dermal substitute also made from neonatal foreskin that was approved by the FDA in September 2001. Results from the pivotal study demonstrated that by week 12, the proportion of wounds that healed in the Dermagraft group was greater as compared to the control group.[65] Ulcers treated with Dermagraft were 1.7 times more likely to close than those in the control group at any time in the study. Time for wound closure was also significantly faster in the Dermagraft group.

Several reports have described the benefit of electrical stimulation to facilitate wound healing in pressure and venous stasis ulcers, and improved survival of ischemic flaps.[76-79] Two studies report improved clinical outcomes in diabetic foot wounds. In 2001, Peters[80] reported the results of a randomized clinical trial of 40 subjects with neuropathic ulcers treated with subsensory electrical stimulation or sham devices. In the electrical stimulation group, 65% of the patients healed compared with 35% of the patients who had received a placebo. Peters[80] and Baker[81] evaluated 80 patients in a prospective study, demonstrating an approximate 60% improvement in healing rates in subjects with electrical stimulation, as compared with controls.

Summary

Diabetic foot ulcer care is a challenge for both the patient and the health care provider. As our population continues to age, the incidence of diabetes will continue to increase. This increased incidence will lead to more diabetic wounds. A team approach with total involvement of the health care system and the necessary compliance of the patient will be the infrastructure for achieving better outcomes of care.

Show what you know

1. According to the ADA (2001), how many people are unaware that they have diabetes mellitus?

A. One-half
B. One-third
C. Three-fourths
D. One-fourth

ANSWER: B. One-third of people with diabetes are unaware of their condition.

2. The single leading cause of lower-extremity amputation is:

A. diabetes mellitus.
B. lymphedema.
C. arterial occlusion.
D. venous disease.

ANSWER: A. Diabetes mellitus is the single leading cause of lower-extremity amputation.

3. According to the ADA, good skin care includes all of the following except:

A. keeping skin clean and dry.
B. applying moisturizers between toes.
C. avoiding very hot showers and tub baths.
D. checking feet daily for cracks or fissures.

ANSWER: B. Moisturizers shouldn't be applied between the toes — fungal infections can occur. All others are ADA recommendations for good skin care.

4. Off-loading strategies must be tailored to the age, strength, activity, and home environment of the patient.

A. True
B. False

ANSWER: A. This statement is true.

References

1. American Diabetes Association: Clinical Practice Recommendations. *Diabetes Care* 21(Suppl 1):1999.
2. American Diabetes Association. *www.diabetes.org,* cited December 2002.
3. Centers for Disease Control and Prevention: The Public Health of Diabetes Mellitus in the United States. Atlanta: Department of Health and Human Services, 1997.
4. Reiber, G.E., et al. "Lower Extremity Foot Ulcers and Amputations in Diabetes," in Mi, H., ed. *Diabetes in America,* 2nd ed. National Institutes of Health 1995.
5. Lavery, L.A., et al. "Increased Foot Pressures After Great Toe Amputation in Diabetes," *Diabetes Care* 18(11):1460-62, November 1995.
6. Lavery, L.A., et al. "Classification of Diabetic Foot Wounds," *Journal of Foot and Ankle Surgery* 35(6):528-31, November-December 1996.
7. Lavery, L.A., et al. "Practical Criteria for Screening Patients at High Risk for Diabetic Foot Ulceration," *Archives of Internal Medicine* 158(2):157-62, January 26, 1998.

8. Miller, A.D., et al. "Diabetes Related Lower-extremity amputation in New Jersey 1979 to 1981," *Journal of the Medical Society of New Jersey* 82(9):723-26, September 1985.

9. Pecoraro, R.E. "Chronology and Determinants of Tissue Repair in Diabetic Lower Extremity Ulcers," *Diabetes* 40(10):1305-13, October 1991.

10. Lavery, L.A., et al. "In-hospital Mortality and Disposition of Diabetic Amputees in the Netherlands," *Diabetic Medicine* 13(2):192-97, February 1996.

11. van Houtum, W.H., et al. "The Impact of Diabetes-Related Lower-Extremity Amputations in the Netherlands," *Journal of Diabetes and Its Complications* 10(6):325-30, November-December 1996.

12. Lavery, L.A., et al. "Diabetes-related Lower-extremity Amputations Disproportionately Affect Blacks and Mexican Americans," *Southern Medical Journal* 92(6):593-99, June 1999.

13. Edmonds, M.E., et al. "Improved Survival of the Diabetic Foot: The Role of a Specialized Foot Clinic," *Quarterly Journal of Medicine* 60(232):763-71, August 1986.

14. Most, R.S., and Sinnock, P. "The Epidemiology of Lower-Extremity Amputations in Diabetic Individuals," *Diabetes Care* 6(1):87-91, January-February 1983.

15. Lavery, L.A., et al. "Variation in the Incidence and Proportion of Diabetes-Related Amputations in Minorities," *Diabetes Care* 19(1):48-52, January 1996.

16. Armstrong, D.G., et al. "Choosing a Practical Screening Instrument to Identify Patients at Risk for Diabetic Foot Ulceration," *Archives of Internal Medicine* 158(3):289-92, February 1998.

17. Calhoun, J.H., et al. "Diabetic Foot Ulcers and Infections: Current Concepts," *Advances in Skin & Wound Care* 15(1):31-42, January-February 2002.

18. Levin, M. "Diabetic Foot Wounds: Pathogenesis and Management," *Advances in Wound Care* 10(2):24-30, March-April 1997.

19. Rith-Najarian, S.J. et al. "Identifying Diabetic Patients at High-Risk for Lower-Extremity Amputation in a Primary Health Care Setting. A Prospective Evaluation of Simple Screening Criteria," *Diabetes Care* 15(10):1386-95, October 1992.

20. Wunderlich, R.P., et al. "Defining Loss of Protective Sensation in the Diabetic Foot," *Advances in Wound Care* 11(3):123-28, May-June 1998.

21. Booth, J., and Young, M.J. "Differences in the Performance of Commercially Available 10-g Monofilaments," *Diabetes Care* 23(7):984-87, July 2000.

22. Young, R., et al. "The Durability of the Semmes-Weinstein 5.07 Monofilament," *Journal of Foot and Ankle Surgery* 39(1):34-38, January-February 2000.

23. Needleman, R.L. "Successes and Pitfalls in the Healing of Neuropathic Forefoot Ulcerations with the IPOS Postoperative Shoe," *Foot & Ankle International* 18(7):412-17, July 1997.

24. Tooke, J.E., and Brash, P.D. "Microvascular Aspects of Diabetic Foot Disease," *Diabetic Medicine* 13(Suppl 1):S26-S29, 1996.

25. LoGerfo, F.W., and Coffman, J.D. "Current Concepts, Vascular and Microvascular Disease of the Foot in Diabetes. Implications for Foot Care," *NEJM* 311(25): 1615-19, December 20, 1984.

26. LoGerfo, F.W., and Misare, F.D. "Current Management of the Diabetic Foot," *Advances in Surgery* 30:417-26, 1997.

27. Mulder, G.D. "Evaluating and Managing the Diabetic Foot: An Overview," *Advances in Skin & Wound Care* 13(1):33- 36, January-February 2000.

28. Catanzariti, A.R., et al. "Off-loading Techniques in the Treatment of Diabetic Plantar Neuropathic Foot Ulceration," *Advances in Wound Care* 12(9):452-58, November-December 1999.

29. Gibbons, G.W., and Habershaw, G.M. "Diabetic Foot Infections: Anatomy and Surgery," *Infectious Diseases Clinics of North America* 9(1):131-42, March 1995.

30. Frykberg, R.G. "The Team Approach in Diabetic Foot Management," *Advances in Wound Care* 11(2):71-77, March-April 1998.

31. Lavery, L.A., and Gazewood, J.D. "Assessing the Feet of Patients with Diabetes," *Journal of Family Practice* 49(11 Suppl):S9-S16, November 2000.

32. Lavery, L.A., et al. "Ankle Equinus Deformity and Its Relationship to High Plantar Pressure in a Large Population with Diabetes Mellitus," *Journal of the American Podiatric Medical Association* 92(9):479-82, October 2002.

33. Holstein, P., et al. "Decreasing Incidence of Major Amputations in People with

Diabetes," *Diabetologia* 43(7):844-47, July 2000.

34. Larsson, J., et al. "Decreasing Incidence of Major Amputation in Diabetic Patients: A Consequence of a Multidisciplinary Foot Care Team Approach?" *Diabetic Medicine* 12(9):770-76, September 1995.

35. Patout, C.A., et al. "Effectiveness of a Comprehensive Diabetes Lower-Extremity Amputation Prevention Program in a Predominantly Low-Income African-American Population," *Diabetes Care* 23(9):1339-42, September 2000.

36. Runyan, J.W. Jr., et al. "The Memphis Diabetes Continuing Care Program," *Diabetes Care* 3(2):382-86, March-April 1980.

37. Pinzur, M.S., et al. "Guidelines for Diabetic Foot Care," *Foot & Ankle International* 29(11):695-702, November 1999.

38. Frykberg, R.G., et al. "Role of Neuropathy and High Foot Pressures in Diabetic Foot Ulceration," *Diabetes Care* 21(10):1714-19, October 1998.

39. Lavery, L.A., et al. "Reducing Plantar Pressure in the Neuropathic Foot: A Comparison of Footwear," *Diabetes Care* 20(11):1706-10, November 1997.

40. Lavery, L.A., et al. "A Novel Methodology to Obtain Salient Biomechanical Characteristics of Insole Materials," *Journal of the American Podiatric Medical Association* 87(6):260-65, June 1997.

41. Armstrong D.G., et al. "Lengthening of the Achilles Tendon in Diabetic Patients Who Are at High Risk for Ulceration of the Foot," *Journal of Bone & Joint Surgery, American Volume* 81(4):535-38, April 1999.

42. Peters, E.J., and Lavery, L.A. "Effectiveness of the Diabetic Foot Risk Classification System of the International Working Group on the Diabetic Foot," *Diabetes Care* 24(8):1442-47, August 2001.

43. Armstrong, D.G., et al. "Validation of a Diabetic Wound Classification System: The Contribution of Depth, Infection and Ischemia to Risk of Amputation," *Diabetes Care* 21(5):855-59, May 1998.

44. Meggitt, B. "Surgical Management of the Diabetic Foot," *British Journal of Hospital Medicine* 227-32, 1976.

45. Wagner, F.W., Jr. "The Dysvascular Foot: A System for Diagnosis and Treatment," *Foot & Ankle* 2(2):64-122, September 1981.

46. Steed, D.L. "The Wound Healing Society (WHS) Evaluation of the Science to Arrive at Guidelines," *Wounds* 13(5 Suppl. E): 15E-16E, 2001.

47. Steed, D.L., et al. Diabetic Ulcer Study Group. "Effect of Extensive Debridement and Treatment on the Healing of Diabetic Foot Ulcers," *Journal of the American College of Surgery* 183(1):61-64, July 1996.

48. Sheehan, P. "American Diabetes Association (ADA): Presentation of Consensus Development Conference on Diabetic Foot Wound Care," *Wounds* 13(5 Suppl. E):6E-8E, 2001.

49. Lavery, L.A., et al. "Total Contact Casts: Pressure Reduction at Ulcer Sites and the Effected on the Contralateral Foot," *Archives of Physical Medicine & Rehabilitation* 78(11):1268-71, November 1997.

50. Myerson, M., et al. "The Total-Contact Cast for Management of Neuropathic Plantar Ulceration of the Foot," *Journal of Bone & Joint Surgery, American Volume* 74(2):261-69, February 1992.

51. Helm, P.A., et al. "Total Contact Casting in Diabetic Patients with Neuropathic Foot Ulcerations," *Archives of Physical Medicine & Rehabilitation* 65(11):691-93, November 1984.

52. Sinacore, D.R., et al. "Diabetic Plantar Ulcers Treated by Total Contact Casting: A Clinical Report," *Physical Therapy* 67(10):1543-49, October 1987.

53. Walker, S.C., et al. "Total Contact Casting and Chronic Diabetic Neuropathic Foot Ulcerations: Healing Rates by Wound Location," *Archives of Physical Medicine & Rehabilitation* 68(4):217-21, April 1987.

54. Lavery, L.A., et al. "Healing Rates of Diabetic Foot Ulcers Associated with Midfoot Fracture Due to Charcot's Arthropathy," *Diabetic Medicine* 14(1):46-49, January 1997.

55. Armstrong D.G., et al. "Off-loading the Diabetic Foot Wound: A Randomized Clinical Trial," erratum in *Diabetes Care* 24(8):1509, August 2001.

56. Mueller, M.J., et al. "Total Contact Casting in Treatment of Diabetic Plantar Ulcers. Controlled Clinical Trial," *Diabetes Care* 12(6):384-88, June 1989.

57. Knowles, E.A., et al. "Off-loading Diabetic Foot Wounds Using the Scotchcast Boot: A Retrospective Study," *Ostomy/Wound*

Management 48(9):50-53, September 2002.

58. Chantelau, E., et al., "Outpatient Treatment of Unilateral Diabetic Foot Ulcers with 'Half Shoes'," *Diabetic Medicine* 10(3):267-70, April 1993.

59. Boninger, M.L., and Leonard, J.A. Jr. "Use of Bivalved Ankle-foot Orthosis in Neuropathic Foot and Ankle Lesions," *Journal of Rehabilitation Research & Development* 33(1):16-22, February 1996.

60. Lavery, L.A., et al. "Reducing Dynamic Foot Pressures in High-Risk Diabetic Subjects with Foot Ulcers: A Comparison of Treatments," *Diabetes Care* 19(8):818-21, August 1996.

61. Sinacore, D.R. "Total Contact Casting for Diabetic Neuropathic Ulcers," *Physical Therapy* 76(3):296-301, March 1996.

62. Caputo, G.M., et al. "The Total Contact Cast: A Method for Treating Neuropathic Diabetic Ulcers," *American Family Physician* 55(2):605-11, February 1, 1997.

63. Veves, A., et al. "Graftskin, A Human Skin Equivalent, Is Effective in the Management of Noninfected Neuropathic Diabetic Foot Ulcers: A Prospective Randomized Multicenter Clinical Trial," *Diabetes Care* 24(2):290-95, February 2001.

64. Veves, A., et al. "A Randomized, Controlled Trial of Promogran (A Collagen/Oxidized Regenerated Cellulose Dressing) Versus Standard Treatment in the Management of Diabetic Foot Ulcers," *Archives of Surgery* 137(7):822-27, July 2002.

65. Gentzkow, G.D., et al. "Use of Dermagraft, A Cultured Human Dermis, to Treat Diabetic Foot Ulcers," *Diabetes Care* 19(4):350-54, April 1996.

66. Wieman, T.J., et al. "Efficacy and Safety of a Topical Gel Formulation of Recombinant Human Platelet-Derived Growth Factor-BB (Becaplermin) in Patients with Chronic Neuropathic Diabetic Ulcers. A Phase III Randomized Placebo-Controlled Double-Blind Study," *Diabetes Care* 21(5):822-27, May 1998.

67. Lair, G. *Use of the Ipos Shoe in the Management of Patients with Diabetes Mellitus.* Cleveland: Cleveland Clinic Foundation, 1992.

68. Sugaman, J.R., et al. "Use of the Therapeutic Footwear Benefit among Diabetic Medicare Beneficiaries in Three States," *Diabetes Care* 21(5):777-81, May 1998.

69. Lipsky, B.A., et al. "The Diabetic Foot: Soft Tissue and Bone Infection," *Infectious Diseases Clinics of North America* 4(3):409-32, September 1990.

70. Lipsky, B.A. "Infections of the Foot in Patients with Diabetes," in *The Diabetic Foot,* 6th ed. Pfeifer, M.A., and Bowker, J.H. (eds). St. Louis: Mosby–Year Book, Inc., 2001.

71. Silver, I.A. "The Measurement of Oxygen Tension in Healing Tissue," *Progress in Respiratory Research* 3:124, 1969.

72. Stone, J.A., and Cianci, P. "The Adjunctive Role of Hyperbaric Oxygen Therapy in the Treatment of Lower Extremity Wounds in Patients with Diabetes," *Diabetes Spectrum* 10:1, 1997.

73. Hammarlund, C., and Sundberg, T. "Hyperbaric Oxygen Reduced Size of Chronic Leg Ulcers: A Randomized Double-Blind Study," *Plastic & Reconstructive Surgery* 93(4):829-33, April 1994.

74. Wunderlich, R.P., et al. "Systemic Hyperbaric Oxygen Therapy: Lower-Extremity Wound Healing and the Diabetic Foot," *Diabetes Care* 23(10):1551-55, October 2000.

75. Johnson, P.C. "The Role of Tissue Engineering," *Advances in Skin & Wound Care* 13(2 Suppl 1):12-14, May-June 2000.

76. Kjartansson, J., Lundeberg, T. "Effects of Electrical Nerve Stimulation (ENS) in Ischemic Tissue," *Scandinavian Journal of Plastic & Reconstructive Hand Surgery* 24(2):129-34, 1990.

77. Feedar, J.A., et al. "Chronic Dermal Ulcer Healing Enhanced with Monophasic Pulsed Electrical Stimulation," *Physical Therapy* 71(7):639-49, July 1991.

78. Gault, W.R. "Use of Low Intensity Direct Current in Management of Ischemic Skin Ulcers," *Physical Therapy* 56(3):256-69, March 1976.

79. Lundeberg, T., et al. "Effect of Electrical Nerve Stimulation on Healing of Ischaemic Skin Flaps," *Lancet* 242(8613):712-14, September 1988.

80. Peters, E.J., et al. "Electric Stimulation as an Adjunct to Heal Diabetic Foot Ulcers: A Randomized Clinical Trial," *Archives of Physical Medicine & Rehabilitation* 82:721-25, June 2001.

81. Baker, L.L., et al. "Effects of Electrical Stimulation on Wound Healing in Patients with Diabetic Ulcers," *Diabetes Care* 20(3):405-12, March 1997.

CHAPTER 16

Sickle cell ulcers

Angela Colette Willis, RN, CWS, CDE
Marc Gibber, BA
Sarah Weinberger, BS, DEC
Harold Brem, MD

OBJECTIVES

After completing this chapter, you'll be able to:

- understand the pathogenesis of sickle cell disease

- differentiate sickle cell ulcers from arterial and venous ulcers

- discuss the pathogenesis of sickle cell ulcers

- implement protocol for treatment of complications of sickle cell ulcers (such as infection)

- implement wound care treatment and pain management strategies that facilitate healing of sickle cell ulcers.

Sickle cell anemia

Sickle cell disease is an inherited hemoglobinopathy characterized by the predominance of hemoglobin S. Sickle cell disease was first reported in 1910 by J.B. Herrick, an American physician.[1] Worldwide more than 100,000 neonates per year are born with sickle cell disease.[2] In the United States, 3 in 1,000 African-American neonates have some form of sickle cell disease; in Africa, approximately 200,000 neonates have sickle cell disease.[3]

The sickling of red cells is caused by inheritance of homozygous hemoglobin S, compound heterozygosity for hemoglobin S and hemoglobin C, or a beta thalassemia.[4]

Prevalence and incidence

Two observational studies, the Cooperative Study of Sickle Cell Disease in the United States[5] and the Jamaica Cohort Study in Jamaica,[6] have provided the most reliable information on the clinical course and complications of sickle cell disease in the context of sickle cell ulcers. Each study followed several hundred patients for at least 10 years.

The Cooperative Study found males were more likely to have ulcers than females. Approximately 5% of patients age 10 and older with sickle cell anemia

Sickle cells

The diagrams below show a normal red blood cell and a sickled cell.

NORMAL RED BLOOD CELL

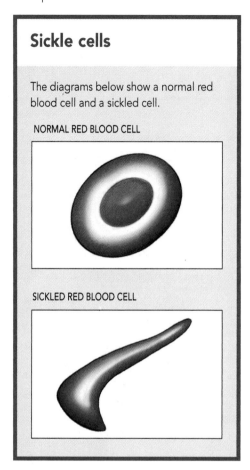

SICKLED RED BLOOD CELL

is indicated by the presence of 80,000 patients in the United States alone.[2]

Complications

The defective properties of the sickle hemoglobin lead to abnormal erythrocyte adhesiveness with reflexive vasoconstriction. Intimal proliferation leading to segmental narrowing of medium-size arteries and degenerative changes of the media, as well as obstruction of the vasa vasorum, all contribute to the vaso-occlusive events that characterize the sickle cell crisis. These pathological changes in vessel walls predispose the patient to superimposed thrombosis or embolization blocking the arterial supply to all or part of the affected organ. Patients with homozygous sickle cell anemia are plagued by recurrent vaso-occlusive crises with ischemic tissue damage causing pain and, eventually, organ failure.[4]

Sickled cells have a shortened life span. The hemolytic anemia they produce is responsible for aplastic crises, megaloblastic anemia, leg ulcers, gallstones, and gout.[9] Erythrostasis develops when sickled red cells are trapped in small vessels, resulting in vaso-occlusion. The hemolytic anemia and vaso-occlusion are linked by the presence of "sticky" short-lived sickle cells and reticulocytes. (See *Sickle cells*.)

Diagnosis

Any African-American patient who doesn't have proven venous reflux disease or who had an ulcer develop prior to age 30 should be tested for sickle cell disease. The threshold for testing should be negligible and the overall sensitivity is 100% for sickle cell disease. The most widely used diagnostic test for sickle cell disease and traits is hemoglobin electrophoresis. Definitive diagnosis may require more specific hemoglobin analysis,

had leg ulcers on entry into the study; however, leg ulcers weren't present in patients with sickle beta thalassemia and sickle hemoglobin C disease. Low steady-state hemoglobin is associated with a higher incidence of ulcer formation in sickle cell anemia patients. According to the genotype of sickle cell disease, in patients age 20 and older with sickle cell anemia, the incidence rates ranged from 15 to 20 per 100 person-years.[7]

The Jamaica Sickle Cell Cohort Study found that chronic leg ulceration has been a major cause of morbidity in homozygous sickle cell disease. The cumulative involvement of leg ulceration reached 75% in patients age 30 and older.[8] The significance of sickle cell disease

Secondary systemic complications

Affected organ	Pathogenesis
Spleen	• Sickled cells produce vaso-occlusion.[10]
Acute chest syndrome	• Abnormal nitric oxide metabolism occurs.[11] • Pulmonary infarction is caused by necrotic bone marrow, sickled cells, or occlusion of small bronchial blood vessels.[12]
Lung	• Lung lesions decrease arterial pressure, causing microinfarction or occlusion of small vessels [9]
Kidneys	• Local production and secretion of vasodilatory prostaglandins occurs in response to microvascular obstruction.[13]
Brain	• Sickled cells alter blood flow, producing occlusion of the large and small vessels, red cell sludging, and distal field insufficiency.[14]
Musculoskeletal (bone)	• Sickling of the red cells produces thromboembolic infarcts in bone leading to pain, crises and, occasionally, osteomyelitis.[15] • Increased destruction of sickled red cells produces hemolysis, increased erythroblastic activity, and expansion of the bone marrow cavity.[15]
Liver	• Ischemia, transfusion-related viral hepatitis, iron overload, or gallstones may occur.[16]
Gastrointestinal	• *Helicobacter pylori* infection occurs due to preexisting anemia, increased nonsteroidal anti-inflammatory drug use, and alloimmunization.[17]
Hypertension	• Salt-losing state may occur, as may a defect in vascular tone.[13]
Leg ulcers	• Marginal blood supply to the skin, local edema, and minor trauma may occur.[18] • Chronic damage to the microcirculation caused by sickling, capillary wall injury and proliferation, and abnormal permeability to macromolecules may occur.[19]

including family studies, red-cell indices, and DNA studies.[4]

PRACTICE POINT

Be aware that ulcers developing in young African-American patients might be due to undiagnosed sickle cell disease.

All patients should be evaluated for the more common systemic complications. (See *Secondary systemic complications*.)

Organs commonly affected by microcirculatory vascular occlusions are bone marrow, spleen, lungs, and kidneys. The brain is usually affected at the level of the large blood vessels.[20] Therefore, the status of the lungs, kidney, brain (such as stroke), bones, and liver should be documented by the wound care practitioner upon patient's entry into the wound program.

Pathogenesis of sickle cell ulcers
In some instances, the same pathology that causes sickle cell disease complica-

tions also causes the ulcer. For example, blood vessel occlusion in the spleen and liver is similar to vascular infarcts in the skin, muscle, or bone of the leg. The latter three sites can contribute significantly to nonhealing ulcers.

Vascular infarcts in the leg are directly related to musculoskeletal problems involved in sickle cell complications presenting with bone pain. Red blood cell sickling, which is advanced by slow circulation in the bone marrow, is the primary contributor to bone complications suffered by patients with sickle cell disease. Two pathogenic pathways have been described for causing these bone complications, both involving an abnormal red blood cell shape. In the first pathway, sickling of the red cells produces thromboembolic infarcts in bone leading to pain, crises and, occasionally, osteomyelitis. In the other pathway, increased destruction of sickled red cells produces hemolysis, an increase in erythroblastic activity, and expansion of the bone marrow cavity. Osteomyelitis, retardation of growth, dactylitis, described as avascular necrosis — particularly of the head of the femur — and leg ulcers are commonly encountered.[15]

Impaired blood flow in the bone commonly results in infarcts in the leg, which in turn causes pain in a sickle cell patient's extremities. Damage to the microcirculation caused by sickling may be chronic.

PRACTICE POINT

Because debridement treats only the ulcer without treating the underlying sickle cell disease (which causes the pain), in-office debridement usually isn't practical for the sickle cell patient.

The high blood flow indicated by a higher ankle brachial index may contribute to capillary wall injury and proliferation and an abnormal permeability of macromolecules, preventing oxygen and nutrients from entering the periphery. These events contribute to the high prevalence of leg ulcers in patients with sickle cell disease.[19] The cumulative damage caused by sickle cells and abnormal blood flow may result in residual decreased angiogenic response, compounding the patient's predisposition to leg ulcers.

Sickle cell ulcers are frequently — and mistakenly — attributed to venous reflux disease[18] because the symptoms are similar to those of venous stasis ulcers. Both sickle cell ulcers and venous stasis ulcers occur near the ankle and show hyperpigmentation and, frequently, dermatitis.[8]

PRACTICE POINT

Misdiagnosis — and thus, mistreatment — sickle cell ulcer as a venous stasis ulcer is extremely dangerous.

Physical examination

Patients with sickle cell ulcers often present with massive ulcers (greater than 10 cm) because treatment was delayed, thereby resulting in extreme morbidity (such as pain) and delayed healing. However, all sickle cell ulcers should heal if they're recognized and treated early.

PRACTICE POINT

Sickle cell ulcers won't become massive ulcers if treated early.

The ulcers usually begin as small, elevated, crusting wounds on the lower third of the leg, around the medial or lateral malleolus. They can also occur over the pretibial area or the dorsum of the foot. They can be single, multiple, unilateral, or bilateral. The patient will usually report some form of minor trauma or insect bite as the precipitating factor. However, the history is often insignificant because the ulcers may occur spontaneously. The emphasis is to understand that as soon as a patient with sickle cell disease presents with a break in the epidermis, treatment should begin immediately.

It's now recognized that the pathogenesis of leg ulcers in sickle cell disease isn't attributable to arterial or venous insufficiency, but is the result of multiple infarcts of the microcirculation. Therefore, arterial testing and venous reflux testing are mandatory to rule out other contributing wound healing impairments. Osteomyelitis and cellulitis must also be diagnosed immediately and treated. Drainage is absolutely not part of a sickle cell ulcer and nearly always represents infection.

PRACTICE POINT

Because sickle cell ulcers don't commonly exhibit drainage, the presence of drainage usually signals infection.

Assessment

"It started off as a tiny little thing," is a phrase frequently heard from patients with sickle cell ulcers that began as wounds of less than 1 cm and developed into substantial leg wounds. Many facilities have established comprehensive wound management programs that provide coordinated, multidisciplinary teams comprised of nurses, physicians, podiatrists, and technologists with specialized experience in wound healing.[21] The establishment of and adherence to a clinical pathway, which includes affiliated services such as physical therapists, radiologists, nutritionists, pain specialists, hematologists, and social workers, allows assessment of the patient and his

wounds to proceed efficiently, thereby promoting successful healing.

All sickle cell ulcers lasting longer than 2 months should be examined by biopsy prior to treatment to rule out malignancy. In addition to determining malignancy, a biopsy can also reveal other histologic features related to diagnosis. Cultures of the deep tissue must always be taken following tissue debridement to determine the presence and type of bacteria in the tissue.

It's important to describe the pathophysiology of sickle cell disease as it manifests in bone to better understand the emergence of sickle cell ulcers from sickle cell disease. In this context, a radiological workup is important to differentiate bone disorders. X-rays are used to determine the presence of osteomyelitis and bone infarcts. Sickle cell disease manifests in the bones with marrow hyperplasia, growth disturbances, and osteonecrosis, which may appear on X-rays as patchy areas of sclerosis and osteopenia, with a "bone-within-a-bone" appearance, cortical thickening, and periosteal reaction. Magnetic resonance imaging (MRI) may demonstrate the striking marrow reconversion with low signal-intensity marrow replacement.

Extensive superimposed infarcts involving diaphysis and metaphysis, as well as epiphysis, may be detected on MRIs before being apparent on plain film. The pattern of signal alteration is variable, with ringlike low signal intensity on T1-weighted images and bright on water-sensitive sequences, central fatty marrow, edema, fibrosis, and hemorrhage.

Patients with sickle cell disease are susceptible to bacterial infection of bone due to hematogenous dissemination and spread from contiguous ulcers, particularly in the lower extremities. Infarcts and osteomyelitis may have similar clinical presentations, requiring imaging for differentiation. Osteomyelitis manifests

EVIDENCE-BASED PRACTICE

Pain management guidelines

The nation's first evidence-based clinical practice guideline concerning pain was released in August 1999.[23] The major recommendations are that:
- Clinicians should ask patients about pain. Patient self-reports should be the primary source of assessments.
- Patients should be reassessed at each visit and asked if pain management measures have been effective.
- Pain therapy should be tailored to the patient's individual needs.
- Pain management should ease pain, enable the patient to tolerate treatments, and attain maximal functional ability.

on MRIs with inflammation replacing normal, reconverted, or ischemic marrow. The finding of associated soft tissue tracts, phlegmon, or abscess is helpful in differentiating intramedullary infarcts from abscesses.

Differentiation of osteomyelitis from acute marrow infarct on MRIs may not always be possible. Follow-up MRI, when performed, may assist in establishing the chronicity of bony changes, or demonstrate subtle new changes requiring intervention.

Pain assessment

Sickle cell ulcers are extremely painful and successful healing can be severely compromised by inadequate pain management. The patient with sickle cell disease will experience pain from childhood, and the added pain of leg ulcers

can affect the quality of life so adversely that therapeutic wound interventions will be completely rejected.

EVIDENCE-BASED PRACTICE

Painful crises have been reported to correlate with early death in adult patients with sickle cell disease.[22] Pain should, therefore, be assessed and treated as early as possible to prevent physical and psychological debilitation and facilitate local wound care.

The most effective pain assessment tool in clinical practice is the analogue scale, which is a simple measurement of pain intensity. At each visit, the patient is asked: "How would you rate your pain on the scale of 0 to 10, with 0 representing no pain and 10 representing the worst pain imaginable?" Because patients often manage pain at home and don't report it, home pain diaries are useful in understanding and managing the pain. To provide education for patients, families, and health care providers, a multidisciplinary panel of experts designed guidelines for the pain management of sickle cell disease.[23] (See *Pain management guidelines*.)

Treatment

The most commonly prescribed dressing for the sickle cell ulcer has been the ubiquitous "wet-to-dry" dressing with instructions to pull off the dry dressing in the effort to remove devitalized tissue. However, this debridement method is nonselective and has a limited role in contemporary wound healing.

Today, dressings are used to accelerate the wound-healing process in addition to covering wounds and facilitating debridement. A multitude of wound care products are now available, the use of which is based on scientific evidence, and many of these products are superior alternatives to wet-to-dry dressings. (See chapter 9, Wound treatment options.)

Allowing a gauze dressing to dry and then pulling it off not only produces acute pain but also causes reinjury to the wound, removing natural growth factors and enzymes near the wound's surface.[24] Adherent dressings should be moistened with normal saline and lifted gently from around the edges of the wound. The patient may prefer to remove the dressing himself. Slow-release silver topical medications provide broad-spectrum antibacterial coverage for long periods of time. Iodosorb or Cadexomer iodine is an alternative that's antimicrobial and stimulates granulation tissue.

Topical anesthetic agents, such as lidocaine (Xylocaine) jelly 2% or lidocaine solution 2% to 5% compresses, are available to assist in wound care. Allow 10 to 15 minutes for the anesthetic to take effect. The patient usually will have taken oral analgesics prior to the dressing change — opioids, in particular, are frequently prescribed for pain management. Lidocaine patches are also useful for the periwound skin. The use of topical opioids, dissolved in 1 to 2 ml of water and mixed with a debriding ointment, has been reported to provide complete pain relief in two patients.[25] However, the outcome of wound care for these patients wasn't reported and more research is needed.

Wounds with infections must be treated with antibiotics. Wounds are defined as being infected if they exhibit:
- positive deep culture
- cellulitis
- foul-smelling drainage
- copious drainage.

Due to poor vascularization, oral antibiotics may not be successful. In these patients, antibiotics administered parenterally may be more efficacious.

Hemoglobin F, at all levels of total hemoglobin, has been documented [7,26] for its protective effect against many of the complications of sickle cell anemia (such as leg ulceration) as well as its ability to increase survival rate. Hydroxyurea increases fetal hemoglobin (HbF) and has been shown to reduce pain, and is therefore recommended as part of the treatment for sickle cell disease.

PRACTICE POINT

Hydroxyurea has been documented to contribute to the formation of skin ulcers;[27,28] therefore, patients with leg ulcers shouldn't be treated with this medication.

Short-chain fatty acid such as butyrate[26,29] have resulted in increased hemoglobin F in some studies. However, butyrate is also known to inhibit cell proliferation in multiple cell types, including erythroid cells, and experiments in animal and clinical trials showed that butyrate loses its ability to induce hemoglobin F after prolonged administration in high doses.

A novel approach to treating sickle cell disease was developed by Atweh and colleagues,[30] who designed a regimen in 1999 consisting of intermittent therapy. In the trial, arginine butyrate was administered for 4 days, followed by 10 to 24 days with no drug exposure. After a mean therapy course of 29.9 weeks, 9 of 11 patients had induced hemoglobin F gene expression with the mean hemoglobin F increase from 7.2% to 21.0% ($p < .002$). A parallel increase in F cells and F reticulocytes was also detected. The total hemoglobin level also increased 1 g/dl to a mean of 8.8 g/dl ($p < .006$) and was sustained in all patients. This regimen, which demonstrated marked and sustained increase in HbF levels in more than two-thirds of adult patients with sickle cell disease, was well-tolerated with no adverse effects.

Surgical debridement should be performed on all sickle cell ulcers lasting longer than 2 months if the wound isn't contracting by a minimum of 10% over a 2-week period as measured by planimetry.

"Most patients are able to tolerate chronic hemoglobin levels of 5 to 7 g/dl exceptionally well." [31] However, debridement can result in a hemoglobin level that can't be tolerated. It's essential that the patient's hemoglobin is raised prior to surgery to compensate for any significant blood loss, common vasodilation, and subsequent hypotension, which may result from the effects of general anesthesia. The ability to debride in the office is often limited due to pain, and adequate pain management is always required. Definitive closure of a clean sickle cell ulcer is an important option to consider.[32] For example, an autologous skin graft may be beneficial to some patients.

Summary

The chronic and acute pain associated with sickle cell disease is well-documented, and the added suffering and reduced quality of life inflicted by chronic leg ulceration provides impetus for the ongoing research in this area, specifically as it relates to treatment.

Many features of the pathophysiology of sickle cell disease-related ulcers are finally being recognized. In particular, major developments are being made in wound healing and in the management of leg ulcers. Understanding the pathogenesis and differentiating the etiology of sickle cell leg ulcers is a prerequisite to understanding the treatment of these wounds. The multifactorial nature of sickle cell wounds requires the services of an interdisciplinary team of specialists to heal

them, as well as the entire spectrum of actions necessary for the healing process. In and of themselves, therapeutic intervention without debridement, maintenance of moist wound-healing environments, infection ablation, and patient education won't produce a healed wound.

Validated treatments for nonhealing wounds, such as living skin equivalents and growth factors, are now available. Initial and repeated assessments of the wound and the patient will help the clinician select the appropriate treatment choice. Wet-to-dry dressings and Unna boots aren't the optimal treatment choice. A moist wound environment and control of edema can be established using appropriate dressings (such as the newer silicone-coated absorbents). Multilayer compression wraps or patient-adjustable compression systems are more efficient methods of edema control.

Alternative and adjunctive physical treatments are additional options for nonhealing wounds (negative pressure wound healing, hyperbaric oxygen, pulsed electromagnetic stimulation, and normothermia), and clinical research will doubtless define their efficacy through evidence-based outcomes. However, none of these interventions has yet been proven to give consistently successful results.

Minor leg trauma must be treated immediately using validated wound-care interventions. Lower extremity vessels shouldn't be accessed for I.V. infusions. Skin turgor and nutrition must be maintained. When wounds are healed, preventive measures and instructions should be reinforced.

The process of healing sickle cell leg ulcers is holistic. Thus, wound care should be implemented in the systematic, comprehensive manner described in this chapter.

Acknowledgment

This work was supported by the Eastern Paralyzed Veterans Association and the

National Institute of Health (NIDDK 59424) (HB).

Show what you know

1. The following are characteristic of sickle cell ulcers except:

A. The microvascular circulation is adversely affected.
B. Ulcers can exhibit characteristics of arterial and venous disease such as severe pain or lower extremity edema.
C. Venous duplex and pulse volume recordings are usually within normal limits.
D. Ulcers are usually "punched out" with round, symmetric wound borders, and located around the medial and lateral malleolus.

ANSWER: D. Ulcers may be located anywhere on the lower leg and, unlike arterial wounds, are often irregular in shape. Round symmetrical wound borders are generally characteristic of an arterial ulcer.

2. Which of the following statements about sickle cell ulcers is correct?

A. The pathophysiology of sickle cell leg ulcers has been well documented.
B. There's no consensus regarding the pathogenesis of sickle cell leg ulcers.
C. Venous and arterial insufficiency are significant factors in the pathogenesis of sickle cell leg ulcers
D. Leg ulcers usually develop in early childhood.

ANSWER: B. Many questions still exist regarding the pathogenesis of sickle cell leg ulcers. It's now known that arterial and venous insufficiencies aren't the underlying factor in the development of sickle cell ulcers. Vascular testing is usually within normal limits and the ulcers occur in the teenage years.

3. Which three of the following five steps are included in treatment to insure the healing of sickle cell ulcers?

A. Objectively rule out venous reflux and arterial insufficiency by ultrasound.
B. Provide a moist wound healing environment.
C. Cure the underlying problem, which is sickle cell disease.
D. Remove nonviable tissue and fibrous exudate.
E. Superoxygenate the wound with hyperbaric oxygen therapy.

ANSWERS: A, B, D. Differentiating the etiology is an important factor in determining the treatment. Debridement of the wound is mandatory. At this time, there's no easily attainable cure for sickle cell disease and there's no scientific evidence that hyperbaric oxygen is effective in the treatment of sickle cell ulcers.

References

1. Herrick, J.B. "Peculiar Elongated and Sickle-shaped Red Blood Corpuscles in a Case of Severe Anemia, 1910," *The Yale Journal of Biology and Medicine* 74(3):179-84, May-June 2001.
2. Clair, B. *Sickle Cell Disease: An Overview, Epidemiology.* Augusta, Ga.: Medical College of Georgia Sickle Cell Center, 2002.
3. Diallo, D., and Tchernia, G. "Sickle Cell Disease in Africa," *Current Opinion in Hematology* 9(2):111-16, March 2002.
4. Eckman, J. *Sickle Cell Information Center Guidelines: Introduction.* Atlanta: The Sickle Cell Information Center 2002.
5. Gill, F.M., et al. "Clinical Events in the First Decade in a Cohort of Infants with Sickle Cell Disease. Cooperative Study of Sickle Cell Disease," *Blood* 86(2):776-83, July 1995.
6. Bainbridge, R., et al. "Clinical Presentation of Homozygous Sickle Cell Disease," *Journal of Pediatrics* 106(6):881-85, June 1985.
7. Koshy, M., et al. "Leg Ulcers in Patients with Sickle Cell Disease," *Blood* 74(4):1403-408, September 1989.

8. Mohan, J.S., et al. "Abnormal Venous Function in Patients with Homozygous Sickle Cell (SS) Disease and Chronic Leg Ulcers," *Clinical Science* 98(6):667-72, June 2000.

9. Charache, S. "One View of the Pathogenesis of Sickle Cell Diseases," *Bulletin Europeen de Physiopathologie Respiratoire* 19(4):361-66, July-August 1983.

10. de Chadarevian, J.P., et al. "Splenic Arteries and Veins in Pediatric Sickle Cell Disease," *Pediatric and Developmental Pathology* 4(6):538-44, November-December 2001.

11. Sullivan, K.J., et al. "Low Exhaled Nitric Oxide and a Polymorphism in the NOS I Gene is Associated with acute Chest Syndrome," *American Journal of Respiratory Critical Care Medicine* 164(12):2186-90, December 2001.

12. Charache, S., et al. "'Acute Chest Syndrome' in Adults with Sickle Cell Anemia. Microbiology, Treatment, and Prevention," *Archives of Internal Medicine* 139(1):67-69, January 1979.

13. Bruno, D., et al. "Genitourinary Complications of Sickle Cell Disease," *Journal of Urology* 166(3):803-11, September 2001.

14. Moser, F.G., et al. "The Spectrum of Brain MRI Abnormalities in Sickle Cell Disease: A Report from the Cooperative Study of Sickle Cell Disease," *American Journal of Neurology* 17(5):965-72, May 1996.

15. Onuba, O. "Bone Disorders in Sickle-Cell Disease," *International Orthopaedics* 17(6):397-99, December 1993.

16. Teixeira, A.L., et al. "Sickle Cell Disease: A Clinical and Histopathologic Study of the Liver in Living Children," *Journal of Pediatric Hematology Oncology* 24(2):125-29, February 2002.

17. Woods, K.F., et al. "*Helicobacter pylori* Infection in Sickle Cell Disease," *Journal of the National Medical Association* 92(7):361-65, July 2000.

18. Billett, H.H., et al. "Venous Insufficiency is not the Cause of Leg Ulcers in Sickle Cell Disease," *American Journal of Hematology* 37(2):133-34, June 1991.

19. "Leg Ulceration and Abnormalities of Calf Blood Flow in Sickle-Cell Anemia," *European Journal of Haematology* 46(3):188-90, March 1991.

20. Gofrit, O.N., et al. "Segmental Testicular Infarction Due to Sickle Cell Disease," *Journal of Urology* 160(3 Pt 1):835-36, September 1998.

21. Gottrup, F., et al. "A New Concept of a Multidisciplinary Wound Healing Center and a National Expert Function of Wound Healing," *Archives of Surgery* 136(7):765-72, July 2001.

22. Reed, W., and Vichinsky, E.P. "New Considerations in the Treatment of Sickle Cell Disease," *Annual Review of Medicine* 49:461-74, 1998.

23. *Guidelines for the Management of Acute and Chronic Pain in Sickle Cell Disease.* Glenview, IL: American Pain Society, 1999.

24. Bolton, L. "The Science of Wound Healing," *Continuing Education Lecture: Theory and Practice in Wound Healing.* New York: New York University, 2002.

25. Ballas, S.K. "Treatment of Painful Sickle Cell Leg Ulcers with Topical Opioids," *Blood* 99(3):1096, February 2002.

26. Sher, G.D., and Olivieri, N.F. "Rapid Healing of Chronic Leg Ulcers During Arginine Butyrate Therapy in Patients with Sickle Cell Disease and Thalassemia," *Blood* 84(7):2378-80, October 1994.

27. Young, H.S., et al. "Aggressive, Extensive, Vasculitic Leg Ulceration Associated with Hydroxyurea Therapy and a Fatal Outcome," *Clinical and Experimental Dermatology* 26(8):664-67, November 2001.

28. Olesen, L.H., and Pedersen, B.B. "Hydroxyurea-induced Leg Ulcers in Patients with Chronic Myeloproliferative Disorders," *Ugeskrift for Laeger* 163(49):6908-11, December 2001.

29. Glauber, J.G., et al. "5'-flanking Sequences Mediate Butyrate Stimulation of Embryonic Globin Gene Expression in Adult Erythroid Cells," *Molecular and Cellular Biology* 11(9):4690-97, September 1991.

30. Atweh, G.F., et al. "Sustained Induction of Fetal Hemoglobin by Pulse Butyrate Therapy in Sickle Cell Disease," *Blood* 93(6):1790-97, March 1999.

31. Ohene-Frempong, K., and Steinberg, M.H. "Clinical Aspects of Sickle Cell Anemia in Adults and Children, in Steinberg, M.H., et al., eds., *Disorders of Hemoglobin: Genetics, Pathophysiology, and Clinical Manifestation.* Cambridge, U.K.: Cambridge University Press, 2001.

32. Weinzweig, N., et al. "Simultaneous Reconstruction of Extensive Soft-tissue Defects of Both Lower Limbs with Free Hemiflaps Harvested from the Omentum," *Plastic Reconstructive Surgery* 99(3):757-62, March 1997.

CHAPTER 17

Wounds in special populations

OBJECTIVES

After completing this chapter, you'll be able to:

- identify the unique risk factors for pressure ulcer development in the patient who is critically ill

- describe risk assessment tools and methods appropriate for use with the patient who is critically ill

- list special considerations for pressure ulcer treatment in the patient who is critically ill

- describe successful strategies for reducing the incidence of pressure ulcers in the patient who has a spinal cord injury

- identify risk factors of pressure ulcers in the patient who has a spinal cord injury

- discuss the major health complications of spinal cord injury

- describe the impact of highly active antiretroviral therapy on the prevalence of skin disorders in the patient with human immunodeficiency virus (HIV) or acquired immunodeficiency syndrome (AIDS)

- describe six common infectious skin disorders and two common noninfectious skin disorders in the patient with HIV or AIDS that results in altered skin integrity

- discuss two of the neoplastic skin disorders seen in the patient with HIV or AIDS.

Intensive care population

Janet E. Cuddigan, PhD, RN, CWCN

Pressure ulcer incidence is higher in patients in the intensive care unit (ICU) than in patients in other areas. Studies have reported the incidence of pressure ulcers in intensive care as:

- 40% in 22 patients on intraaortic balloon pumps[1]
- 30.6% in 36 trauma patients[2]
- 14% in 57 surgical intensive care patients on a ventilators or experiencing hemodynamic instability[3]
- 12% in 136 medical, surgical, and respiratory ICU patients[4]

Pressure ulcer risk factors in intensive care patients

Epidemiologic studies of critically ill patients show the following individual risk factors are associated with the development of pressure ulcers:

- longer length of stay[6,12]
- low albumin levels[12]
- use of vasoconstrictive agents[11]
- being "too unstable to turn"[17] or "turned less often"[10]
- days in bed and days without nutrition[6]
- low body mass index on admission[5]

Many of these risk factors can be included under the more general categories of the Braden Scale. For example, "too unstable to turn" could fit into the Braden subscale of mobility. None of these individual risk factors carry enough "statistical weight" to be included in a risk assessment scale; however, keep them in mind as you're assessing the unique risks of critically ill patients.

- 12.4% (stage II or greater ulcers) in 186 patients in a neurologic ICU[5]
- 8% (stage II and greater ulcers) in 412 surgical ICU patients[6]
- 8% in 110 patients randomly assigned to one of three support surfaces.[7]

Similar pressure ulcer incidence rates have been found in pediatric ICU (PICU) patients. In a recent multisite study of 322 PICU patients, the incidence was 27%.[8] These patients tend to develop pressure ulcers on the occiput more often than adult patients because a higher proportion of body weight resides in the head.[8,9]

Risk factors

All too often, the critically ill patient survives a life-threatening illness with the aid of advanced technology, yet faces weeks or months of additional treatment for a painful, disfiguring, and potentially preventable complication — pressure ulcers. The intensive care population encompasses a broad range of physiologically unstable patients.

The key component of a pressure ulcer prevention program for patients in the ICU is an initial risk assessment to identify the specific level and type of risk the patient faces. Frequent follow-up assessments are also essential for prevention. If pressure ulcers develop, supplement aggressive treatment with continued preventive measures, including frequent reassessment.

The Braden Scale for pressure ulcer risk (described in detail in chapter 13, Pressure ulcers) isn't as predictive for the intensive care population as it is for long-term care and general acute care populations. In a prospective study of 186 neurological ICU patients, the Braden Scale was a better predictor of pressure ulcers than any other factors, except low body mass index on admission.[5] With a cutoff score of 16, all patients developing stage II or greater pressure ulcers were considered at risk; however, the false positive rate was 81.9%. The high false positive may be due to over-prediction by the Braden Scale, or the staff may have succeeded in preventing pressure ulcers in some patients whose scores indicated risk. In the same study, a cutoff score of 13 more accurately predicted pressure ulcers, with a sensitivity of 91.4%, but a false negative rate of 1.8%. Other authors have recommended different Braden Scale cutoff scores.[2,10]

Individualize the Braden Scale cutoff score to your patient population, but remember — the total score is only part of the picture. Effective risk-based prevention programs should focus on remedying the unique risks identified by subscale scores. Several investigators have developed risk assessment scales specific to the intensive care population.[6,11-16] These tools show varying levels of accuracy, yet none have undergone the degree of validation testing of the Braden Scale, nor proven superior to the Braden Scale.

The risk factors assessed by the Braden Scale (activity, mobility, sensory perception, moisture, nutrition, and friction and shear), are found in the intensive care population, just as in other patient populations. However, patients in the ICU have additional risk factors; for example, sicker and older patients develop pressure ulcers more often. Several studies correlate higher Acute Physiological Assessment and Chronic Health Evaluation (APACHE) II or III scores among intensive care patients with pressure ulcer development.[4,12,17] The scale is based on physiologic factors, age, and chronic health conditions. It's predictive of patient mortality, so it isn't surprising that the scale that predicts the death of a patient would also predict the tissue death associated with pressure ulcers. (See *Pressure ulcer risk factors in intensive care patients*.)

Several authors have looked for the "one or two additional risk factors" that would make the Braden Scale more predictive of pressure ulcer development in the critically ill patient, yet none have developed a tool that has clinical utility and predictive validity. The most validated is Quigley and Curley's study of PICU patients. Quigley and Curley adapted the descriptions in the Braden Scale for the pediatric population and added a tissue perfusion and oxygenation subscale. Recent findings demonstrate high predictive validity for PICU patients.[8]

Risk assessment depends on a finely integrated combination of risk assessment tools, research-based evidence, and clinical judgment. To develop a successful preventive plan, each risk factor or abnormal Braden subscore should be ad-dressed comprehensively, given the patient's physiologic condition. Risk assessment should be conducted daily and reassessed with major changes in the patient's condition.

Risk-based prevention

Although allocating resources according to the overall level of risk estimated by a total Braden score is useful, a risk-based prevention program should be based on each patient's unique level and type of risk. Target your interventions to address low subscale scores. For example, if mobility and activity subscores are low (1 or 2) and moisture subscores are high (4), focus your interventions on mobility and activity issues.

Mobility subscale

If the patient's condition prevents position changes, provide a bed that allows additional pressure relief. If the patient can't be turned completely due to hemodynamic instability, small shifts in position may be effective.[18] Too frequently, the memory of a patient desaturating or becoming hypotensive during turning prevents us from resuming a turning schedule. Reassess to determine when you can resume turning.

> **PRACTICE POINT**
>
> Watch the tubes when turning! Is the patient lying on any tubes or medical devices? Are endotracheal tubes putting pressure on the lips or mouth?

Patients in respiratory distress are often placed in the prone position to improve partial pressure of arterial oxygen to fraction of inspired oxygen ratios. Prone positioning creates a whole new set of pressure points, including the chin, jaw, breasts, anterior ribs, pelvic bones, male genitalia, anterior knees, and toes. Ensure that pressure is off-loaded in these areas. Pressure-reducing mattresses and "bridging" to off-load pressure points may be helpful. Significant facial edema may develop. Without proper oral care, skin around the mouth and cheeks may become macerated from saliva. Assess the patient for tubes, devices, or positioning strategies that may increase pressure in this position. Respiratory patients may also be placed on rotation beds to improve pulmonary status. Make sure that the patient is secure in the bed and friction and shear injuries don't occur with rotation.

Bed selection

It may be cost-effective to have pressure-relieving mattresses on all beds in an ICU if patient acuity and pressure ulcer incidence tend to be high.[19-21] The cost-benefit ratio may vary according to the overall patient acuity in your unit. The decision to order a pressure-reducing bed should be triggered by low scores on the Braden mobility-activity subscales or in the presence of conditions, such as pharmacological paralysis and sedation.

PRACTICE POINT

• Don't counteract the pressure-relieving effects of these specialized beds by using extra layers of sheets and underpads. Don't use padding because this increases pressure
• Use incontinence pads recommended by the bed manufacturer for patients who need moisture management.
• Above all, make sure that any powered specialty bed is turned on and adjusted for maximum pressure relief for each individual patient. Specialty beds don't replace turning and positioning, nor do they adequately relieve heel pressure.

Positioning

Although the sacrum and the coccyx are the most frequent sites of pressure ulcers, heels are a close second and the incidence of heel ulcers is increasing. Therefore, vigilant protection of heels in the critically ill patient is essential.[22] Your patient assessment should include signs that alert you to vascular insufficiency (pulses—palpated or Doppler, capillary refill, color, warmth, shiny hairless skin, ankle-brachial pressure index, toe pressure, pulse wave-form analysis, and vascular studies). Patients in shock experience constricted vessels in their extremities, accentuating the problem. Rooke boots may keep the heels warm (supporting perfusion) and protected, but they don't relieve pressure. Likewise, cloth heel protectors may decrease the risk of skin injury from friction without relieving pressure. A number of commercial heel protectors are designed to relieve heel pressure by "suspending" the heel. Correct placement is essential to prevent additional rubbing or pressure. Heel protectors should be removed regularly for a careful skin inspection. Placing a pillow or bath blanket under the calves to elevate the heels is an effective technique in patients who aren't agitated.

Activity subscale

Getting a critically ill patient into a chair—even a stretch or Cadillac chair—can be challenging due to the potential problems with postural hypotension, oxygenation, coordination of multiple tubes and invasive lines, and dependence on ventilators. Some bed manufacturers make beds that adjust to a sitting position, which may be an effective alternative for improving early activity, but the patient should progress to sitting in a chair.

PRACTICE POINT

If you can get the patient into a chair, don't forget a seat cushion! A 3″ to 4″ (7.5 to 10 cm) thick foam cushion is usually adequate. In a study involving interface pressure measurement, sheepskin and gel cushions were found to have little pressure-reducing effect.[23]

Remember that skin injury from shear is a possibility when placing a patient with respiratory difficulty in an elevated position to facilitate breathing. Placing pillows under his arms may help support him in the upright position and assist with respiratory excursion. In a study involving interface pressure testing in healthy volunteers, the seating position with the lowest interface pressure was the sitting back (seat tilted) posture with lower legs on a rest. If the seat can't be tilted back, an upright seating posture with feet on the ground is preferable.[24] Check for slouching and reposition the patient as needed. Periodically adjust his position (for example, with lift-offs) and don't leave him in the chair more than 1 hour at a time. When the patient has returned to bed, check his skin carefully for areas of redness.

Sensory perception subscale

Patients scoring low on the sensory perception subscale include those with spinal cord injuries, head trauma, pharmacological paralysis, heavy sedation, and coma. Carlson's[4] Braden Scale validation study of 136 critically ill patients found the sensory perception subscale to be the most predictive of pressure-ulcer risk. Patients with a low sensory score may not feel pressure-induced discomfort and may not be able to change position. As long as the patient lacks this ability, the nursing staff must assume the responsibility for anticipating pressure-induced discomfort and ensuring routine repositioning and pressure reduction.

Moisture subscale

Moisture comes from numerous sources in the critically ill patient, the most obvious being fecal and urinary incontinence. Typical measures include correcting incontinence (when possible), using pads or briefs that wick moisture away from the skin, using moisture barrier creams, frequent changing and cleansing, and assessing skin for maceration and yeast infections.

Don't underestimate other sources of moisture damage that may macerate skin and increase the risk of pressure ulcers. Wound drainage may be excessive and require absorptive dressings, such as foams and alginates. Intensive care patients may exhibit massive, generalized edema. Small injuries such as skin tears may lead to leakage of large amounts of exudates and serum proteins, particularly in patients with low serum albumin levels. Absorptive dressings and pads should be used to wick moisture away from the skin. Skin protectants may be appropriate for some patients.

Nutrition subscale

Poor nutrition is another risk factor for pressure ulcer development in the critically ill patient.[6] Initiate oral or enteral feeding as soon as possible. If these methods of feeding aren't feasible, weigh the risks and benefits of total parenteral nutrition. Recommend a dietary consult within 48 hours of admission if the patient's Braden nutrition subscale score is 3 or less. Even if nutritional supplementation is provided, be aware that it may be inadequate to meet the increased metabolic needs of a critically ill patient despite your best efforts.

Friction and shear subscale

Friction injury may occur with agitation or with insufficient help with turning. Shear injury in the sacrum is a problem when the patient slides down in the bed or chair. Make sure you have enough help when turning and positioning. Use lift sheets and slide boards. When the patient is sitting in a chair or in bed, place pillows under his arms to support his weight and lessen the chance of shear injury.

Skin assessment

Total skin assessment should be performed on every shift with precise documentation of all breaks in skin integrity. The AHCPR guideline recommends that pressure ulcers be assessed and measured weekly. Pressure ulcers may deteriorate more rapidly in the medically unstable, critically ill patient; therefore he should be assessed more frequently.

PRACTICE POINT

Pressure ulcers can be a source of sepsis in a critically ill, immuno-compromised patient.

Be aware of unusual sites of pressure injury, such as under medical devices (casts, splints, external pelvic fixators, pins, traction devices, or heel lifters). Bipap masks, indwelling catheter tugging, and endotracheal tubes — common sources of pressure injury in the intensive care environment — can also be easily overlooked as a potential site for pressure ulcer development. Check anterior surfaces for the patient who has been placed in a supine position.

Pressure injuries can occur internally from tracheostomy and endotracheal tubes; use the minimal occlusive volume to prevent tracheal damage. Assess the intubated patient's oral cavity and lips with a flashlight by shifting his position

slightly without disrupting the tube's level. Tape or commercial tube tamers may be used. Likewise, inspect the site of tracheostomy stoma; excessive exudate around the tracheostomy stoma can cause skin breakdown. Consider more absorptive dressings, such as foam or alginates, under tracheostomy tubes with a lot of mucous and drainage rather than a low absorptive split-gauze dressing. Whenever you can, avoid using rigid equipment on the critically ill patient; for example, switch to a soft cervical collar when possible.

PRACTICE POINT

Always provide thorough oral care for the intubated patient to prevent pressure-related wounds.

Deep-tissue injury

The exact nature of deep-tissue injury is still being investigated. (See chapter 13, Pressure ulcers, for information about the NPUAP task force.) Be careful when assessing early deep tissue injuries, which can be mistaken for stage I pressure ulcers. For example, a patient who develops a deep purple area on his buttocks following a sustained period of hypotension and immobility might not have a stage I pressure ulcer, even if the skin is intact. Such a wound is consistent with deep-tissue damage, which will become apparent as dead superficial tissues slough off. The area should be off-loaded to prevent further damage; it should also be reassessed frequently, with the expectation that the wound may continue to show signs of deterioration.

Spinal cord injury population

Susan L. Garber, MA, OTR, FAOTA, FACRM

Between 183,000 and 230,000 people in the United States have spinal cord injuries and approximately 11,000 new cases are reported every year.[25] The veteran population comprises 22% of the spinal cord injury population.[26] The National Spinal Cord Injury Database documents five major categories of etiology:

- motor vehicle crashes (44.5%)
- falls (18%)
- acts of violence (17%)
- recreational sporting activities (13%)
- causes that don't fit into any of the categories above (8%).[27]

Spinal cord injury occurs most frequently in males ages 16 to 30 (55%).[25] Although the average age is 32 and the most frequently occurring age at injury is 19, the median age is 25 years. More than 82% of the patients in the spinal cord injury database are male. Among patients injured since 1990, 59% are White, 28% are Black, 8% are Hispanic, 2% are Asian, 0.4% are American Indian ethnicity, 0.5% are unknown of unknown ethnicity, and 2.5% are unclassified.[1] Almost half of the spinal cord injury population had completed high school at the time of injury. Given the young age at onset of spinal cord injury, more than half are single. Although most were employed at the time of injury, more than 14% were unemployed.[27]

Pulmonary complications are the most common cause of death during both the acute and chronic phases after spinal cord injury.[28] Other potential complications arising soon after injury — some of which may become lifelong problems— include pressure ulcers, urinary tract infections, osteoporosis, fractures, and heterotopic ossification.

Pressure ulcers are among the most common long-term secondary medical complications found at annual follow-up visits.[29] As such, they're a serious, costly, and potentially lifelong complication of spinal cord injury. Clinical observations and research studies have confirmed staggering costs and human suffering, including a profound negative impact on the patient's general physical health, socialization, financial status, and body image, compounded by his loss of independence and control.[30] Reliable and current data on the incidence and prevalence of pressure ulcers in patients with spinal cord injuries has been difficult to obtain, primarily because limitations of the methods used prevent standardization of the statistics. These limitations include the use of different classification systems to stage pressure ulcers, the inability to compare varied populations (for example, acute or chronic spinal cord injury) presenting with or developing pressure ulcers, and the use of different methods of obtaining data (such as direct observation or retrospective chart review).[31]

Some available data reflect the scope of the problem; the database of the Spinal Cord Injury Model Systems is one of the most reliable. The National Institute on Disability and Rehabilitation Research sponsors the Model Systems Program, a federal extramural grant program of selected research and demonstration sites. Model System sites provide exemplary, state-of-the-art care from the time of injury through acute medical care, comprehensive rehabilitation, and long-term follow-up and health maintenance services. An individual can be included in the database only if he was admitted to a system facility within 24 hours of trauma. As far back as 1981,[32] the Model System database included statistics on pressure ulcers in patients with spinal cord injuries. According to the 1998 National Spinal Cord Injury Statistical Center Annual Report, 34% of patients admitted to a Model System facility within 24 hours of spinal cord injury developed at least one pressure ulcer during acute care or rehabilitation.[33] On follow-up, 15% had a pressure ulcer at their first annual examination, 20% at year 5, 23% at year 10, 24% at year 15, and 29% at year 20. These numbers are based on 4,065 patients of whom 2,971 developed pressure ulcers. Other investigators have reported prevalence rates that ranged from 17% to 33% in populations of patients with spinal cord injuries residing in the community.[32,34,35]

High rates of pressure ulcer recurrence also have been reported, with rates ranging from 21% to 79% regardless of treatment.[36-38] A number of epidemiological studies have found that 36% to 50% of all patients with spinal cord injuries who develop pressure ulcers will develop a recurrence within the first year after initial healing.[34,35,38-40] Niazi and colleagues[38] reported a recurrence rate of 35% regardless of type of treatment (medical or surgical). Holmes et al.[41] found that 55% of their sample, most of which had a history of severe previous ulcers, experienced recurrence within 2 years after surgical repair. In a 20-year study in Canada (1976 to 1996), Schryvers and colleagues[36] found recurrence rates of 31% at the same site for severe ulcers, requiring surgery in 168 patients with spinal cord injuries. Goodman et al.[37] observed a recurrence or new ulcer development rate of 79% within a 1- to 6-year follow-up.

The financial burden of pressure ulcers is undoubtedly immense, although estimates of the cost of preventing and treating pressure ulcers in the patient with spinal cord injury isn't readily available. Miller and DeLozier[42] reported that the total cost of treating stage II, III, and IV pressure ulcers in hospitals, nursing homes, and home care was approximately $1.335 billion per year. One could extrapolate from these data the financial implications of pressure ulcers for patients with spinal cord injuries. However, the financial burden of pressure ulcers doesn't begin to reflect the personal and social costs experienced by the patient and his family. These include loss of independence and self-esteem; time away from work, school, or family; and, ultimately, diminished quality of life.

Risk factors

There are more than 200 risk factors for the development of pressure ulcers. Most of the risk factors that have been described in the literature were derived from studying elderly nursing home residents. Many of the risk factors for these patients differ from those experienced by patients with spinal cord injuries. Immobility increases the risk of pressure ulcer development in both populations; unlike nursing home residents, however, patients with spinal cord injuries typically oversee or direct their own daily care and are expected to take primary responsibility for pressure ulcer prevention. The literature is often contradictory regarding the effects of a particular risk factor or set of factors potentially responsible for the development of pressure ulcers. These contradictions occur due to the limitations imposed by the variables among studies. Different populations (for example, acute or chronic spinal cord injury), inadequate sample sizes, different ways of standardizing the dependent measures, and poor or uncontrolled study designs all add confusion to the interpretation of study results.[43,44]

Despite these limitations, a number of pressure ulcer risk factors specific to the patient with spinal cord injury have been identified and described in the literature.

Byrne and Salzberg's[43] study (1996) summarized the major pressure ulcer risk factors for patients with spinal cord injuries as:

- severity of spinal cord injury (immobility, completeness of spinal cord injury, urinary incontinence, and severe spasticity)
- preexisting conditions (advanced age, smoking, lung and cardiac disease, diabetes and renal disease, and impaired cognition)
- residence in a nursing home
- nutrition (malnutrition and anemia).

The Consortium for Spinal Cord Medicine Clinical Practice Guidelines (Pressure Ulcer Prevention and Treatment Following Spinal Cord Injury)[31] categorized pressure ulcer risk factors in spinal cord injury as:

- demographic factors (age, gender, ethnicity, marital status, and education)
- physical or medical and spinal cord injury-related factors (level and completeness of spinal cord injury, activity and mobility, bladder, bowel and moisture control, and comorbidities such as diabetes and spasticity)
- psychological and social factors (psychological distress, financial problems, cognition, substance abuse, adherence, and health beliefs and practices).[31]

As far back as 1979, Anderson and Andberg[45] identified psychological factors associated with the development of pressure ulcers, including the patient's unwillingness to take responsibility in skin care, low self-esteem, and dissatisfaction with life activities. Gordon and colleagues[46] found poor social adjustment in patients with spinal cord injuries and pressure ulcers.

Recurrence of pressure ulcers in the patient with spinal cord injury has been associated with gender (male), age (younger), ethnicity (black), unemployment, residence in a nursing home, and previous pressure ulcer surgery.[38,47,48]

Most of the literature describing recurrence following surgery focuses on surgical techniques.[49-52] Investigators have reported recurrence rates of 11% to 29% in cases with postoperative complications and 6% to 61% in cases without postoperative complications.[48,53-55] Of these investigators, Relander and Palmer[54] recommended that social factors be studied to determine the causes of pressure ulcer recurrence after surgical repair and suggested that the patient who doesn't display the appropriate knowledge regarding pressure ulcer prevention should be counseled before consideration for surgery. Disa and colleagues[48] reported that high recurrence rates among patients with traumatic paraplegia were associated with substance abuse and the absence of an adequate social support system; they suggested developing more effective educational programs for both patients and caregivers. In other studies by Mandrekas and Mastorakos,[55] Baek et al.,[56] and Rubayi et al.,[57] investigators reported that inadequate patient education with regard to pressure ulcer prevention contributed to the recurrence rates.

PRACTICE POINT

Innovative educational programs are needed to provide the patient with spinal cord injury with information and the motivation necessary to regain some measure of control over their lives.

Risk-based prevention

The patient with spinal cord injury is at risk for the development of pressure ulcers from the moment of injury. Prolonged immobilization during the hours and days immediately after injury significantly increases the risk. Pressure reduction strategies to protect vulnerable anatomical areas of the body should be implemented soon

PATIENT TEACHING

Preventing pressure ulcers at home

Patients with spinal cord injuries are at risk for developing pressure ulcers even after they leave your care. Teach the patient and his family the following strategies to help him prevent pressure ulcers after he has returned home.

- Perform daily visual and tactile skin inspection.
- Maintain good personal hygiene.
- Perform frequent turning and repositioning, including frequent weight shifts.
- Use support surfaces for the bed and wheelchair.
- Maintain adequate nutrition.

after emergency medical interventions and spinal stabilization.

PRACTICE POINT

Pressure ulcer development is a lifelong concern for the patient with spinal cord injury.

Preventing pressure ulcers is a major component of both informal and formal educational sessions during rehabilitation. A regimen of preventive strategies is developed for each patient and includes information and instructions that traditionally have been imparted to the patient and his family following spinal cord injury.[58] (See *Preventing pressure ulcers at home.*)

Printed materials or videos are frequently used to augment the educational sessions, some of which may go with the patient when he's discharged. Because most patient education programs are hospital-based, little is known about what information the patient retains, which behaviors or activities are practiced routinely, and the compatibility of the patient's lifestyles with prevention strategies. In the 1970s and 1980s, a number of spinal cord injury centers established comprehensive pressure ulcer prevention education programs.[59-61] Both inpatient and outpatient programs advocated multidisciplinary, coordinated, structured, and wide-ranging approaches to prevention. Some of these programs serve as models for practice today.[62]

Skin assessment

The patient with spinal cord injury and a pressure ulcer should undergo two assessment phases. The first phase is a comprehensive evaluation and examination, including:

- complete patient history
- physical examination
- laboratory tests
- assessment of psychological health, behavior, and cognitive status
- information on social and financial resources and the availability and utilization of personal care assistance
- assessment of positioning, posture, and related equipment.[31]

The second phase of assessment consists of a detailed description of the pressure ulcer itself and surrounding tissues, including the following factors:

- anatomical location and general appearance
- size in terms of length, width, depth, and wound area
- stage or severity
- exudate
- odor
- necrosis
- undermining
- sinus tracts
- infection

- granulation and epithelialization
- wound margins and surrounding tissue.[31]

Photographs can also be useful.

PRACTICE POINT

Patients with darkly pigmented skin are particularly vulnerable to undetected pressure ulcers. Although areas of damaged skin appear darker than the surrounding skin, tactile information must be used in addition to visual data when assessing patients with darker skin. The skin may be taut and shiny, indurated, and warm to the touch. Color changes may range from purple to blue. Remember, pressure-damaged dark skin doesn't blanch when compressed.[63]

Treatment

Prevention and treatment are inextricably linked across the continuum of care for the patient with a pressure ulcer.[64] During rehabilitation following spinal cord injury, the patient is exposed to a great deal of information about the major physiological changes that have occurred as well as how to prevent or manage the potential secondary complications such as pressure ulcers and urinary tract infections. Unfortunately, much of this information isn't absorbed during this early posttraumatic phase, resulting in episodes of potentially life-threatening conditions once the patient returns to his home and community. Coupled with nonretention of information is the significant decrease in length of stay that precludes structured education sessions during hospitalization. The treatment of pressure ulcers is a complex process, based on a number of patient- and pressure ulcer-related factors.

Nonsurgical treatment

Nonsurgical treatment for pressure ulcers is a multistep process. The elements of a comprehensive treatment plan include cleansing, debridement, applying dressings, and assessing the need for (and appropriateness of) new technologies aimed at wound healing. Education, in the form of printed materials or discussions with health professionals, is intended to prevent recurrence in the patient with spinal cord injury.

Surgical treatment

Stage III and IV pressure ulcers are frequently treated surgically in the patient with spinal cord injury. The goals of surgical closure include:

- preventing protein loss through the wound
- reducing risk of progressive osteomyelitis and sepsis
- preventing renal failure
- reducing costly and lengthy hospitalization
- improving hygiene and appearance
- expediting time to healing.[31,65,66]

The surgical process includes:

- excision of the ulcer and surrounding scar, underlying bursa, and soft-tissue calcification removal of underlying necrotic or infected bone
- filling dead space with fascia or muscle flaps
- improving vascularity and distribution of pressure over bony prominences
- resurfacing the area with large flap so that the suture line is away from areas of direct pressure
- providing a flap that leaves options for future surgeries.[65,66]

Preoperatively, the rehabilitation and surgical teams coordinate their efforts to control local wound infection, improve and maintain nutrition, regulate the bowels, control spasms and contractures, and address comorbid conditions. Previous pressure ulcer surgery, smoking, urinary

Support surface characteristics

PERFORMANCE CHARACTERISTICS	DYNAMIC SUPPORT DEVICES			STATIC SUPPORT DEVICES		
	Air-fluidized	Low-air-loss	Alternating-air	Static flotation (air or water)	Foam	Standard mattress
Increased support area	Yes	Yes	Yes	Yes	Yes	No
Pressure reduction	Yes	Yes	Yes	Yes	Yes	No
Shear reduction	Yes	Questionable	Yes	Yes	No	No
Low moisture retention	Yes	Yes	No	No	No	No
Reduced heat accumulation	Yes	Yes	No	No	No	No
Transfers	Difficult	Routine	Routine	Routine	Routine	Routine
Cost per day	Highest	High	Moderate	Low	Low	Lowest

Adapted with permission from the Paralyzed Veterans of America (PVA). *Prevention and Treatment of Pressure Ulcers Following Traumatic Spinal Cord Injury: A Clinical Practice Guideline for Health-Care Professionals.* Washington, D.C.: Paralyzed Veterans of America, 2000.

tract infection, and heterotopic ossification could affect surgical outcomes.[31]

 EVIDENCE-BASED PRACTICE

Pain care includes keeping the surgical site pressure-free, using specialty beds to maximize pressure reduction, mobilizing the patient progressively, and providing patient and family education.[31]

Support surfaces

Support surfaces are devices or systems intended to reduce the interface pressure between a patient and his bed or wheelchair.[64] Support surfaces don't heal pressure ulcers; rather, they're prescribed by a clinician and incorporated into a comprehensive pressure ulcer prevention and management program. Static or dynamic mattresses, mattress overlays, or specialty beds may be used at various times to reduce the patient's risk of developing pressure ulcers. Materials such as foams and gels, alone or in combination, and elements such as air and water, also alone or in combination, are being used across patient-care and home environments. Wheelchair cushions and seating systems of various materials and designs are intended to reduce pressure and maximize balance and stability when a patient is in a wheelchair. (See *Support surface characteristics* and *Support surface pros and cons.*)

Support surface pros and cons

This chart presents the major categories of support surfaces with their advantages and disadvantages.

Major types	Common applications	Advantages	Disadvantages
Static support surface	• Pressure ulcer prevention • Individual may be kept off pressure ulcer	• Reduces interface pressure • Is cost-effective when properly matched to individual • Does not consume power	• May result in shearing • Moisture and heat build up
Alternating pressure surface	• Individual who requires more pressure reduction than a static mattress	• Relieves pressure intermittently	• Intermittent elevated pressure • Moisture retention possible
Low air-loss surface	• Individual who has more than 1 turning surface impaired due to multiple pelvic pressure ulcers or other factors	• Reduces interface pressure • Manages moisture and heat	• Shear reduction depends on design; possible noise • Complicated activities of daily living maneuvers and transfers
Air-fluidized bed	• Postoperative flap surgery • Deterioration of multiple pelvic pressure ulcers	• Reduces interface pressure below capillary closing pressure • Manages moisture	• Most expensive • Vulnerable to respiratory or dehydration problems • Premature drying of moist dressings • Significant electric energy requirement • Noise • Limited ability to elevate head of the bed

Adapted with permission from the Paralyzed Veterans of America (PVA). *Prevention and Treatment of Pressure Ulcers Following Traumatic Spinal Cord Injury: A Clinical Practice Guideline for Health-Care Professionals.* Washington, D.C.: Paralyzed Veterans of America; 56-57, 2000.

PRACTICE POINT

No single product meets every patient's needs, or all the needs of a single patient. Use your experience and your judgment in concert with objective selection of products to match the device to the patient.

New interventions

A number of adjunctive therapies have been reported in the literature with varying degrees of success in treating pressure ulcers in the patient with spinal cord injury, including:

• electrical stimulation
• ultraviolet and laser therapy

- normothermia
- hyperbaric oxygen and ultrasound
- subatmospheric pressure therapy (vacuum-assisted closure)
- nonantibiotic drugs
- topical agents
- skin equivalents
- growth factors.

Among these, only electrical stimulation has enough scientific evidence supporting it to justify its use as a treatment for pressure ulcers in the patient with spinal cord injury.[67-68]

HIV/AIDS population

Carl A. Kirton, MA, RN, APRN,BC

The skin is the most commonly affected organ in patients infected with HIV. In fact, in the early 1980s it was the identification of an unusual skin lesion in young homosexual men that prompted the search for the virus that causes AIDS.

A broad range of infectious and noninfectious skin lesions may develop during both the asymptomatic and symptomatic course of the disease. Alteration in the skin is often the first manifestation of an impaired immune system and may be a harbinger of a serious opportunistic infection. Skin alterations can also indicate advancing disease.

Several points regarding HIV, skin disease, and its treatments are noteworthy. Lesions that are common in the non–HIV-infected adult population may present atypically in HIV-infected persons. In addition, skin disorders often aren't responsive to the usual treatments, may be present for longer than expected, and may develop into chronic, disfiguring disorders. Skin lesions may also be the harbinger of a life-threatening illness.

PRACTICE POINT

Prompt and accurate investigation of skin lesions in the HIV-infected patient is essential and often warrants collaboration with an HIV specialist.

The use of combination drug regimens that often include a protease inhibitor, also known as highly active antiretroviral therapy (HAART), suppresses viral replication with consequent repletion of CD4+-positive lymphocyte counts. HAART-based regimens have contributed to a significant decline in HIV-associated morbidity and mortality. Some skin disorders also decreased in incidence with HAART, including Kaposi's sarcoma, eosinophilic folliculitis, molluscum contagiosum, bacillary angiomatosis, and condylomata acuminate. Although HARRT and regimens that treat opportunistic infections have improved the quality of life for patients infected with HIV, adverse reactions to drugs have increased. Such severe adverse reactions are much more frequent in HIV-infected patients than in noninfected patients. Drugs often implicated include sulfonamides, cotrimoxazole, and tuberculostatics as well as nucleoside-type reverse transcriptase inhibitors.

Infectious skin disorders

The immunocompromised status of patients with HIV or AIDS puts them at greater risk for infectious bacterial or viral skin disorders.

Herpes virus

Breakouts of grouped blister-like lesions typically caused by the common herpes virus are easily recognized and common in patients with HIV at all stages of the disease. Herpes infection may occur on the oral and genital mucosa as well as the perianal region. Lesions typically manifest as painful, grouped vesicles on an erythematous base that rupture and become crusted. History and clinical presentation are often all that's necessary to establish the disorder; therefore, confirmatory tests, such as the Tzanck smear preparation, biopsy, or viral culture are rarely necessary. In patients with advanced HIV, a herpetic infection may develop into chronic ulcers and fissures with a substantial degree of edema.

Herpes zoster occurs with higher frequency among HIV-seropositive patients than among those who are seronegative. A longitudinal study demonstrated an incidence of 29.4 cases of herpes zoster per 1,000 person-years among HIV-seropositive patients, as compared with 2.0 cases per 1,000 person-years among HIV-seronegative controls.[69] Uncomplicated zoster outbreaks should be treated with acyclovir (Zovirax), famciclovir, or valacyclovir, all for 10 days. Painful atrophic scars, persistent ulcerations, and acyclovir-resistant chronic verrucous lesions may also develop. (See *Herpes virus teaching tips*.)

PATIENT TEACHING

Herpes virus teaching tips

- Scrupulous hand washing helps prevent the spread of infection.
- Use individual washcloths and linens.
- Mild analgesics may be necessary for pain associated with herpes infection.
- Topical soaks (such as Domeboro solution) can be used to help dry wet lesions.
- Impetiginization of skin lesions may be treated with warm compresses.

PRACTICE POINT

Healing is usually complete in less than 2 weeks. If the lesions haven't healed within 3 to 4 weeks, the patient may have a drug-resistant virus. Acyclovir-resistant cases of varicella-zoster virus or herpes simplex virus infection require treatment with intravenous foscarnet.

PRACTICE POINT

A patient with zoster-involving V1, the ophthalmic division of the trigeminal nerve, should be referred to an ophthalmologist immediately due to the risk of corneal ulceration. Signs or symptoms of this condition, such as painful vesicular lesions on the tip of the nose or lid margins, should be considered an ocular emergency.

Cytomegalovirus

Up to 90% of patients with AIDS develop acute, active cytomegalovirus infection at some point during their illness.[70] When the skin is involved, cytomegalovirus may cause a number of different clinical manifestations including ulcers, verrucous lesions, and palpable purpuric papules. Cytomegalovirus commonly affects the GI tract in advanced disease and patients often develop perianal ulcerations. Cytomegalovirus is treated with intravenous ganciclovir, foscarnet, or cidofovir.

PRACTICE POINT

Ulcers are commonly secondarily colonized with cytomegalovirus and many patients have combined herpes simplex and cytomegalovirus infections.

Human papillomavirus infections

The most common skin complaint of HIV-positive patients is warts caused by the human papillomavirus. It has been shown that immune deficiency is associated with increased frequency of human papillomavirus infections, suggesting

PATIENT TEACHING

Postprocedure care for human papillomavirus infection

Lesions associated with human papillomavirus typically require either chemical or surgical excision following treatment of the viral cause. Postprocedure patient teaching should include the following.

- Medication usually isn't needed after removal of lesions. Topical anesthetic ointments may be used to minimize discomfort. Sitz baths may aid resolution when large areas are treated; silver sulfadiazine (Silvadene) ointment or antibiotic ointment may not only be soothing, but may also reduce the possibility of superficial infection. No dressing is required, but some patients may request a sanitary napkin for treated genital lesions. Ice packs are helpful.
- Cryonecrosed lesions will progress from erythema to edema, and then will turn black. The lesions will disappear within a few days, and healing should be complete in 7 to 8 days. For chemically cauterized lesions, the healing process is usually less than 1 week.
- Treated areas should be washed and dried gently each day of the healing process. Postcryotherapy management is similar to a superficial partial thickness burn.
- Counsel the patient to report excessive discomfort or any signs of infection.[71]

These dull-colored papules erupt anywhere on the skin, including the anal mucous membrane, vagina, scrotum, penis, and mouth. Their appearance, size, and number vary with the site. Warts can range in size from less than 1 mm to 2 cm "cauliflower lesions." Treatment, although effective, rarely eradicates human papillomavirus entirely. Destructive measures—such as the application of topical chemicals (for example, salicylic or trichloroacetic acid), cryotherapy with liquid nitrogen, and ablative surgery—are standard measures used for common verrucae. Condylomata acuminata can be treated by using podophyllin resin 10% to 50% in tincture of benzoin, 3% cidofovir ointment, intralesional interferon-alpha, liquid nitrogen cryotherapy, electrodissication and curettage, or carbon dioxide laser.

PATIENT TEACHING

Instruct the patient to apply imiquimod (Aldara) 5% to his warts at night three times per week for up to 16 weeks.

Plantar verrucae are generally treated with topical 40% salicylic acid plaster applied daily, with paring of hyperkeratotic areas, although intralesional bleomycin and liquid nitrogen therapy have also been used. Verruca plana and filiform verrucae are commonly treated with topical tretinoin alone or in combination with 5-flurouracil. Light electrodessication and liquid nitrogen application may be used as an adjunct therapy. Verrucous carcinoma requires excision surgery. (See *Postprocedure care for human papillomavirus infection*.)

Molluscum contagiosum

Molluscum contagiosum is a benign, usually asymptomatic viral skin infection caused by the poxvirus that causes no systemic manifestations. The diagnosis

that the emergence of human papillomavirus is modulated by the patient's immune status.

can usually be made from the characteristic appearance of dome-shaped, umbilicated translucent papules that may develop on any cutaneous site, especially the genital areas and the face. In the patient with AIDS, lesions may become widespread, disfiguring, and recalcitrant to treatment. The prevalence of molluscum contagiosum in the patient with AIDS is 5% to 18%.[72] Treatment of molluscum contagiosum is generally by destructive measures. Cryotherapy or curettage are the usual methods of treatment. (See *Molluscum contagiosum teaching tips*.)

Staphylococcus or Streptococcus

In general, most bacterial infections are caused by *Staphylococcus* and *Streptococcus* organisms and are commonly encountered in immunocompetent patients. Primary bacterial lesions manifest as vesicles, papules and pustules, and are often pruritic. It's the pruritic feature that often leads the patient to scratching, subsequently resulting in a break in the epithelial surface with subsequent excoriation of the lesion. Some lesions (such as impetigo) may contain purulent fluid. Diffusely red, warm, tender areas in the skin suggest soft-tissue cellulitis or a deep-seated infected wound. Treatment with dicloxacillin, cephalexin, or ciprofloxacin is indicated in bacterial infections. Wounds caused by bacterial infections should be assessed regularly and treated accordingly. (See chapter 7, Wound bioburden.)

Bacillary angiomatosis

Bacillary angiomatosis is a bacterial infection caused by organisms of the genus *Bartonella* (formerly *Rochalimaea*), specifically *B. quintana* and *B. henselae*. These cutaneous vascular lesions are characteristically small reddish to purple papules that are tender to touch. Lesions may ulcerate and then be covered by a

PATIENT TEACHING

Molluscum contagiosum teaching tips

- Molluscum contagiosum can be transmitted through direct contact.
- The lesions are prone to autoinoculation, and in male patients, shaving the beard area has been reported to cause particularly severe infections, with lesions encompassing the entire face.
- Cryonecrosed lesions will progress from erythema to edema, and then will turn black. The lesions will disappear within a few days, and healing should be complete in 7 to 8 days.
- For chemically cauterized lesions, the healing process is usually less than 1 week.

crust. Complicated bacillary angiomatosis infections occur when the lesion is located deep in the subcutis, extending to involve soft tissue and bone. Infection with bacillary angiomatosis leads to systemic involvement. Biopsy and special staining is often necessary to definitely identify the organism. Treatment with erythromycin or doxycycline provides a prompt response. (See *Bacillary angiomatosis teaching tips*, page 360.)

PRACTICE POINT

With the advent of HAART, bacillary angiomatosis infections are rarely seen. Bacillary angiomatosis infections may mimic Kaposi's sarcoma, which should therefore remain in the differential diagnosis until the actual causative agent is identified.

PATIENT TEACHING

Bacillary angiomatosis teaching tips

The most common reservoirs for the bacilli that cause bacillary angiomatosis are domestic cats and cat fleas. Clients with AIDS should avoid rough play with cats and situations in which scratches from cats are likely to occur. Cats shouldn't be allowed to lick open wounds or cuts. All cats should be treated for fleas, or other flea control measures should be followed.[74]

Noninfectious skin disorders

The immunocompromised status of patients with HIV and AIDS also puts them at greater risk for noninfectious skin disorders.[73]

Porphyria cutanea tarda

Porphyria cutanea tarda has been reported to be increasing in incidence in patients with HIV infection. Porphyrias result from inherited or acquired deficiencies in any one of several enzymes that synthesize heme. When a given enzyme is absent or in short supply, porphyrins are shunted away from heme synthesis into pathways that produce porphyrin by-products. These by-products, in turn, build up in tissues and cause the clinical manifestations of porphyria. In HIV, the deficiencies may be acquired as a consequence of abnormal liver function secondary to liver disease such as hepatitis C. The lesions associated with this disorder generally appear on the dorsal surfaces of the hands, with numerous intact and ruptured bullae that become painful erosions that heal as atrophic scars and milia. The face and forehead are often covered with thickly wrinkled, hyperpigmented skin. Patients may describe the excretion of dark urine. The diagnosis is made on the basis of clinical findings as well as demonstration of elevated porphyrins and coproporphyrins in the urine.

PRACTICE POINT

The usual treatment of porphyria cutanea tarda is repeated phlebotomy until the patient's hemoglobin and serum iron are normalized; however, this treatment isn't appropriate in HIV-infected patients, who are often anemic.

Treatment with low-dose chloroquine phosphate (Aralen) until porphyrin levels become normal is recommended. Oral administration twice weekly is typically required for about 1 year. (See *Porphyria cutanea tarda teaching tips*.)

PRACTICE POINT

Several drugs in HIV can induce or exacerbate porphyrias, including:
- barbiturates (various)
- erythromycin
- pyrazinamide
- rifampin
- sulfonamides (various).

Cutaneous drug eruptions

Cutaneous drug-induced eruptions are common manifestations of drug hypersensitivity in HIV-infected patients. Bactrim (trimethoprim-sulfamethoxazole), the most efficacious drug in the prevention and treatment of *Pneumocystis carinii* pneumonia, is known for causing cutaneous eruption in patients with HIV infection.

Approximately 50% to 60% of HIV-positive patients have been shown to develop a cutaneous eruption from Bactrim. A Bactrim drug eruption is characterized by widely disseminated spread eruptions of fine pink to red macules and papules involving the trunk and extremities.

In its severe form, Stevens-Johnson syndrome and toxic epidermal necrolysis may also develop. Stevens-Johnson syndrome is characterized by fever, widespread blisters of the skin, and mucous membranes of the eye, mouth, or genitals. Toxic epidermal necrolysis is a more serious manifestation, which involves widespread areas of the skin with confluent bullae that can lead to loss of skin in massive sheets.

PRACTICE POINT

Toxic epidermal necrolysis may lead to secondary infection with sepsis, volume depletion, and high output cardiac failure as a consequence of widespread denudation of the skin. Patients who develop toxic epidermal necrolysis must be treated aggressively in an acute care setting.

PRACTICE POINT

Because Bactrim is the most efficacious drug in the prevention and treatment of *Pneumocystis carinii* pneumonia, it's advised that the patient with cutaneous reactions be desensitized in a controlled setting (such as a hospital or clinic).

Neoplastic disorders

Patients with HIV and AIDS are at risk for a variety of neoplastic disorders.[73]

PATIENT TEACHING

Porphyria cutanea tarda teaching tips

- Advise the patient to minimize sun exposure by regularly applying a sunscreen with a high sun protectant factor (SPF), covering exposed skin with clothing, and finding an indoor occupation.
- Counsel the patient to abstain from drinking alcohol, which can exacerbate the disease.

Lymphoma

Although lymphomas generally start in the lymph nodes or collections of lymphatic tissue in organs such as the stomach or intestines, the skin may be affected. Non-Hodgkin's lymphoma is usually manifested as pink to purplish papules or nodules. Deeply seated soft-tissue involvement may expand superficially, forming dome-shaped nodules that often ulcerate. Cutaneous Hodgkin's disease appears similar to non-Hodgkin's lymphoma. The diagnosis is made by the identification of atypical cells having a Reed-Sternberg-like morphology. Treatments include methotrexate, prednisone, bleomycin, adriamycin, cyclophosphamide, and vincristine.

Kaposi's sarcoma

Kaposi's sarcoma is a vascular neoplastic disorder. Prior to the use of HARRT, Kaposi's sarcoma was the most common skin disorder seen in men who have sex with men with AIDS. The pathogenesis of Kaposi's sarcoma has now been identified as a Human herpesvirus type 8. This virus is transmitted sexually, which, in part, explains the epidemiology of Kaposi's sarcoma predominantly in the men who have sex with men population.

Clinically, Kaposi's sarcoma skin lesions may be pink, red, brown, or purple macules, patches, plaques, nodules, or tumors and can appear almost anywhere on the body, including the mucous membranes. The appearance of many cutaneous lesions typically predicts visceral organ involvement. When pressure-bearing areas such as the base of the spine are involved, lesions often ulcerate. When tumors involve the lymphatics, marked edema may develop leading to diffuse swollen areas of the skin and subsequent breaks in the skin.

Diagnosis is usually based on the finding of purplish skin lesions. Biopsy is rarely necessary, but may be performed because bacillary angiomatosis mimics Kaposi's sarcoma lesions. Effective HAART therapy is considered the first-line treatment for Kaposi's sarcoma lesions, and when CD4 cells improve, lesions tend to regress. Other treatments include liquid nitrogen cryotherapy for small cutaneous lesions; radiation treatment and electron-beam therapy are used in selected cases. Radiotherapy is effective for painful lesions of the palms and soles. Intralesional injections of vinblastine sulfate at biweekly intervals are also effective, especially if the patient has only a few small lesions; however, the injections are often associated with pain. With more advanced disease, systemic therapy with interferon and liposomally encapsulated doxorubicin and daunorubicin are effective agents.

Summary

Some pressure ulcers may be unavoidable in the intensive care setting. Vigilant monitoring is necessary to find and treat these ulcers as soon as they develop.

Remember, pressure ulcers may be a source of sepsis in an already compromised patient. Assess the patient and determine his, and his family's, wishes, and adapt your goals accordingly. Aggressive treatment may be necessary to minimize tissue damage and relieve pain. Some patients may be too physiologically unstable for interventions such as turning. In cases such as this, the priority is saving the patient, sometimes at the expense of the skin.

Patients with spinal cord injuries are at lifelong risk for the development of pressure ulcers. Although mostly preventable, pressure ulcers are a deterrent to achieving rehabilitation goals, may contribute to a loss of independence, and interfere with the pursuit of educational, vocational, and leisure activities after spinal cord injury. It's now possible to identify patients at the highest risk for pressure ulcers so that effective prevention strategies can be incorporated into the lifestyle of patients with spinal cord injuries.

Skin disorders are common in patients with HIV and AIDS. Accurate identification of the skin lesions is critical so appropriate treatment can be implemented. Consultation with an HIV or AIDS clinician is helpful in the comprehensive care of these patients.

Show what you know

1. Risk assessment for pressure ulcer development in the critically ill patient should be done:

    A. weekly.
    B. every shift.
    C. daily.
    D. on admission and discharge.

ANSWER: C. Critically ill patients have compounding risk factors. Daily assessment is recommended.

2. *A risk-based prevention program for pressure ulcers in the intensive care setting should be based on each subscale of a risk assessment tool.*

    A. True
    B. False

ANSWER: A. Each critically ill patient has a unique level and type of risk. Each subscale should be addressed separately with appropriate interventions.

3. *All of the following are major risk factors for pressure ulcer development in the spinal cord injury population except:*

    A. preexisting conditions.
    B. severity of the spinal cord injury.
    C. gender.
    D. nutrition.

ANSWER: C. Gender isn't a risk factor for pressure ulcer development. Preexisting conditions, severity of the spinal cord injury, and nutrition are all major risk factors.

4. *The most commonly occurring complication of spinal cord injury is:*

    A. fracture.
    B. urinary tract infection.
    C. pressure ulcer development.
    D. osteoporosis.

ANSWER: B. Urinary tract is the most commonly occurring complication of spinal cord injury; pressure ulcer development is second. Fractures and osteoporosis are also other complications that may occur.

5. *Highly active antiretroviral therapy (HAART) has impacted skin disorders in HIV in which one of the following ways:*

    A. Adverse effects of HAART have led to an increase in the number of skin disorders seen in the patient infected with HIV.

    B. There has been a decrease in the incidence of skin disorders seen in the patient with HIV.
    C. There has been an increase in the number of noninfectious skin disorders in the patient with HIV.
    D. Viral infections are the only skin disorders affected by HAART.

ANSWER: B. HAART based regimens have contributed to a significant drop in HIV associated morbidity and mortality, including many of the cutaneous manifestations of HIV infection.

6. *Patients with porphyria cutanea tarda and HIV should be screened for which one of the following disorders?*

    A. *Pneumocystis carinii* pneumonia
    B. Syphilis
    C. Thyroid disease
    D. Hepatitis C

ANSWER: D. Porphyria-associated deficiencies are acquired possibly as a consequence of abnormal liver function secondary to liver disease such as hepatitis C.

References

1. Jesurum, J., et al. "Balloons, Beds, and Breakdown. Effects of Low-air-loss Therapy on the Development of Pressure Ulcers in Cardiovascular Surgical Patients with Intra-aortic Balloon Pump Support," *Critical Care Nursing Clinics of North America* 8(4):423-40, December 1996.
2. Baldwin, K.M., and Ziegler, S.M. "Pressure Ulcer Risk Following Critical Traumatic Injury," *Advances in Wound Care* 11(4):168-73, July-August 1998.
3. Sideranko, S., et al. "Effects of Position and Mattress Overlay on Sacral and Heel Pressures in a Clinical Population," *Research in Nursing & Health* 15(4):245-51, August 1992.
4. Carlson, E.V., et al. "Predicting the Risk of Pressure Ulcers in Critically Ill Patients," *American Journal of Critical Care* 8(4):262-69, July 1999.

5. Fife, C., et al. "Incidence of Pressure Ulcers in a Neurologic Critical Care Unit," *Critical Care Medicine* 29(2):283-90, February 2001.

6. Eachempati, S.R., et al. "Factors Influencing the Development of Decubitus Ulcers in Critically Ill Surgical Patients," *Critical Care Medicine* 29(9):1678-82, September 2001.

7. Ooka, M., et al. "Evaluation of Three Types of Support Surfaces for Preventing Pressure Ulcers in Patients in a Surgical Critical Care Unit," *Journal of Wound Ostomy Continence Nursing* 22(6):271-79, November 1995.

8. Curley, M.A., et al. "Predicting Pressure Ulcer Risk in Pediatric Patients: The Braden Q Scale," *Nursing Research* 51(1):22-33, January-February 2003.

9. Willock, J., et al. "Pressure Sores in Children—the Acute Hospital Perspective," *Journal of Tissue Viability* 10(2):59-62, April 2000.

10. Lewicki, L.J., et al. "Sensitivity and Specificity of the Braden Scale in the Cardiac Surgical Population," *Journal of Wound Ostomy Continence Nursing* 27(1):36-41, January 2000.

11. Batson, S., et al. "The Development of a Pressure Area Scoring System for Critically Ill Patients: A Pilot Study," *Intensive Critical Care Nursing* 9(3):146-51, September 1993.

12. Inman, K.J., et al. "Clinical Utility and Cost-effectiveness of an Air Suspension Bed in the Prevention of Pressure Ulcers," *JAMA* 269(9):1139-43, March 3, 1993.

13. Jiricka, M.K., et al. "Pressure Ulcer Risk Factors in a Critical Care Unit Population," *American Journal of Critical Care* 4(5):361-67, September 1995.

14. Lowery, M.T. "A Pressure Sore Risk Calculator for Critical Care Patients: 'The Sunderland Experience'," *Intensive Critical Care Nursing* 11(6):344-53, December 1995.

15. Weststrate, J.T., et al. "The Clinical Relevance of the Waterlow Pressure Sore Risk Scale in the Critical Care Unit," *Critical Care Medicine* 24(8):815-20, August 1998.

16. Jackson, C. "The Revised Jackson/Cubbin Pressure Area Risk Calculator," *Intensive Critical Care Nursing* 15(3):169-75, June 1999.

17. Theaker, C., et al. "Risk Factors for Pressure Sores in the Critically Ill," *Anesthesia* 55(3):221-24, March 2000.

18. Oertwich, P.A., et al. "The Effects of Small Shifts in Body Weight on Blood Flow and Interface Pressure," *Research in Nursing & Health* 18(6):481-88, December 1995.

19. Hibbert, C.L., et al. "Cost Considerations for the Use of Low-air-loss Bed Therapy in Adult Critical Care," *Intensive Critical Care Nursing* 15(3):154-62, June 1999.

20. Inman, K.J., et al. "Pressure Ulcer Prevention: A Randomized Controlled Trial of Two Risk-directed Strategies for Patient Surface Assignment," *Advances in Wound Care* 12(2):72-80, March 1999.

21. Jastremski, C.A. "Pressure Relief Bedding to Prevent Pressure Ulcer Development in Critical Care," *Journal of Critical Care* 17(2):122-25, June 2002.

22. Burdette-Taylor, S.R., and Kass, J. "Heel Ulcers in Critical Care Units: A Major Pressure Problem," *Critical Care Nursing Quarterly* 25(2):41-53, August 2002.

23. Defloor, T., and Grypdonck, M.H. "Do Pressure Relief Cushions Really Relieve Pressure?" *Western Journal of Nursing Research* 22(3):335-50, April 2000.

24. Defloor, T. and Grypdonck, M.H. "Sitting Posture and Prevention of Pressure Ulcers," *Applied Nursing Research* 12(3):136-42, August 1999.

25. National Spinal Cord Injury Statistical Center, Birmingham, Alabama. "Spinal Cord Injury: Facts and Figures at a Glance," *Journal of Spinal Cord Medicine* 25(2):139-40, Summer 2002.

26. Lasfargues, J.E., et al. "A Model for Estimating Spinal Cord Injury Prevalence in the United States," *Paraplegia* 33(2):62-68, February 1995.

27. Go, B.K., et al. "The Epidemiology of Spinal Cord Injury," in Stover, S.L., et al., eds. *Spinal Cord Injury-Clinical Outcomes from the Model Systems.* Gaithersburg, Md.: Aspen Publishers, Inc., 1995.

28. Ragnarsson K.T., et al. "Management of Pulmonary, Cardiovascular, and Metabolic Conditions after Spinal Cord Injury," in Stover, S.L., et al., eds., *Spinal Cord Injury-Clinical Outcomes from the Model Systems.* Gaithersburg, Md.: Aspen Pubs., Inc., 1995.

29. McKinley, W.O., et al. "Long-term Medical Complications After Traumatic Spinal Cord Injury: A Regional Model Systems Analysis," *Archives of Physical Medicine*

Rehabilitation 80(11):1402-10, November 1999.

30. Langemo, D.K., et al. "The Lived Experience of Having a Pressure Ulcer: A Qualitative Analysis," *Advances in Skin & Wound Care* 13(5):225-35, September-October 2000.

31. Garber S.L., et al. "Pressure Ulcer Prevention and Treatment Following Spinal Cord Injury: A Clinical Practice Guideline for Health-care Professionals," *Consortium for Spinal Cord Medicine Clinical Practice Guidelines*. Washington, D.C.: Paralyzed Veterans of America, 2000.

32. Young, J.S., and Burns, P.E. "Pressure Sores and the Spinal Cord Injured: Part II," *Spinal Cord Injury Digest* 3:11-26, 48, 1981.

33. Yarkony, G.M. and Heinemann, A.W. "Pressure Ulcers," in Stover, S.L., et al., eds., *Spinal Cord Injury: Clinical Outcomes from the Model Systems*. Gaithersburg, Md.: Aspen Pubs., 1995.

34. Fuhrer, M.J., et al. "Pressure Ulcers in Community-resident Persons with Spinal Cord Injury: Prevalence and Risk Factors," *Archives of Physical Medicine Rehabilitation* 74(11):1172-77, November 1993.

35. Carlson, C.E., et al. "Incidence and Correlates of Pressure Ulcer Development After Spinal Cord Injury," *Journal of Rehabilitation Nursing Research* 1(1):34-40, 1992.

36. Schryvers, O.I., et al. "Surgical Treatment of Pressure Ulcers: A 20-year Experience," *Archives of Physical Medicine Rehabilitation* 81(12):1556-62, December 2000.

37. Goodman, C.M., et al. "Evaluation of Results and Treatment Variables for Pressure Ulcers in 48 Veteran Spinal Cord-injured Patients," *Annals of Plastic Surgery* 43(6):572-74, June 1999.

38. Niazi, Z.B., et al. "Recurrence of Initial Pressure Ulcer in Persons with Spinal Cord Injuries," *Advances in Wound Care* 10(3):38-42, May-June 1997.

39. Goldstein, B. "Neurogenic Skin and Pressure Ulcers," in Hammond, M.C., ed., *Medical Care of Persons with Spinal Cord Injury*. Washington, D.C.: DVA Employee Education System and Government Printing Office, 1998.

40. Salzberg, C.A., et al. "Predicting and Preventing Pressure Ulcers in Adults with Paralysis," *Advances in Wound Care* 11(5):237-46, September 1998.

41. Holmes, S.A., et al. "Preventing Recurrent Pressure Ulcers After Myocutaneous Flap in Persons with Spinal Cord Injury," in preparation for submission to *Archives of Physical Medicine and Rehabilitation*.

42. Miller, H., and DeLozier, J. "Cost Implications," in Bergstrom, N., and Cuddigan, J., eds., *Treating Pressure Ulcers: Guideline Technical Report*, Vol II, No. 15, Rockville, Md.: U.S. Department of Health and Human Services, Public Health Service, Agency for Health Care Policy and Research. Publication 96-N015, 1994.

43. Byrne, D.W., and Salzberg, C.A. "Major Risk Factors for Pressure Ulcers in the Spinal Cord Disabled: A Literature Review," *Spinal Cord* 34(5):255-63, May 1996.

44. Rintala, D.H. "Quality-of-life Considerations," *Advances in Wound Care* 8(4):71-83, July-August 1995.

45. Anderson, T.P., and Andberg, M.M. "Psychosocial Factors Associated with Pressure Sores," *Archives of Physical Medicine Rehabilitation* 60(8):341-46, August 1979.

46. Gordon, W.A., et al. "The Relationship Between Pressure Sores and Psychosocial Adjustment in Persons with Spinal Cord Injury," *Rehabilitation Psychology* 27:185-91, 1982.

47. Yasenchak, P.A., et al. "Variables Related to Severe Pressure Sore Recurrence," [Abstract]. Orlando: Annual Meeting of the American Spinal Injury Association (ASIA), 1990.

48. Disa, J.J., et al. "Efficacy of Operative Cure in Pressure Sore Patients," *Plastic Reconstructive Surgery* 89(2):272-78, February 1992.

49. Scheflan, M. "Surgical Methods for Managing Ischial Pressure Wounds," *Annals of Plastic Surgery* 3(3):238-47, March 1982.

50. Romm, S., et al. "Pressure Sores: State of the Art," *Texas Medicine* 78(4):52-60,62, April 1982.

51. Pers, M. "Plastic Surgery for Pressure Sores," *Paraplegia* 25(3):275-78, June 1987.

52. Buntine, J.A., and Johnstone, B.R. "The Contributions of Plastic Surgery to Care of the Spinal Cord Injured Patient," *Paraplegia* 26(2):87-93, April 1988.

53. Hentz, V.R. "Management of Pressure Sores in a Specialty Center—A Reappraisal,"

Plastic Reconstructive Surgery 64(4):683-91, October 1979.

54. Relander, M., and Palmer, B. "Recurrence of Surgically Treated Pressure Sores," *Scandinavian Journal of Plastic Reconstructive Surgery* 2(1):89-92, 1988.

55. Mandrekas, A.D., and Mastorakos, D.P. "Management of Decubitus Ulcers by Musculocutaneous Flaps: A Five-year Experience," *Annals of Plastic Surgery* 28(2):167-74, February 1992.

56. Baek, S., et al. "The Gluteus Maximus Myocutaneous Flap in the Management of Pressure Sores," *Annals of Plastic Surgery* 5(6):471-76, December 1980.

57. Rubayi, S., et al. "Proximal Femoral Resection and Myocutaneous Flap for Treatment of Pressure Ulcers in Spinal Cord Injury Patients," *Annals of Plastic Surgery* 27(2):132-37, August 1991.

58. Garber, S.L., et al. "A Structured Educational Model to Improve Pressure Ulcer Prevention Knowledge in Veterans with Spinal Cord Dysfunction," *Journal of Rehabilitation Research and Development* 39(5): 575-88, September-October 2002.

59. Andberg, M.M., et al. "Improving Skin Care through Patient and Family Training," *Topics in Clinical Nursing* 5(2):45-54, July 1983.

60. Krouskop, T.A., et al. "The Effectiveness of Preventive Management in Reducing the Occurrence of Pressure Sores," *Journal of Rehabilitation R&D* 20(1):7483, July 1983.

61. King, R.B., et al., eds. "The Skin," in *Rehabilitation Guide*. Chicago: The Rehabilitation Institute of Chicago, 1977.

62. Bergstrom, N., et al. "Pressure Ulcers in Adults: Prediction and Prevention," Guideline Report No. 3. Rockville, Md.: U.S. Department of Health and Human Services, Public Health Service, Agency for Health Care Policy and Research. AHCPR Publication No. 93-0013, May 1992.

63. Bennett, M.A. "Report of the Task Force on the Implications for Darkly Pigmented Intact Skin in the Prediction and Prevention of Pressure Ulcers," *Advances in Wound Care* 8(6):34-35, November-December 1995.

64. Bergstrom, N., et al. "Treatment of Pressure Ulcers," Guideline Report No. 15. Rockville, Md.: US Department of Health and Human Services, Public Health Service, Agency for Health Care Policy and Research. AHCPR Publication No. 96-N014, December 1994.

65. Netscher, D., et al. "Surgical Repair of Pressure Ulcers," *Plastic Surgery Nursing* 16:225-33,239, Winter 1996.

66. Clamon, J., and Netscher, D.T. "General Principles of Flap Reconstruction: Goals for Aesthetic and Functional Outcome," *Plastic Surgery Nursing* 14:9-14, Spring 1994.

67. Baker, L., et al. "Effect of Electrical Stimulation Waveform on Healing of Ulcers in Human Beings with Spinal Cord Injury," *Wound Repair and Regeneration* 4(1):21-28, January-February 1996.

68. Wood, J.M., et al. "A Multicenter Study on the Use of Pulsed Low-intensity Direct Current for Healing Chronic Stage II and III Decubitus Ulcers," *Archives of Dermatology* 129(8):999-1009, August 1993.

69. Buchbinder S.P., et al. "Herpes Zoster and Human Immunodeficiency Virus Infection," *Journal of Infectious Disease* 166(5):1153-56, November 1992.

70. Klatt, E.C., and Shibata, D. "Cytomegalovirus Infection in the Acquired Immunodeficiency Syndrome," *Archives of Pathology and Laboratory Medicine* 112(5):540-44, May 1988.

71. Apgar, S.A., and Pfenninger, J.L. "Treatment of Vulvar, Perianal, Vaginal, Penile, and Urethral Condyloma Acuminata," in Pfenninger, J.L., and Fowler, G.C., eds., *Procedures for Primary Care Physicians*, 1st ed. St. Louis: Mosby–Year Book, Inc., 1994.

72. Czelusta, A., et al. "An Overview Of Sexually Transmitted Diseases. Part III. Sexually Transmitted Diseases in HIV-Infected Patients," *Journal of the American Academy of Dermatology* 43(3): 409-32, September 2000.

73. Goldstein, B., et al. "Correlation of Skin Disorders with CD4 Lymphocyte Counts in Patients with HIV/AIDS," *Journal of the American Academy of Dermatology* 36(2, pt. 1): 262-4, February 1997.

74. Zwolski, K., and Talotta, D. "Bacterial Infections," in Kirton, C., *Handbook of HIV/AIDS Nursing*. St. Louis: Mosby–Year Book, Inc., 2001.

CHAPTER 18

Complex wounds

Joyce M. Black, PhD, RN, CPSN, CWCN
Steven B. Black, MD, FACS

OBJECTIVES

After completing this chapter, you'll be able to:

- describe the reconstructive ladder as a process for choosing the type of wound closure

- identify the different types of complex wounds

- discuss methods of reconstruction using skin grafts, myocutaneous flaps, and free flaps

- explain the diagnosis and treatment of patients with necrotizing fasciitis.

Etiology first

Patients may be hospitalized with complex wounds, or they may develop wounds during hospitalization for a seemingly unrelated problem. When first asked to manage these patients, it's imperative that you thoroughly assess the patient and determine the cause of the wound. While many wounds may look similar, if the etiology isn't addressed, misdiagnosis may occur and incorrect treatments implemented. Due to their size or etiology, complex wounds can be a health care challenge.

Goals of care

For acute wounds, wound closure with the return of form and function are the goals of care. Left alone to close via contraction and scar formation, wounds seldom have either form or function and will often recur and look unpleasant. The ability to reach ideal and complete healing without unsightly scarring, such as seen in fetal wounds, is impossible. Therefore the return of acceptable healing with sustained function and anatomic continuity becomes the ideal end point.

Reconstructive ladder

A decision-making process in choosing the type of wound closure is based on the following information and the "rungs" of the reconstructive ladder.

Is the wound missing tissue?

If the wound hasn't lost any tissue, it may be possible to close it primarily. Wounds are capable of healing by primary intention, which ocurs when the wound edges are approximated, pulled together, and retained by sutures, staples, or glue. The dynamics of healing begin, and new tissue synthesis begins to occur. A healing ridge (an induration beneath the skin, extending to approximately 1 cm) forms directly under the suture line between days 5 and 9 after surgery.

What kind of tissue, if any, is missing?

Wounds that only lack portions of skin may be allowed to granulate closed if they're small, or skin may be grafted to speed the healing process. Wounds that lack tendon, muscle, or bone may require transplantation of these tissues to provide form and function. Such operations require flaps of skin, muscle, fascia, or bone. Such flaps are named for their composition, such as an osteocutaneous flap, which is a bone and skin flap. Another type of flap is the free flap, which employs the surgical technique of freely removing tissue from the arm and reanastomosing it to the recipient vessels using a microscope. A radial free-arm flap, for example, contains radius bone, overlying muscle, and skin. This procedure is commonly used to reconstruct the face after wide excision of cancer of the mandible and floor of the mouth.

What donor-site morbidity may occur?

Donor sites have some form of scar and may exhibit loss of function, depending on the tissues removed. Once skin is removed for a skin graft, moist wound-healing techniques should be implemented at the donor site to minimize scarring and postoperative pain. When the breast is reconstructed using the latisimus muscle from the back, the woman may lose some function of the shoulder. Although some patients perceive the loss of function as tolerable, other patients — for example, a tennis player — would undoubtedly perceive it differently. In other words, the degree of loss a patient is willing to experience is proportional to his need for the sacrificed tissue. If a patient lost a thumb, he may opt to transplant the great toe to provide opposition for hand function; however, most people wouldn't want to sacrifice a thumb to replace the great toe.

What's the simplest method to achieve wound closure?

The easiest method available to close the wound is often used first. Wounds that can heal on their own via granulation and epithelialization are allowed to do so. Skin grafting is the next simplest method and is used to treat wounds that are missing only skin. Skin grafting can be full- or partial-thickness, depending on the kinds of tissue missing in the recipient site. Wounds that could close on their own, but with accompanying contracture and loss of function, can also be grafted. If muscle is missing, muscle flaps are used to fill the wound defect or cavity, but the muscle isn't made functional (that is, an insertion, origin, and nerve aren't restored to create a functional muscle). The blood supply to the muscle is restored so that it remains viable. The ample blood flow into muscle is commonly used to treat complex wound problems such as osteomyelitis, where restoring blood flow can be used to transport antibiotics to the wound.

Muscle has been shown to supply islands of skin through a series of vessels that perforate the muscle body. Surgeons can simultaneously transplant a muscle and the island of skin to both fill a wound cavity and provide skin coverage. Such a flap is called a musculocutaneous flap. Often the specific muscle is noted, as in the case of the tensor fascia lata flap, which is used to close a trochanteric pressure ulcer. If a large amount of skin is missing, the muscle may be transplanted and then covered with skin grafting to achieve the same effect. Such an operation is called a muscle-flap and split-thickness skin graft, with the specific muscle being grafted added to the name.

Muscle is brought to the recipient site in one of two ways:
• it's rotated along an arc with its original blood supply left intact
• it's freed from its blood supply and the artery and vein are reattached via the microscope at the recipient site.

Freeing the muscle, skin, and other parts of a flap allows the flap to be used for reconstruction in areas that the muscle normally couldn't reach, such as the lower third of the leg.

It's important to note that as often as possible, tissue is replaced with similar tissue. Similar hair bearing, appearance, and thickness improve aesthetic appearance on the reconstructed wound. This process of choosing a method to close a wound has been called a reconstructive ladder. (See *Reconstructive ladder*.) The easiest method, secondary healing, is at the bottom of the ladder.

Wounds without missing tissues

Some wounds don't require grafts because they aren't missing tissue.

Simple lacerations

Traumatic wounds are often missing little or no tissues and can be closed primarily; however, the full extent of the injury must

---

Reconstructive ladder

The reconstructive ladder is used to determine the method to replace missing tissue from a wound bed. The ladder shows the simplest method — simply allowing the wound to heal on its own — at the bottom of the ladder.

• Free (microscopically anastomosed) flaps
• Rotated muscle flaps

• Full-thickness skin grafts
• Partial-thickness skin grafts
• Primary closure

• Secondary healing

---

be known before any closure is attempted. Laceration of arteries and veins is usually obvious by the amount of bleeding present. Facial lacerations are especially bloody due to the robust blood supply in the face. The patient is assessed for function of nerves and ligaments in the area prior to injection with lidocaine, which would obscure the findings. Repair of these tissues (vessels, tendons, ligaments, and nerves) is commonly completed in the operating room with the benefit of the operating microscope and a sterile environment. Wounds are copiously irrigated to remove any debris. Skin closure is accomplished by undermining surrounding tissues and suturing all layers of tissue with minimal tension. Drains are placed in wounds with large amounts of dead space. The appearance of the wound should ideally mimic the ipsilateral appearance. However, traumatic amputation or extensive debridement may leave appearance less than normal or acceptable.

Removing all forms of tension on the wound reduces the scar. Wounds that must be mobilized to gain function, such as incisions over joints, are often wide and may be disturbing to the patient's self-image. Stinted dressings, immobility (for example, limited chewing or talking with facial lacerations), and thin applications of topical antibiotics may help to minimize scars. Moist wound-healing techniques, used throughout the healing process, will minimize healing time and, potentially, the amount of scarring. However, it's important for the patient, the patient's family, and members of the health care team to realize that scarring is inevitable and only after the scar has matured, which can take more than 1 year, will scar revision be attempted. Silicone-based dressings may be used over healed wounds to help minimize scar build-up during the maturation phase.

Extensive lacerations

Extensive lacerations, even though unsightly, are seldom life-threatening. Lifesaving care of the heart, lungs, and brain precedes definitive wound care. Initial wound care includes debridement of obvious dirt, glass, grass, or other foreign bodies. Massive lacerations are packed with moist dressings to prevent tissue desiccation and, when the patient is stable, the wounds are debrided and surgically closed if possible. Extensive wounds may require multiple debridements until viable tissue is present; these wounds may also require more complex forms of delayed closure, such as flaps.

Wounds requiring tissue transplantation for closure

Some wounds, such as pressure ulcers, may require tissue transplantation for closure.

Pressure ulcer repair

Repairing a pressure ulcer site is a process containing multiple steps that begin prior to surgery.

Preoperative care

After the pressure ulcer bed is clean, it can be surgically closed. However, before any decisions are made for surgery, such plans must be considered in light of the patient's goals. While various surgical options may be technically possible, doing these operations for the right reasons is an essential first step. Surgery shouldn't be entered into lightly. For some patients, not closing the wound surgically may be the final decision. With proper nutrition, pressure relief, and local wound care, deep pressure ulcers may remain stable for the duration of the patient's life. Adjunctive therapies, such as negative pressure wound therapy, electrical stimulation, and the use of bioengineered tissue products, may be considered to help with closure of these chronic wounds. Cases have been reported of patients whose pressure ulcers were present for 35 to 40 years.

Prior to any surgery, the patient's nutritional status and comorbidities must be controlled. Although operative blood loss is usually modest with this type of surgery, general anesthesia is commonly used and the patient must be able to tolerate the stress. If the pressure ulcer is in large part due to malnutrition, surgery should be delayed until the patient has achieved positive nitrogen balance. Calorie counts provide clear data on actual intake of protein and calories, and adjustments can be made to reach ideal levels of intake of 25 to 35 cal/kg of calories and 1.5 to 3.0 g/kg of protein. Monitoring albumin is a reasonable marker, although the half-life of albumin is 20 to 21 days, which seldom reflects current nutritional status. With a half-life of 3 days, prealbumin is now accepted as a better marker for assessing visceral protein status. More accurate nutritional information on protein status can benefit the healing potential for the patient. It's important to recognize that patients who are malnourished are usually deficient in vitamins (especially vitamin C) and minerals (especially zinc and iron); these supplements should also be given throughout the course of care.

If the ulcer is due primarily to pressure (such as ischial ulcers in a paraplegic patient), pressure must be relieved, not just reduced, both before and after surgery. Long-term plans for continued pressure relief must be included in the operative plan, such as fitting the patient for a wheelchair and appropriate off-loading device, and teaching him pressure-relief techniques to avoid high rates of recidivism. If the ulcer is due to a combination of erosion, shear, and pressure (such as ulcers on the sacrum in a patient with dyspnea and incontinence), all contributing factors need to be addressed. Similarly, long-term pressure reduction and proper skin care management must be included in the care plan.

Wound infection may not be evident from the surface appearance of the wound. The presence of osteomyelitis should be considered and ruled out in all stage III and IV ulcers. The workup for suspected osteomyelitis includes a complete blood count, erythrocyte sedimentation rate, and X-rays. This combination of studies has a sensitivity of 73% and specificity of 96%.[1] Biopsy after adequate debridement can also be used if osteomyelitis is still suspected and the above studies are negative.

Other infections must also be controlled prior to surgery. Urinary tract infections are common in people with diabetes, elderly women, patients with catheters, and those with sacral wounds. Urosepsis is a serious complication and should be considered as the cause of changes in mental status, malnutrition,

or changes in vital signs. Chronic urinary antibiotics may be needed for persistent urinary infections. Wound infection can also lead to sepsis. (See chapter 7, Wound bioburden.)

Spasms are often a contributing factor to both shear and friction injuries and may also complicate a postoperative course. Spasms are common after spinal cord injury due to loss of supraspinal inhibitory pathways. The higher the level of spinal cord injury, the more likely spasms will occur. People with cervical injury have almost a 100% chance of spasm compared to those with injury in the lower thoracic or lumbar spine, who have a 50% chance of spasm. Spasm must be controlled prior to surgery with medications such as baclofen (Lioresal) or dantrolene (Dantrium). Botulism toxin (Botox) can also be injected into the muscle to attempt to reduce spasm; however, the efficacy of this treatment is unrecorded. Spastic limbs may lead to wound dehiscence and postoperative wound complications, and therefore must be controlled.

Contracture develops in patients with longstanding denervation due to tightening of the muscle and joint capsules. Because hip flexors are so strong, hip contraction is common and can make positioning difficult, with bony prominences resting upon each other and leading to ulcers. Contractures can be minimized and even prevented with proper, persistent positioning, splinting, and a program of aggressive (often passive) range-of-motion exercises. Patients with significant contracture can't be placed in a supine position; if surgery is performed on one hip, only one side will be available as a turning surface, which will require a sophisticated pressure relief system to prevent complications or undue pressure at the other hip. A defined turning schedule is essential in these cases. If contractures can be released via tenotomy, the wound may heal. However, leaving a limb flaccid after tenotomy may leave the patient more immobile.

Debridement

Wound debridement is most thoroughly completed in the surgical environment. The wound and surrounding tissues should be examined fully to assess for fluid collection, abscess formation, and extensions. Bedside debridement may be used to unroof hard eschar, but can seldom be completed to the level of a clean wound bed. Enzymatic debridement will often provide reasonable wound debridement, but may take many weeks. However, in the patient who is a poor surgical risk, this is a good alternative.

Debridement of nonviable tissue is often seen with full-thickness necrotic pressure ulcers or infected, dehisced surgical wounds. Debridement of adherent eschar in pressure ulcers is advised to reduce the wound bioburden and risk of sepsis. Pressure ulcer can't be determined until adequate debridement has been performed. For example, pelvic pressure ulcers can extend to the scapula and to the vagina or trochanters. Removal of necrotic tissue may enhance the wound healing cascade and diminish the risk of infection. Debridement of necrotic wounds is an important element of wound management. (See chapter 8, Wound debridement.)

Heels are a controversial area in debridement. Most clinicians feel that stable, dry, adherent eschar on the foot shouldn't be debrided. The foot, especially the posterior heel, has very limited blood flow and no subcutaneous tissue. Once the underlying fatty tissue is exposed to the environment, it may quickly become infected. If bone is exposed during debridement, osteomyelitis may be an inevitable occurrence.[1] Stable, dry eschar that has no openings should be left intact, assessed often, and off-loaded completely with pillows under the calves or heels. If the eschar softens or breaks, or the tissue around the ulcer becomes fluctuant or inflamed, the tissue should be excised to prevent deeper bacterial invasion and sepsis. Moist wound-healing techniques should be instituted at this time. Off-loading should continue throughout the course of treatment.

Vascular ulcers are often ischemic due to underlying venous or arterial disease. Arterial ulcers are extremely unlikely to heal without appropriate interventions to provide an increase in arterial flow. They quickly deteriorate, can develop osteomyelitis, and require amputation if not properly managed. The Lower Extremity Amputation Prevention (LEAP) program has compiled a comprehensive program aimed to reduce the number of lower limb amputations. The LEAP Web site is a tremendous source of information (*http://bphc.hrsa.gov/programs/LEAPprog raminfo.htm*).

Flaps for pressure ulcer repair

Using the reconstructive ladder as an assessment tool may reveal large areas of skin or skin and muscle missing from a pressure ulcer. Surgical repair options depend on what kind of tissue needs replacement. If skin is missing on a sacral wound, for example, rotational flaps of skin or skin and fascia can be rotated to close the wound. If muscle is missing, such as in a deep stage IV ulcer, the gluteus may be used to provide padding and protection of the bony structures. The muscle moved into the wound doesn't function as muscle; it atrophies over time due to denervation. Muscle tissue provides padding and robust blood supply to combat osteomyelitis. (See *Flaps for pressure ulcer reconstruction*.)

Flaps for pressure ulcer reconstruction

This chart presents closure options for pressure ulcers at common sites.

Pressure ulcer site	Muscle flap options	Skin or fasciocutaneous flap options
Sacral ulcer	• Gluteus maximus (superiorly or inferiorly based)	• Transverse or vertical lumbosacral
Ischial ulcer	• Gluteus maximus (superiorly based) • Biceps femoris • Semimembranosus • Semitendinosus • Tensor fascia lata (may retain sensation)	• Posterior thigh advancement flap with skin graft of donor site • Posterior V-Y advancement flap • Medial thigh rotation flap
Trochanteric ulcer	• Tensor fascia lata (may retain sensation)	

Postoperative care

The transplanted muscle flap requires adequate perfusion of arterial blood and drainage of venous blood to survive. Because a limited number of flaps are available to reconstruct any wound, the threat of flap failure is great. Early flap failure is most commonly due to arterial spasm or clots in the venous drainage. Flaps that have impaired arterial flow appear pale, have poor to absent capillary refill, and show sluggish bleeding when lanced. These wounds require quick restoration of their arterial supply by opening the wound and examining the arterial anastomosis site. Occasionally, arterial spasm is the culprit. Spasm can be treated by positioning the flap dependently and warming the area. Flaps that have impaired venous drainage appear dark blue and swollen. The problem is seldom a faulty anastomosis site; usually, it results from the sluggish exit of venous blood. Venous congestion can be treated by elevation and application of leeches to drain excess blood from the flap. Negative pressure wound therapy may also be recommended to decrease fluid collection. Drains are commonly used to empty fluid accumulation in dead space, and can be left in place for a week or longer until drainage has subsided.

Tension on the incision line can lead to dehiscence. Bolster dressings are typically used to close the wound with little tension. Suture lines are slow to heal, especially in the denervated patient, and sutures are left in place for at least 3 weeks. Due to poor approximation and tensile strength, great caution must be used when moving the patient to avoid pulling on the suture line. It's possible to tear open a late-stage surgical repair, which commonly leads to complete flap failure.

Pressure relief is crucial following flap repair. Surgeons usually prescribe air-fluidized beds or low-air-loss beds for 2 to 6 weeks. Large skin flaps are especially prone to failure because of tension on the distal edges of the flap. If fecal incontinence is likely, the patient may be placed on low residue diets and constipating medications. Diverting colostomy may be required prior to flap closure in extreme cases to prevent contamination of the surgical site with stool.

The patient must be compliant with off-loading after a surgical flap for wound closure to prevent breakdown of the surgical repair. This involves not only immediate postoperative pressure reduction, but continued pressure reduction after complete healing has occurred, especially in patients confined to wheelchairs. Proper chair cushions and weight shifts are essential.

Chest wall reconstruction

Defects following excision of a tumor, tissue loss from infection of the pleural space, or dehiscence of sternal wounds after coronary bypass grafting are some chest wall wounds that usually require reconstruction. Infected medial sternotomy wounds following cardiac surgery are a dreaded complication. Left untreated, these infections smolder down into the mediastinum and may even extend into aortic suture lines, prosthetic grafts, and intracardiac prosthesis. Early wounds appear like suppurative mediastinitis with cellulitis, purulent wound drainage, and obvious tracking between the skin, sternum, and mediastinum. Stabilization of the patient prior to surgery includes maximizing heart and pulmonary function, improving nutrition, and preparing the wound bed.

Wound-bed preparation may include packing, debridement, or the use of negative-pressure wound therapy. Caution is required when packing deep wounds. One continuous piece of rolled gauze is the preferred method to avoid losing single dressings in the cavities. Furthermore, if wounds require topical application of solutions, the large amount of open tissue will quickly absorb the fluids. Use of products such as povidone-iodine solution in these large wounds has resulted in iodine toxicity due to the large absorptive surface. Wounds that extend to the myocardium or around the myocardium should be gently packed between heartbeats. Packing the wound tightly can constrict myocardial contraction; therefore, the wound must be tucked loosely with gauze.

Several muscles are available for reconstruction, depending on the location of the wound. The latissimus dorsi, pectoralis major, rectus abdominus, and trapezius are the most common muscles used for chest-wall reconstruction.[2]

Leg reconstruction

Tissue defects of the leg can be reconstructed with muscle flap covered with skin grafts, myocutaneous flaps, or free flaps, depending on the location of the wound and available tissue. Attempts are made to salvage the leg unless there is irretrievable nerve or vessel damage. Major soft tissue injuries with or without bone involvement provide an environment favorable for infection. Wound care is commonly completed in the operating room, where debridement can be performed in a sterile atmosphere. Definitive wound coverage often includes rectus abdominus, gluteus, rectus femoris, gastrocnemius, and soleus muscle.

Following surgery, it's imperative to monitor the flap for signs of vascular compromise including pallor, coolness, lack of pulses, pain with movement, slow or absent capillary refill, or lack of ability to move the extremity. These situations are emergent, and without immediate intervention, the limb may be lost due to ischemia. Prompt and accurate reporting of unusual findings must be made to the attending surgeon.

PRACTICE POINT

Monitor for the following to assess vascular compromise and flap survival:
- pallor and coolness
- lack of pulses
- pain with movement
- low or absent capillary refill
- Inability to move extremity.

Necrotizing fasciitis

Necrotizing fasciitis, formerly called streptococcal gangrene, is a rapidly progressive skin infection. Although beta-hemolytic *Streptococcus pyrogenes* is the most common organism, no single organism is responsible for the infection. Frequently, necrotizing fasciitis is caused by two organisms acting in concert, called synergistic gangrene. Gram-positive bacteria (including staphylococcus), gram-negative bacteria, anaerobic (including gas gangrene caused by *Clostridium perfringens*), marine vibrio, and fungi have been identified. Necrotizing fasciitis due to beta-hemolytic streptococcal organisms is highly sensitive to antibiotics. However, antibiotics don't penetrate necrotic tissue so delay in treatment can lead to a 75% mortality.[3] Necrotizing fasciitis is known to the public as "flesh-eating bacteria."

Many conditions increase risk of necrotizing fasciitis. (See *Conditions leading to necrotizing fasciitis.*) Necrotizing fasciitis seems to develop following a breach in the integrity of a mucous membrane barrier, especially in the abdomen and perineum. The extremities are also commonly involved. A portal can also be due to a malignancy. In males, leakage into the perineal region can result in a syndrome called Fournier's gangrene, characterized by massive swelling and tissue loss of the scrotum and penis with extension into the perineum, the abdominal wall, and legs.

Conditions leading to necrotizing fasciitis

The conditions listed below place patients at risk for necrotizing fasciitis.
- Age 50 and older
- Alcoholism
- Anal fissure
- Atherosclerosis
- Diabetes mellitus
- Diverticulum
- Hemorrhoids
- Hypertension
- Immunosuppression
- Intravenous drug use
- Malignancy
- Malnutrition
- Obesity
- Renal failure
- Surgery
- Trauma
- Urethral tear

Adapted with permission from Ault, M.J., et al. "Rapid Identification of Group A Streptococcus as a Cause of Necrotizing Fasciitis," *Annals of Emergency Medicine* 28(2):227-30, August 1996.

A reddened, painful, swollen area of cellulitis accompanied by severe local pain and fever are the most common early signs. More generalized swelling develops and is followed by brawny edema. With progression, dark red induration of the epidermis appears, along with bullae filled with blue or purple fluid. Later, the skin becomes friable and takes on a bluish, maroon, or black color. By this stage, thrombosis of blood vessels in the dermal papillae is extensive. Extension of infection to the level of the deep fascia causes this tissue to take on a brownish-gray appearance of frank gangrene. Skin is a very effective barrier preventing bacteria from invading the body, and likewise, skin is also able to trap organisms within the body leading to rapid spread along fascial planes and through venous channels and lymphatics. Patients in the later stages are toxic and frequently manifest septic shock and multiorgan failure. Skin inflammation is rapidly followed by necrosis of superficial fascia, subcutaneous fat, and in some cases, muscle. Necrotizing fasciitis is commonly seen in conjunction with severe systemic toxicities.

Diagnosis and treatment

Aspiration cultures from the wound edge or punch biopsy with frozen section may be helpful if the results are positive, but false-negative results occur in approximately 80% of cases. There is some evidence that aspiration alone may be superior to injection and aspiration using normal saline solution. However, deep biopsy and frozen section histopathology may confirm diagnosis. Frozen sections are especially useful in distinguishing necrotizing fasciitis from other skin infections such as toxic epidermal necrolysis.

PRACTICE POINT

In cases of suspected necrotizing fasciitis, myositis, or gangrene, early, aggressive surgical exploration is necessary to:
- visualize deep structures
- remove necrotic tissue
- open compartments to decrease pressure
- obtain tissue for Gram stain for aerobic and anaerobic organisms
- repeat debridements.

Repeated debridements are usually necessary until all devitalized tissue is removed. Broad-spectrum antibiotics are started intravenously pending more specific culture results.

Appropriate empirical antibiotic treatment for necrotizing fasciitis from group A streptococcal organisms is commonly clindamycin plus penicillin G and

cephalosporin (first- or second-generation). Mixed aerobic-anaerobic infections can be treated with ampicillin and sulbactam, cefoxitin, or combinations of clindamycin, metronidazole, ampicillin, or ampicillin, sulbactam, and gentamicin. Group A streptococcal and clostridial infection of the fascia or muscle carries a mortality rate of 20% to 50% even with penicillin treatment. Hyperbaric oxygen treatment may also be useful as many of these infections have an anaerobic or micro-aerophilic component. Antibiotic treatment should be continued until all signs of systemic toxicity have resolved, all devitalized tissue has been removed, and granulation tissue has developed.

Following debridement, the wounds are packed open. The packing can be extensive and may be completed in the operating room with daily debridement. Definitive treatment may include amputation and extensive skin grafting after the infection is under control and the wounds show evidence of granulation. It's essential that the dressings stay moist to prevent desiccation of tissue. It may be helpful to use products with a higher absorptive capacity than gauze to manage fluid from draining wounds.

Calciphylaxis

Calciphylaxis is a rare, life-threatening disorder associated with chronic renal failure, diabetes, or advanced HIV disease, presenting with ulcerating plaques leading to death by sepsis in 60% of patients. Patients with hyperparathyroidism are also at risk. Calcification of tunica media of small arteries associated with intimal fibrosis and thrombus formation leads to the development of painful livedo reticularis-like purpuric patches and plaques, vesicles, irregularly shaped ulcers, and black eschar with subcutaneous tissue necrosis. Super-infection of skin lesions is a common consequence of this syndrome.

Treatment is multifocal and may include management of comorbidities, aggressive wound debridement, wound excision, and various methods of achieving closure. Parathyroidectomy has been shown to aid healing and prolong life in those patients with parathyroid disease, and has also been suggested for patients with renal failure, but the procedure has never been shown to improve outcomes in more than a few of these patients. There is a fatal outcome in a majority of cases due to septicemia. Despite treatment, fulminant sepsis as a consequence of secondary infection of necrotic and gangrenous tissue is a frequent cause of patient morbidity and mortality.

Coumadin necrosis

Warfarin-induced skin necrosis is a rare complication of anticoagulant treatment. The incidence of this complication has been estimated to occur between 1:100 and 1:10,000 of patients treated with anticoagulants. Coumadin skin necrosis occurs almost exclusively between the 1st and 10th day after beginning anticoagulation, in association with the administration of a large initial loading dose of the drug. Although the precise nature of the disease is still unknown, advances in knowledge about protein C, protein S, and antithrombin III anticoagulant pathways have led to a better understanding of the mechanisms involved in pathogenesis.[4,5]

Postpartum women have a unique risk due to reduced levels of free protein S during the antepartum and immediate postpartum periods.[6] Manifestations range from ecchymoses and purpura, hemorrhagic necrosis, and maculopapular, vesicular urticarial eruptions to purple toes.

Wounds are painful and usually evolve into full-thickness skin necrosis within a few days. Differential diagnosis between warfarin induced skin necrosis and necrotizing fasciitis, gangrene and other causes of skin necrosis may be difficult.[7]

Local wound care can be conservative, but may include debridement and grafting, depending on the extensiveness of the wound. Previously uncomplicated courses of warfarin therapy don't obviate the possibility of skin necrosis with future warfarin administrations. Initiation of low-dose warfarin with heparin can reduce the likelihood of this disorder.

Extravasation

Solutions of calcium, potassium, bicarbonate, hypertonic dextrose, cardiac drugs, chemotherapeutic drugs, cytotoxic drugs, and antibiotics can lead to extravasation injury. Tissue loss can evolve into extensive wounds. Local wound care with debridement and eventual skin grafting is usually required for extensive skin and tissue loss. Wounds with less tissue loss can be managed conservatively with the same outcome.[8] Because many extravasation injuries occur on the hands, scar management and return of function remains a problem. Proper administration through the correct needle size (small), vein size (large), and dilution of the medication is best. Infusion should be performed as slowly as possible to allow adequate dilution into the blood. Any complaints of pain during infusion warrant immediate cessation of the solution, assessment of the IV site, and adherence to treatment protocols for extravasation as deemed necessary. Calcium gluconate is less likely to extravasate and should be used instead of calcium chloride for the management of low serum levels, especially those levels that aren't life-threatening. Since many of these cases may elicit external review and sometimes legal review, documentation is crucial to determine what care was given prior to, and after, the medication was given. Nurses need to be especially vigilant when administering medications prone to extravasation.

Radiation necrosis

Wounds following irradiation can be acute or chronic. Immediate reactions to irradiation are due to inflammation. Acute irradiation wounds are erythematous and due to dilation of the vessels in the irradiated area. These wounds mimic a superficial partial-thickness burn and should be treated in a like manner. Dressings such as hydrogels serve to rehydrate the skin. Pain may be reduced by applying dressings that have been cooled in the refrigerator.

Irradiation may also lead to desquamation. Wet and painful wounds should be covered to prevent evaporative fluid loss, control pain, and reduce the risk of infection. Hydrocolloids, hydrogels, and absorptive dressings may be used to maintain a moist wound environment. Severe irradiation wounds may require skin grafting or application of growth factors alone or embedded in dressings.[9] Bioengineered tissue products may also be an alternative to skin grafting.

Chronic changes in the skin are seen due to sclerosis, with a reduction in the actual number of blood vessels. The etiology of the burn wound hasn't been well defined, but is presumed to be from ischemia due to obliteration of the microvasculature. Histologically there is little angiogenesis or inflammatory response. The skin is usually pigmented, dry from loss of sebaceous glands, and hairless. The epidermis is thin due to loss of rete pegs. Irradiated skin is easily damaged and can lead to nonhealing wounds. The wound bed is commonly covered with fibropurulent material. These wounds don't heal spontaneously due to a lack of functional fibroblasts

and altered migratory ability of cells. Tissue remains relatively ischemic, increasing the risk of infection, which further slows healing.

Treatment of irradiation wounds begins with ruling out a new malignancy in the area. After malignancy is ruled out, the wound may be excised, commonly leaving a larger than anticipated wound. Reconstruction with arterialized tissue to bring in a new blood supply, such as a flap, is ideal and usually reduces pain almost immediately. Irradiation wounds of the chest wall can be repaired with the omentum, the fatty drape of the abdomen. This will provide padding and the necessary blood supply. Since surgery can be extensive, it may be in the patient's best interest to continue with local wound care. Wounds due to irradiation are typically difficult and very slow to heal. However, utilizing the concept of moist wound healing and debriding agents, these wounds may close without surgical intervention.

Marjolin's ulcer

Marjolin's ulcer is an aggressive squamous-cell carcinoma that develops in long-standing scar tissue (older than 30 years), particularly a burn scar. Any bizarre looking ulcer with thick and rolled up edges should be subject to biopsy for diagnosis. Treatment is wide excision. The prognosis is relatively poor.

Summary

Understanding the etiology of complex wounds is a critical first step in developing an effective treatment plan. Recognition of unique characteristics of each of these wound categories will enable the clinician to correctly identify the wound. The goal of care for acute wounds is wound closure with the return of form and function. Use of the reconstructive ladder can assist clinicians in the decision-making process. Surgical management may be part of the care plan for complex acute and chronic wounds.

Show what you know

1. Which of the following situations depicts the use of the simplest method for closure of the wound described?

A. A skin graft of a venous stasis ulcer
B. Secondary healing of a calcium extravasation
C. Primary closure for a sternal incisional dehiscence
D. A free fasciocutaneous flap for a stage III pressure ulcer

ANSWER: B. Secondary healing is the simplest method for any wound, but in many deep wounds secondary healing will require excessive scar and time. Venous stasis ulcers and sternal dehiscence can sometimes heal secondarily, so skin grafting would be more complex. A stage III ulcer should be able to heal with other methods than free flaps, which are the "top of the line" for surgical options.

2. Which of the following wounds might require a musculocutaneous flap for closure?

A. A large burn on the face
B. Calciphylaxis of the lower legs
C. Radiation necrosis of the chest wall
D. A stage II pressure ulcer on the trochanter

ANSWER: C. Only the radiation of the chest wall is a wound with muscle involvement. In addition, the additional blood supply brought into the area by the muscle will often be used to treat any osteomyelitis.

3. Which of the following signs might indicate arterial impairment in a flap?

A. Pain and coolness
B. Pallor and warmth
C. Slow capillary refill and pain
D. Slow capillary refill and pallor

ANSWER: D. The loss of arterial inflow will render a flap pulseless (often only by Doppler), so delays in capillary refill are seen first, and pallor. If the early signs are not recognized, the flap can become cyanotic and eventually lose tissue.

4. You dismissed a patient with ischial ulcers from the hospital after 6 weeks of local wound care. Upon return to the clinic, the wounds have recurred and are necrotic. Which of these causes of recurrence should be investigated first?

A. Presence of urinary incontinence
B. Inadequate pressure relief in seating
C. Deterioration of nutritional status
D. Development of ischial osteomyelitis

ANSWER: B. A hospitalized patient often has pressure reduction via beds and chair cushions. In addition, the nurses remind the patient to off load. Once dismissed, the lack of these devices and cues can quickly lead to deterioration. The other factors can contribute and should be considered too.

References

1. Lewis, V.L., et al. "The Diagnosis of Osteomyelitis in Patients with Pressure Sores," *Plastic and Reconstructive Surgery* 81(2):229-32, February 1988.
2. Seyfer, A. "Chest Wall Reconstruction," in Achauer, B. ed., *Plastic Surgery: Indications, Operations and Outcomes.* St. Louis: Mosby–Year Book, Inc., 2001.
3. Chapnick, E.K., and Albert, E.I. "Necrotizing Soft Tissue Infections," *Infectious Disease Clinics of North America* 10(4):835-55, December 1996.
4. Porock, D., et al. "Management of Radiation Skin Reactions: Literature Review and

Clinical Application," *Plastic Surgical Nursing* 19(4):185-92, Winter 1999.

5. Sallah, S., et al. "Recurrent Warfarin-induced Skin Necrosis in Kindreds with Protein S Deficiency," *Haemostasis* 28(1):25-30, January-February 1998.

6. Cheng, A., et al. "Warfarin Skin Necrosis in a Postpartum Woman with Protein S Deficiency," *Obstetrics and Gynecology* 90(4 pt 2):671-72, October 1997.

7. Chan, Y.C., et al. "Warfarin Induced Skin Necrosis," *British Journal of Surgery* 87(3):266-72, March 2000.

8. Kumar, R.J., et al. "Management of Extravasation Injuries," *Austrlia and New Zealand Journal of Surgery* 71(5):285-89, May 2001.

9. Mendelsohn, F., et al. "Wound Care After Radiation Therapy," *Advances in Wound Care* 15(5):216-24, September-October 2002.

CHAPTER 19

Atypical wounds

Tami de Araujo, MD
Robert S. Kirsner, MD

OBJECTIVES

After completing this chapter, you'll be able to:

- recognize the importance of identifying atypical wounds

- state the need for wound biopsies in determining the etiology of an atypical wound

- describe the various clinical manifestations of atypical wounds.

Types of atypical wounds

Prolonged pressure (pressure ulcers), venous insufficiency (venous leg ulcers), complications of longstanding diabetes mellitus (diabetic foot ulcers), or poor vascular supply (arterial ulcers) are the most common causes of chronic wounds. Wounds due to uncommon etiologies, called atypical wounds, are less frequently encountered and less well-understood. Their prevalence hasn't been studied extensively, but it's estimated that, of the more than 500,000 leg ulcers in the United States, 10% may be due to unusual causes.[1] A variety of etiologies may cause atypical wounds,[2] such as infections, external or traumatic causes, metabolic disorders, genetic diseases, neoplasms, or inflammatory processes.

It's critical to recognize when a wound is caused by an etiology other than prolonged pressure, neuropathy, or abnormal vascular supply so that a correct diagnosis can be made and the appropriate therapy provided. A wound should be evaluated for an atypical etiology if:

- it's present in a location different from that of a common chronic wound
- its appearance varies from that of a common chronic wound
- it doesn't respond to conventional therapy.

Potential etiologies of atypical wounds

Although not all-inclusive, this list presents some of the most commonly encountered etiologies for an atypical wound.

Inflammatory causes
- Vasculitis
- Pyoderma gangrenosum

Infections
- Atypical mycobacteria
- Deep fungal infections

Vasculopathies
- Cryoglobulinemia
- Cryofibrinogenaemia
- Antiphospholipid antibody syndrome

Metabolic and genetic causes
- Calciphylaxis
- Sickle cell anemia

Malignancies
- Squamous cell carcinoma
- Basal cell carcinoma
- Lymphoma
- Kaposi's sarcoma

External causes
- Burns
- Bites
- Stings
- Radiation

For example, the thigh is an atypical location for a pressure, venous, arterial, or diabetic ulcer, and should raise the suspicion of an atypical cause. A wound on the medial aspect of the leg but extending deep to the tendon would be considered atypical despite being a common location, because the depth of this wound is atypical for venous ulcers. Finally, any wound that isn't healing after 3 to 6 months of appropriate treatment should raise the consideration of an atypical cause, even if the distribution and clinical appearance are classic for a common chronic wound.

Once a wound is deemed atypical, a tissue sample is critical to include histology evaluation with special stains, tissue culture (for infectious causes), and immunofluorescence testing (for some inflammatory or immune-based causes).

 EVIDENCE-BASED PRACTICE

Tissue samples are mandatory for atypical wounds because many of the unusual causes of wounds can resemble each other, making visual diagnosis alone difficult and risky.

Etiologies of atypical wounds

Some of the most commonly encountered etiologies for an atypical wound include inflammatory causes, infections, vasculopathies, metabolic and genetic causes, malignancies, and external causes. (See *Potential etiologies of atypical wounds.*) However, a thorough medical history, including epidemiological exposure, family history, personal habits, and concomitant systemic diseases, along with a thorough physical examination in combination with histologic evaluation and laboratory testing, will provide critical information necessary for a correct diagnosis of an atypical wound.

Potential etiologies of vasculitis

Although not all-inclusive, the most common causes of vasculitis are listed below.

Infections
- *Streptococcus spp.*
- *Mycobacterium tuberculosis*
- *Staphylococcus spp.*
- *Mycobacterium leprae*
- Hepatitis viruses A, B, and C
- Herpes virus
- Influenza virus
- *Candida spp.*
- *Plasmodium spp.*
- Schistosomiasis

Medications
- Penicillin
- Sulfonamides
- Tamoxifen
- Streptomycin
- Oral contraceptives
- Thiazides

Chemicals
- Insecticides

- Petroleum products

Foods
- Milk
- Gluten

Connective tissue and other inflammatory diseases
- Systemic lupus erythematosus
- Dermatomyositis
- Sjogren's syndrome
- Rheumatoid arthritis
- Behçet's syndrome
- Cryoglobulinemia
- Scleroderma
- Primary biliary cirrhosis
- Human immunodeficiency virus infection

Malignancies
- Lymphomas
- Leukemias
- Multiple myeloma

Inflammatory causes

Among the most interesting — and probably more common — causes of atypical wounds are the inflammatory ulcers. Although a variety of inflammatory and immunologic diseases affect the skin, two relatively common causes of inflammatory ulcers are vasculitis and pyoderma gangrenosum.

Vasculitis

Vasculitis is defined as inflammation and necrosis of the blood vessels, which can ultimately result in end organ damage.[3] Often idiopathic, vasculitis is a reaction pattern that may be triggered by certain reactants, among these are underlying infections, malignancy, medications, and connective tissue diseases. (See *Potential etiologies of vasculitis*.) Clinically, vasculitis varies depending on the size of the underlying vessel affected. For example, lesions may include a reticulated erythema due to disease of the superficial cutaneous plexus, or may present as widespread purpura, necrosis, and ulceration due to disease in larger, deeper vessels. Patients may also have similar involvement of different end organs (such as the kidney, lung, central nervous system, and the GI tract).[4]

Circulating immune (antibody-antigen) complexes, which deposit in blood vessel walls, are the cause of many types of vasculitis.[5] Tissue biopsies will confirm the presence of vasculitis if performed

Diagnostic tests for vasculitis

Use the following tests to determine the etiology of vasculitis.
- Anti-neutrophilic cytoplasmic antibody
- Rheumatoid factor
- Anti-nuclear antibody
- Hepatitis A, B, C profile
- Complete blood count
- Anti-streptolysin O titer
- Cryoglobulin level
- Serum protein electrophoresis
- Chest radiograph
- Purified protein derivative test
- Throat culture
- Tissue culture.

To determine the extent of disease, use these tests:
- Urinalysis
- Stool guaiac
- Chest radiograph
- Renal function tests
- Liver function tests
- Complete blood count.

is based on the extent of the disease. (See *Diagnostic tests for vasculitis*.) Mild disease that's limited to the skin can be treated with only supportive care, for example, leg elevation and dressings. Treatments with limited side effects, such as colchicine, dapsone, antihistamines, or nonsteroidal anti-inflammatory agents, may also be used. If skin disease is extensive or systemic involvement is present, more aggressive treatment including systemic steroids, anti-inflammatory agents, or immunosuppressants may be needed.[6] (See *Vasculitis treatment options*.)

Pyoderma gangrenosum

The term pyoderma gangrenosum is actually a misnomer; pyoderma gangrenosum is neither infectious nor gangrenous. Rather, it's an inflammatory process of unknown etiology that leads to painful skin ulcers. Pyoderma gangrenosum is characterized by the appearance of one or more chronic ulcerations with violaceous undermined borders.[7] Pyoderma gangrenosum mainly affects adults and its usual course is that of recurring, destructive ulcers, which begin as pustules and resolve with cribriform scars. Several clinical variants of pyoderma gangrenosum have been described including ulcerative, pustular, bullous, vegetative, and peristomal types.

PRACTICE POINT

Because a diagnostic test to confirm pyoderma gangrenosum doesn't exist and a number of other conditions may resemble it clinically, a correct diagnosis relies on the clinical presentation and exclusion of other causes.

early, and biopsies of perilesional skin may detect the type of immunoglobulin involved in the process. Biopsies performed later in the course of lesion development may fail to reveal immunoreactants as inflammatory cells, and their by-products will degrade immunoglobulins. Tissue culture may aid by determining if the vasculitis is due to an infectious process. Once a diagnosis is confirmed histologically, evaluation of other organ systems and an attempt to determine the eliciting factor is mandated.

If identified — and if possible — the causative agent should be addressed. Additionally, treatment of the vasculitis

It's important for the clinician to search for underlying diseases when a diagnosis of pyoderma gangrenosum is rendered because pyoderma gangrenosum is associated with other conditions in up to 75% of patients.[8] (See *Systemic diseases associated with pyoderma gangrenosum,* page 386.) Among these are inflammatory bowel disease, arthritis (seropositive and seronegative), monoclonal gammopathies, and other hematologic disorders and malignancies.

The mechanism by which pyoderma gangrenosum lesions develops is unknown; however, it's believed that pathergy (defined as development of lesions in areas of trauma) plays a role. In susceptible people, even minimal trauma to the skin can result in the production of pyoderma gangrenosum lesions such as pustules or ulcers.

Curative treatment doesn't exist and the course pyoderma gangrenosum waxes and wanes; however, corticosteroids are usually helpful.[9] For limited or mild disease, topical or intralesional steroids may be used. For more severe or widespread disease, systemic steroids can be used, although their side effects limit long-term use. A variety of systemic therapies can be used including antibiotics with anti-inflammatory properties or systemic steroids. Immunosuppressant or anti-inflammatory agents may also be useful; for example, cyclosporine also appears quite effective in treating pyoderma gangrenosum. (See *Pyoderma gangrenosum treatment options,* page 387.) Infliximab (Remicade) a monoclonal antibody to tumor necrosis factor alpha, has been reported to be useful.[10] Infliximab is FDA-approved to treat Crohn's disease and rheumatoid arthritis. A randomized study evaluating the efficacy of different treatment modalities for pyoderma gangrenosum hasn't been done.

Infectious causes

Infectious causes of atypical wounds may be due to a variety of different or-

ganisms, some of which aren't commonly encountered in the United States. For example, atypical mycobacteria (other than leprosy and tuberculosis) and fungi (other than dermatophytes and candida) infections are occasionally detected upon diagnostic testing. Infection caused by *Vibrio vulnificus* may be responsible for lower leg ulcers in geographic areas where there's warm salt water.

Atypical mycobacterial infection

Atypical mycobacteria are ubiquitous in the environment and weren't generally

---

Vasculitis treatment options

Extent of disease	Treatment options
Mild	• Leg elevation • Compression dressings • Antihistamines • Nonsteroidal anti-inflammatory drugs • Anti-inflammatory antibiotics • Topical steroids • Support stockings • Dapsone • Colchicine • Potassium iodide
Extensive or systemic	• Dapsone • Systemic steroids • Stanozolol • Cyclophosphamide • Methotrexate • Azathioprine • Cyclosporin • Plasmapheresis • Mycophenolate mofetil • Tacrolimus • Other anti-inflammatory or immunosuppressant drugs

Systemic diseases associated with pyoderma gangrenosum

No diagnostic test exists to confirm the presence of pyoderma gangrenosum. In addition, pyoderma gangrenosum is typically associated with other conditions.[8] Reported associations are listed below.

Inflammatory bowel disease
- Ulcerative colitis
- Regional enteritis
- Crohn's disease

Arthritis
- Seronegative arthritis
- Rheumatoid arthritis
- Osteoarthritis
- Psoriatic arthritis

Hematologic abnormalities
- Myeloid leukemia
- Hairy cell leukemia
- Myelofibrosis
- Myeloid metaplasia
- Immunoglobulin A monoclonal gammopathy
- Polycythemia rubra, polycythemia vera
- Paroxysmal nocturnal hemoglobinuria
- Myeloma
- Lymphoma

Immunologic abnormalities
- Systemic lupus erythematosus
- Complement deficiency
- Hypogammaglobulinemia
- Hyperimmunoglobulin E syndrome
- Acquired immunodeficiency syndrome

viewed as human pathogens until the 1950s, when several cases of disease caused by these organisms were reported.[11] Cutaneous infection usually results from exogenous inoculation, and predisposing factors include a history of preceding trauma, immunosuppression, or chronic disease. While *Mycobacteria marinum* is the most common agent of skin infection by atypical mycobacteria,[12] many others have been reported in recent decades. (See *Mycobacteria species that cause skin ulcers,* page 388.) The cutaneous lesions vary depending on the causative agent, and may present as granulomas, small superficial ulcers, sinus tracts, or large ulcerated lesions localized in exposed areas.

Histologically, mycobacterial infections present as granulomas and abscesses that are hard to distinguish from those of leprosy and cutaneous tuberculosis. Diagnosis will invariably depend on tissue culture or more recent techniques, such as polymerase chain reaction and gene rearrangement studies.

The appropriate therapy will depend on the causative agent because susceptibility to antibiotics varies. In some cases, simple excision of the cutaneous lesions or a combination of excision and chemotherapy often is most beneficial to the patient.

Deep fungal infections

Deep fungal infections of the skin can be divided into subcutaneous and systemic mycosis. The subcutaneous mycoses result from traumatic implantation of the etiologic agent into the subcutaneous tissue, development of localized disease, and eventual lymphatic spread. In rare instances, hematogenous dissemination can occur, especially in immunocompromised hosts. As may occur with sporotrichosis or chromomycosis, ulcers from deep fungal infections are found worldwide and can present in a wide variety of clinical settings.[13,14]

Systemic mycoses are the result of systemic penetration of pathogenic fungi, the lungs being the most common port of entry. These infections are restricted to the geographic areas where the fungi occur, especially tropical countries such as Central and South America. After an initial pulmonary infection, the fungi can spread hematogenously or via lymphatic vessels to other organs, including the skin. A decrease in immunity will lead to expression of the fungal infection, as is commonly observed in HIV-infected patients.

PRACTICE POINT

A thorough patient history assists in allowing a clinician to consider a diagnosis of systemic mycoses because of the limited area in which the causative fungi occur.

Sporotrichosis

Sporotrichosis is a subacute or chronic fungal infection caused by the fungus *Sporothrix schenckii*. Occurring as a consequence of traumatic implantation of the fungus into the skin, it's often associated with lymphangitis. Less commonly, inhalation of the conidia can lead to pulmonary infection and subsequently spread to the bones, eyes, central nervous system, and viscera. Systemic disease is seen in individuals with impaired immunity, such as alcoholics and HIV-infected patients.[15]

S. schenckii, a saprophyte in the environment, has been isolated in a variety of plants and other fauna, as well as animals (bites or scratches from animals, such as armadillos and cats). Individuals whose professional or leisure activities

Pyoderma gangrenosum treatment options

Type of treatment	Treatment options
Topical	• Topical steroids • Topical tacrolimus • Nicotine patch • Intralesional steroids
Systemic	• Steroids • Antibiotics (dapsone and minocycline) • Cyclosporin • Clofazamine • Azathioprine • Methotrexate • Chlorambucil • Cyclophosphamide • Thalidomide • Tacrolimus • Mycophenalate • Mofetil • Intravenous immunoglobulin • Plasmapheresis • Infliximab

expose them to the environment are at greater risk of acquiring the infection. Sporotrichosis is treated with systemic medications, including saturated solution of potassium iodide, itraconazole, fluconazole, terbinafine, and amphotericin B. Topically applied heat may also be used because the organism grows at low temperatures.

EVIDENCE-BASED PRACTICE

Because it's difficult to distinguish the presence of sporotrichosis directly from host tissues, culture on Sabouraud medium should be performed.[14,15]

Mycobacteria species that cause skin ulcers

Mycobacterium species	Clinical manifestations	Diagnosis	Treatment
M. marinum	• Swimming pool granuloma	Tissue culture	• Antituberculous drugs
M. ulcerans	• Subcutaneous nodule • Deep ulcers	Tissue culture	• Surgical excision
M. scrofulaceum	• Cervical lymphadenitis • Fistulae	Tissue culture	• Surgical excision
M. avium-intracellulare	• Small ulcers with erythematous borders	Tissue culture	• Surgical excision • Chemotherapy
M. kansaii	• Crusted ulcerations	Tissue culture	• Antituberculous drugs • Minocycline
M. chelonei	• Painful nodules and abscesses • Surgical wound infection	Tissue culture	• Erythromycin • Tobramycin • Amikacin • Doxycycline
M. fortuitum	• Painful nodules and abscesses • Surgical wound infection	Tissue culture	• Amikacin • Doxycycline • Ciprofloxacin • Sulfamethoxazole

Chromoblastomycosis

Chromoblastomycosis is a subcutaneous mycosis caused by several pigmented fungi including *Fonsecaea pedrosoi*, *Fonsecaea compacta*, *Phialophora verrucosae*, *Cladosporium carinii*, and *Rhinocladiella aquaspera*. These fungi are acquired through inoculation of the causative agents in the skin, after which infection mycosis develops at the site of inoculation. These microorganisms can be found in soil throughout the world; however, the disease is most common in tropical and subtropical climates, with the majority of cases seen in South America.[16]

Primarily affecting men ages 30 to 50, the principal lesion is a slow-growing papule that eventuates into a verrucous nodule. Exposed areas are involved with extremities being affected in 95% of the cases, especially the lower limbs.[17] The surface of the lesion may be covered by scales or may be ulcerated with serosanguinous crusts. Black dots can be often observed; these dots are rich in fungi and represent the site of transepidermal elimination of necrotic tissue.

Diagnostic examinations should include scrapings from the lesion with potassium hydroxide 20%; tissue samples should be obtained from biopsies for tissue culture and histology.

The disease tends to be chronic and difficult to treat, and may lead to lymphedema and elephantiasis. Ulcerated and cicatricial lesions have been reported to develop into carcinoma. Small lesions can be cured by surgical excision; however, chronic lesions are often resistant to treatment.

Systemic antifungic agents, such as ketoconazole, itraconazole, terbinafine, and amphotericin B, have been utilized, alone or in combination, with variable results.[18,19] Itraconazole is perhaps the most effective. Cryosurgery has also been used alone and in combination with itraconazole. Local heat therapy and flucytosine can also be effective therapeutic modalities.

Paracoccidioidomycosis

Paracoccidioidomycosis (South American blastomycosis) is a chronic, infectious disease caused by the fungus *Paracoccidioides brasiliensis*, a saprophyte of soil and decaying vegetation found in tropical and subtropical climates. Infection occurs via a respiratory route with occasional dissemination to other organs, including the skin. Patients present with painful ulcerative lesions of the mouth, face or, less frequently, the extremities. Involvement of regional lymphatics is characteristic.[20]

Diagnosis can be established by isolation and identification of the etiologic agent in culture. Treatment includes Amphotericin B and the azoles derivatives, such as itraconazole and ketoconazole.

Mycetoma

Mycetoma is a chronic infection of the skin and subcutaneous tissues characterized by local edema, sinus tract formation, and the presence of grains—hard concretions representing colonies of the etiologic agent. It occurs worldwide, but most commonly in tropical and subtropical regions. The most common agent in Central and South America is *Nocardia brasiliensis*, which is found in soil.[21] This agent is rarely found in the United States but when it does occur, *Pseudallescheria boydii* is the most commonly isolated agent.

Men ages 20 to 40 are most frequently affected. After trauma, a slow-growing, painless nodule develops, which may discharge purulent material and grains. Neighboring lesions may interconnect with each other, giving rise to the sinus tracts that are characteristic of the disease.

Diagnosis can be rendered based on clinical findings; additional examinations may include biopsy and tissue culture. On ultrasonographic evaluation, the mycetoma grains, capsules, and the resulting inflammatory granulomas have characteristic appearances.[22] Treatment is difficult. Surgical excision, commonly in combination with chemotherapy, may be effective. Sulfonamides, tetracycline, erythromycin, rifampin, oral azoles and Amphotericin B may be used,[23,24] depending on sensitivities of the etiologic agent.

Vibrio vulnificus infection

Vibrio vulnificus, a bacteria, is found widely in Atlantic Coast waters and raw shellfish.[25] It produces extracellular proteolytic and elastolytic enzymes and collagenases that favor tissue invasiveness. Wound infection with *V. vulnificus* occurs when contaminated seawater enters the body through a break in the epidermal barrier, commonly during fishing or water sports activities. Pustular lesions, lymphangitis, lymphadenitis, and cellulitis may ensue; in some cases, rapid progression to myositis and skin necrosis follows. Treatment of *V. vulnificus* wound infections consists of antibiotics, such as tetracycline and an aminoglycoside, and wound care.[26]

Primary septicemia from *V. vulnificus* occurs 24 to 48 hours after the ingestion of raw oysters, especially in patients with hepatic cirrhosis, diabetes, renal failure, or immunosuppression. Clinically, fever and hypotension may be present, along with the development of bullous cellulitis and necrotic skin ulcers.

Vasculopathies

A heterogeneous group of disorders are classified under this category. Vasculopathy is characterized by occlusion of small vessels within the skin due to thrombi or emboli, which leads to tissue hypoxia and the clinical manifestations of purpura, livedo reticularis, and painful ulcers. Cryofibrinogenemia, monoclonal cryoglobulinemia, and antiphospholipid antibody syndrome are among the vasculopathy causes that commonly present as atypical skin ulcerations of the lower extremities.

Cryofibrinogenemia

Cryofibrinogenemia occurs as a primary (idiopathic) disorder or in association with underlying diseases, such as infectious processes, malignancy, or collagen, vascular, or thromboembolic disease. The clinical presentation is of painful cutaneous ulcerations located on the leg and foot; these lesions are usually unresponsive to treatment. Other cutaneous findings include livedo reticularis (a net-like erythema), purpura, ecchymoses, and gangrene. The pathogenesis of the lesions is related to the in vivo occlusion of small blood vessels initiated in the distal extremities by the abnormal precipitate. This hypothesis is corroborated by the pathology findings of cryofibrinogen, consisting of thrombi within superficial dermal vessels due in part to protein deposition. Cryofibrinogen is a circulating complex of fibrin, fibrinogen, and fibronectin along with albumin, cold-insoluble globulin, and factor VIII. The complex is soluble at 98.6° F (37° C) but forms a cryoprecipitate at 39.2° F (4° C.)[27] Additionally, this complex can be made to clot with thrombin. The mechanism by which cryofibrinogen is produced isn't well-understood.

Treatment is symptomatic or, in secondary disease, directed to the underlying cause.[28] Agents which lyse fibrin thrombi are helpful. Stanozolol, streptokinase, and streptodornase have been used with success.

Cryoglobulinemia

Cryoglobulinemia occurs when deposits of cryoglobulins lead to the formulation of thrombi in medium and small vessel walls.[29] Three types of cryoglobulins have been identified; type I or monoclonal cryoglobulinemia may be seen in patients with malignant diseases, such as myeloma, or benign lymphoproliferative conditions, such as Waldenström's macroglobulinemia. This classically leads to thrombotic phenomena but can clinically resemble vasculitis. Type II, or mixed, cryoglobulinemia combines polyclonal and a monoclonal immunoglobulin; this type of cryoglobulinemia is seen less often in association with malignancies and is more often associated with infectious or inflammatory diseases. Type III is comprised of only polyclonal immunoglobulin and is most commonly associated with hepatitis C infection and the monoclonal component is IgM kappa. Both type II and III cryoglobulinemia cause vasculitis, which can lead to skin ulcers.[30] Other skin manifestations include acral cyanosis, Raynaud's phenomenon, livedo reticularis, altered pigmentation of involved skin, and palpable purpura, which may progress to blistering and frank ulceration. Some patients may have systemic manifestations, such as arthritis, peripheral neuropathy and glomerulonephritis. Diagnosis is based on skin biopsies, which show either vasculopathy or vasculitis, and subsequent detection of cryoglobulin by electrophoresis.

 PRACTICE POINT

Evaluate the patient with vasculitis for type II or III cryoglobulinemia; these conditions can cause vasculopathy.

Treatment should be directed to the underlying cause when cryoglobulinemia is associated with hepatitis C. Interferon alpha-2b is used to treat hepatitis C and may result in resolution of the associated cryoglobulinemia. Plasmapheresis alone or in combination with prednisone or immunosuppressive drugs (cyclophosphamide or chlorambucil) has also been used to treat cryoglobulinemia.[31,32]

Antiphospholipid antibody syndrome

Antiphospholipid antibody syndrome is characterized by elevated titers of antiphospholipid antibodies in association with venous or arterial thrombosis, recurrent fetal loss, and thrombocytopenia. Antiphospholipid antibodies are immunoglobulins (IgG, IgM, or both). The lupus anticoagulant, anticardiolipin antibodies, and Venereal Disease Research Laboratories (VDRL) test (false positive) are all antiphospholipid antibodies and any or all may be present as part of the syndrome.[33,34] Antiphospholipid antibody syndrome may present as primary disease or may be secondary to an underlying autoimmune disease such as systemic lupus erythematosus (seen in about 50% of cases). The syndrome has also been associated with malignancy and infectious states. The exact pathogenic mechanism of antiphospholipid antibody syndrome remains unknown.

The clinical hallmark of the disease is the presence of livedo reticularis. Arterial and venous thrombosis may elicit a variety of skin lesions, including ulcerations (most commonly), superficial thrombophlebitis, and cutaneous infarcts. Any organ system can be affected. Placental vessel thrombosis and ischemia can eventuate in miscarriage precipitated by placental insufficiency. The proposed mechanism responsible for this is a reduction of annexin V (a cell-surface protein with anticoagulant properties) on the trophoblast cells promoting a procoagulant state that leads to thrombosis at the maternal-fetal interface, and subsequent damage to the placenta and fetal loss.[35]

Treatment includes the use of aspirin, warfarin, and prednisone, but response isn't uniform.

Metabolic disorders

Metabolic diseases are uncommon causes of chronic wounds. One condition, called calciphylaxis, is commonly seen in a subset of patients undergoing chronic hemodialysis who developed secondary hyperparathyroidism.[36] This leads to deposition of calcium within soft tissue and the vasculature and, eventually, tissue death.

Calciphylaxis

Calciphylaxis is a rare, often fatal condition, characterized clinically by progressive cutaneous necrosis, which frequently occurs in patients with end-stage renal disease. Many eliciting factors have been suggested but the most common linking phenomenon is the development of secondary hyperparathyroidism.[36,37] Secondary hyperparathyroidism causes elevated calcium-phosphate product and development of vascular, cutaneous, and subcutaneous calcification that, in turn, leads to tissue death. Calciphylaxis typically develops after beginning dialysis and is seen in approximately 1% of patients with chronic renal failure and 4.1% of patients receiving hemodialysis.[38] The prognosis for patients who develop calciphylaxis is grim, with an estimated 5-year survival rate of less than 50%.[39] In addition to skin involvement, the pathophysiologic process may also occur within internal organs which, along with sepsis from infected skin wounds, is a major cause of morbidity and mortality.

Calciphylaxis treatment options

Medical treatment options
- Phosphate binders
- Decreased calcium in dialysate
- Antibiotics
- Low phosphate diet
- Calcitriol
- Diphosphonates
- Avoidance of challenging agents
- Avoidance of systemic steroids
- Hyperbaric oxygen
- Anticoagulation
- Cyclosporine
- Stanozolol

Surgical treatment options
- Parathyroidectomy
- Wound care and debridement
- Amputation
- Renal transplantation
- Skin grafting using either autologous or tissue engineered skin

specific agent, such as parathyroid hormone, hyperphosphatemia, or hypercalcemia, among other sensitizing agents. Once a patient is sensitized, the hypersensitivity reaction is induced in response to a challenging agent such as systemic steroids, infusion of albumin, iron dextran, immunosuppression, or trauma. The hypersensitivity reaction leads to the development of calcinosis, inflammation, and sclerosis associated with calciphylaxis.

Diagnosis can usually be based on clinical grounds. Although vascular processes may present similarly, laboratory evaluation looking for the presence of an elevated calcium, phosphate, or calcium x phosphate product confirms calciphylaxis. An elevated intact parathyroid hormone level along with radiographic evidence and confirmatory histology is also diagnostic. Calcification of the intima and media of small- and medium-sized vessels in the dermis and subcutaneous tissue are characteristic of calciphylaxis. Radiographic findings include pipe-stem calcifications due to the calcium deposits outlining the vessels in these patients.

As secondary infections may have tragic sequelae, treatment of infected ulcers is critical. Swab and tissue cultures from the wound may aid in guiding antibiotic therapy.

The treatments used to treat patients with calciphylaxis can be divided into either medical or surgical therapies[36-42] and are often used in tandem. (See *Calciphylaxis treatment options.*)

Malignancies

Malignancies may present either as wounds or developing from wounds. Nonmelanoma skin cancer, lymphomas, and sarcomas may ulcerate as they outgrow their blood supply. Alternatively, chronic wounds may develop into a malig-

The cutaneous manifestations begin as red or violaceous mottled plaques, in a livedo reticularis-like pattern. This signifies a vascular pattern and these early ischemic lesions often progress to gangrenous, ill-defined, black plaques. With time, these gangrenous plaques will ulcerate and become tender, indurated ulcers that can lead to auto-amputation. The ulcers of calciphylaxis are usually bilateral and symmetric, and may extend deep into muscle. Vesicles frequently appear at the periphery of the ulcers.

It's believed that patients develop this condition as a result of a hypersensitivity reaction.[36,40-42] In certain circumstances, a patient may be sensitized by a

nancy, most commonly squamous cell carcinoma. This phenomenon is termed Marjolin's ulcer after the author who first described cells from an edge of a chronic wound that have undergone malignant change, an occurrence that can be seen in up to 2% of chronic wounds.[43] A similar phenomenon may also occur in scars, burn wounds, sinus tracts, chronic osteomyelitis, and even vaccination sites.

The precise mechanism of malignant degeneration in chronic wounds isn't known, although several theories have been proposed.[44-46] In addition to squamous cell carcinoma, basal cell carcinomas and other neoplasms, such as Kaposi's sarcoma and lymphoma, have also been found in chronic wounds.

Early identification of malignancy, typically via biopsy of suspected lesions, is critical. Treatment of biopsy-confirmed neoplasia includes excision with margins; amputation of the affected limb may be necessary in some cases. Mohs surgery (to ensure complete removal of the primary lesion) has been used successfully to treat malignancy arising from chronic osteomyelitis.[43]

External causes

External causes of atypical wounds include spider bites, chemical injury, chronic radiation exposure, trauma, and factitial ulcers.[47] A thorough patient history is the most valuable tool in determining the etiologic agent in ulcers caused by external factors.

Spider bites

At least 50 spider species in the United States have been implicated in causing significant medical conditions; however, the *Loxosceles* (brown recluse or violin spider) and the *Latrodectus* (black widow) species are the most well-known to cause skin necrosis and ulcers in the Americas.

Loxoscelism

The bite of *L. reclusae* is usually painless and often goes unnoticed; however, 10% of patients will experience progression to more significant wounds.[48] In these patients, enlargement of the bite site occurs within 6 to 12 hours, with associated pain and general symptoms such as fever, malaise, headaches, and arthralgias. As the disease progresses, a pustule, blister, or large plaque forms at the bite site. These wounds may present as a deep purple plaque surrounded by a clear halo (vasoconstriction) and surrounding erythema — the so-called red, white, and blue sign.

With bites occurring in areas of greater fat content, such as the abdomen, buttocks, and thighs, necrosis develops more frequently. When the eschar is shed, an ulcer may result. Healing of the ulcer is generally very slow and may take up to 6 months.

The differential diagnosis includes foreign body reaction, infections, trauma, vasculitis, and pyoderma gangrenosum. Treatment consists of cooling the bite site, elevation (if possible), and analgesics. The use of systemic steroids may prevent the enlargement of the necrotic areas. Dapsone has also been recommended at a dose of 100 mg per day in adults.

Latrodectism

The black widow spider, or *Latrodectus mutans,* is easily recognized by a bright red hour-glass on the abdomen. The painless bite is followed by severe pain, swelling, and tenderness at the site where the bite occurred. Systemic symptoms such as headaches and abdominal pain may follow, but they subside in 1 to 3 days. Treatment includes local ice, calcium gluconate, and the administration of specific antivenin. Black widow bites are rarely fatal; death may occur in children, those with comorbidities, or elderly people.

Chemical burns

A variety of chemical products are capable of producing skin wounds.[49] Cutaneous injury caused by caustic chemicals progresses continually after the initial exposure and, if not properly cared for, may produce painful ulcers that are difficult to heal. The lesions caused by alkalis are usually more severe than those caused by acids; however, the severity of the burn is determined by the mode of action and concentration of the chemical as well as the duration of contact before treatment is initiated.[49] Prolonged irrigation with water for 30 minutes or more is the most important initial treatment, followed by standard burn care.

Certain chemicals possess unique properties that require special additional therapy, such as hydrofluoric acid (application of 25% magnesium sulphate), chromic acid (excision of the affected area), and phenol (application of polyethylene glycol mixed with alcohol 2:1).[47]

Radiation dermatitis

After exposure to ionizing radiation exceeding 10 Gy, local skin reactions characterized by mild erythema, edema, and pruritus may occur.[50] This acute radiation dermatitis usually begins 2 to 7 days after exposure, peaks within 2 weeks, and gradually subsides. With exposure to higher doses, intense erythema with vesiculation, erosion, and superficial ulceration may ensue. Postinflammatory pigmentary abnormalities, teleangiectasia, and atrophy are common.

Excision of the affected area and hyperbaric oxygen have been suggested as possible treatment options.

Factitial dermatitis

The term factitial dermatitis denotes a self-imposed injury. The clinical appearance of these ulcers is usually particular, with sharp or linear edges in an area of easy access such as the extremities, abdomen, and anterior chest.

Treatment includes evaluation and treatment of underlying psychological diseases and limitation of accessibility to the wound, such as placing a dressing or cast over the wound.

Summary

Treating the underlying cause, when possible, is the initial step in caring for patients with atypical wounds. Anti-infective agents may be used for infectious ulcers, malignancies may require surgical removal, and anti-inflammatory agents may be used for inflammatory ulcers. In addition, the use of a moist healing environment, compression dressings (in the absence of arterial insufficiency) for leg lesions, off-loading areas at risk for prolonged pressure, and maximizing patients' nutritional status are essential.

Despite these measures, healing is often slow in patients with atypical wounds. Prolonged healing leads to increased morbidity and decreased quality of life as well as an increase in direct and indirect costs of care. Adjunctive therapies are often used, aimed at both increasing the number of patients who will heal (effectiveness of therapy) and the speed at which they heal (cost-effectiveness of therapy).

Show what you know

1. Which of the following is the most important reason to recognize a wound as atypical?

A. The wound may be contagious.
B. Treatment varies based on etiology.
C. Standard wound healing therapies don't apply.
D. To bill correctly.

ANSWER: B. It's critical to recognize when a wound is caused by an etiology other than prolonged pressure, neuropathy, or abnormal vascular supply, so that appropriate measures may be undertaken to make a correct diagnosis and provide appropriate therapy. Although an infectious agent that's contagious may be a cause of an atypical ulcer, this isn't common. Although oftentimes specific therapies for atypical wounds exist, these are usually coupled with principles of good wound care, such as compression, off loading, moist wound healing, and others. Billing for medical therapies is based on Evaluation and Management Codes as opposed to CPT codes.

2. Which of the following may be performed on tissue biopsies of wounds?

A. Histology
B. Culture
C. Immunofluorescence
D. All of the above

ANSWER: D. As a variety of etiologies cause atypical wounds, a variety of techniques are used to confirm these etiologies. Histology is critical for diagnosing inflammatory, malignant, and infectious causes. Biopsies for tissue culture aid in diagnosing infectious causes and biopsies for immunofluorescence will aid in diagnosing some inflammatory and autoimmune diseases.

3. Which of the following shouldn't typically be debrided?

A. Diabetic foot ulcer
B. Ulcers due to infectious causes
C. Pyoderma gangrenosum ulcers
D. Ulcers due to vasculitis

ANSWER: C. In susceptible people, even minimal trauma to the skin can result in the production of pyoderma gangrenosum lesions, such as pustules and ulcers. This phenomenon is called pathergy. Therefore, debridement of an ulcer secondary to pyoderma gangrenosum may lead to severe worsening of the ulcer.

4. Sporotrichosis is a fungal infection caused by:

A. *Sporothrix schenckii.*
B. *Mycobacterium ulcerans.*
C. *Fonsecaea pedrosoi.*
D. *M. marinum.*

ANSWER: A. *Sporothrix schenckii* causes sporothrichosis. *M. ulcerans* and *M. marinum* are species of mycobacteria. *Fonsecaea pedrosoi* is a pigment fungi related to chromoblastomycosis.

5. Cryofibrinogenemia is classified as a:

A. mycobacterium.
B. pyoderma gangrenosum.
C. vasculopathy.
D. metabolic disease.

ANSWER: C. Cryofibrinogenemia is a painful cutaneous ulceration classified as a vasculopathy. Mycobacterium is a bacteria. Pyoderma gangrenosum is an inflammatory ulcer, and metabolic disease is an uncommon cause of chronic wounds.

6. Which type of wound is a rare, often fatal condition characterized by progressive cutaneous necrosis that occurs in patients with end stage renal disease?

    A. Calciphylaxis
    B. Vasculopathy
    C. Radiation dermatitis
    D. Chemical burn

ANSWER: A. Vasculopathy, radiation dermatitis, and chemical burns are all other types of atypical wounds.

7. Factitial dermatitis is a:

    A. rare condition.
    B. self-imposed injury.
    C. red rash.
    D. dry, scaly scab.

ANSWER: B. Factitial dermatitis is a self-imposed injury usually found in easily accessible areas such as the extremities, abdomen, and anterior chest.

References

1. Phillips, T.J., and Dover, J.S. "Leg Ulcers," *Journal of the American Academy of Dermatology* 25(6 Pt 1):65-87, December 1991.
2. Falabella, A., and Falanga, V. "Uncommon Causes of Ulcers," *Clinics in Plastic Surgery* 25(3):467-79, July 1998.
3. Lotti, T., et al. "Cutaneous Small-Vessel Vasculitis," *Journal of the American Academy of Dermatology* 39(5 Pt 1):667-87, November 1998.
4. Gibson, L.E. "Cutaneous Vasculitis: Approach to Diagnosis and Systemic Associations," *Mayo Clinic Proceedings* 65(2):221-29, February 1990.
5. Jennette, J.C., and Falk, R.J. "Small-vessel Vasculitis," *New England Journal of Medicine* 337(21):1512-23, November 20, 1997.
6. Scott, D.G., and Watts, R.A. "Systemic Vasculitis: Epidemiology, Classification and Environmental Factors," *Annals of Rheumatic Disease* 59(3):161-63, March 2000.
7. von den Driesch, P. "Pyoderma Gangrenosum: A Report of 44 Cases with Follow-Up," *British Journal of Dermatology* 137(6):1000-1005, December 1997.
8. Callen, J.P. "Pyoderma Gangrenosum," *Lancet* 351(9102):581-85, February 1998.
9. Powell, F.C., and Collins, S. "Pyoderma Gangrenosum," *Clinics in Dermatology* 18(3):283-93, May-June 2000.
10. Geren, S.M., et al. "Infliximab: A Treatment Option for Ulcerative Pyoderma Gangrenosum," *Wounds* 15(2): 49-53, May 2003.
11. Groves R. "Unusual Cutaneous Mycobacterial Diseases," *Clinics in Dermatology* 13(3):257-63, May-June 1995.
12. Hautmann, G., and Lotti, T. "Atypical Mycobacterial Infections of the Skin," *Dermatologic Clinics* 12(4):657-68, October 1994.
13. Rivitti, E.A., Aoki, V. "Deep Fungal Infections in Tropical Countries," *Clinics in Dermatology* 17(2):171-90, March-April 1999.
14. Kauffman, C.A. "Sporotrichosis," *Clinical Infectious Disease* 29(2): 231-36, August 1999.
15. Davis, B.A. "Sporotrichosis," *Dermatologic Clinics* 14(1):69-76, January 1996.
16. Bonifaz, A., et al. "Treatment of Chromoblastomycosis with Itraconazole, Cryosurgery, and a Combination of Both," *International Journal of Dermatology* 36(7):542-47, July 1997.
17. Guerriero, C., et al. "A Case of Chromoblastomycosis due to Phialophora Verrucosa Responding to Treatment with Itraconazole," *European Journal of Dermatology* 8(3):167-68, April-May 1998.
18. Tanuma, H., et al. "Case Report. A Case of chromoblastomycosis Effectively Treated with Terbinafine. Characteristics of Chromoblastomycosis in the Kitasato Region, Japan," *Mycoses* 43(1-2):79-83, 2000.
19. Kumarasinghe, S.P., and Kumarasinghe, M.P. "Itraconazole Pulse Therapy in Chromoblastomycosis," *European Journal of Dermatology* 10(3):220-22, April-May 2000.

20. Bernard, G., and Duarte, A.J. "Paracoccidioidomycosis: A Model for Evaluation of the Effects of Human Immunodeficiency Virus Infection on the Natural History of Endemic Tropical Diseases," *Clinical Infectious Disease* 31(4):1032-39, October 2000.

21. Salinas-Carmona, L.C. "Nocardia Brasiliensis: From Microbe to Human and Experimental Infections," *Microbes and Infection* 2(11):1373-81, September 2000.

22. Fahal, A.H., et al. "Ultrasonographic Imaging of Mycetoma," *British Journal of Surgery* 84(8): 1120-2, August 1997.

23. Young, B.A., et al. "Mycetoma," *Journal of the American Podiatric Medical Association* 90(2):81-84, February 2000.

24. Boiron, P., et al. "Nocardia, Nocardiosis and Mycetoma," *Medical Mycology* 36(S1):26-37, 1998.

25. Kumamoto, K.S., and Vukich, D.J. "Clinical Infections of Vibrio Vulnificus: A Case Report and Review of Literature," *Journal of Emergency Medicine* 16(1):61-66, January-February 1998.

26. Serrano-Jaen, L., and Vega-Lopez, F. "Fulminating Septicaemia Caused by Vibrio Vulnificus," *British Journal of Dermatology* 142(2):386-87, February 2000.

27. Brungger, A., et al. "Cryofibrinogenemic Purpura," *Archives of Dermatological Research* 279(Suppl):S24-S29, 1987.

28. Falanga, V., et al. "Stanozolol in Treatment of Leg Ulcers due to Cryofibrinogenaemia," *Lancet* 338(8763):347-48, August 1991.

29. Piette, W.W. "Hematologic Associations of Leg Ulcers," *Clinics in Dermatology* 8(3-4):66-85, July-December 1990.

30. Rallis, T.M., et al. "Leg Ulcers and Purple Nail Beds. Essential Mixed Cryoglobulinemia," *Archives of Dermatology* 131(3):342-46, March 1995.

31. Yancey Jr., W.B., et al. "Cryoglobulins in a Patient with SLE, Livedo Reticularis, and Elevated Level of Anticardiolipin Antibodies," *American Journal of Medicine* 88(6):699, June 1990.

32. Karlsberg, P.L. et al. "Cutaneous Vasculitis and Rheumatoid Factor Positivity as Presenting Signs of Hepatitis C Virus-induced Mixed Cryoglobulinemia," *Archives of Dermatology* 131(10):1119-23, October 1995.

33. Smith, K.J., et al. "Cutaneous Histopathologic Findings in Antiphospholipid Antibody Syndrome," *Archives of Dermatology* 1990(9):126, 1176-83, September 1990.

34. Selva, A., et al. "Pyoderma-gangrenosum-like Ulcers Associated with Lupus Anticoagulant," *Dermatology* 1994(2):189, 182-84.

35. Rote, N.S. "Antiphospholipid Antibodies, Annexin V, and Pregnancy Loss," *New England Journal of Medicine* 337(22):1630-31, November 27, 1997.

36. Smiley, C.M., et al. "Calciphylaxis in Moderate Renal Insufficiency: Changing Disease Concepts," *American Journal of Nephrology* 20(4):324-28, July-August 2000.

37. Roe, S.M., et al. "Calciphylaxis: Early Recognition and Management," *The American Surgeon* 60(2):81-86, February 1994.

38. Kim, Y.J., et al. "Calciphylaxis in a Patient with End-Stage Renal Disease," *Journal of Dermatology* 28(5):272-75, May 2001.

39. Budisavljevic, M.N., et al. "Calciphylaxis in Chronic Renal Failure," *Journal of the American Society of Nephrology* 7(7):978-82, July 1996.

40. Kang, A.S., et al. "Is Calciphylaxis Best Treated Surgically or Medically?" *Surgery* 128(6):967-72, December 2000.

41. Oh, D.H., et al. "Five Cases of Calciphylaxis and a Review of the Literature," *Journal of the American Academy of Dermatology* 40(6 Pt 1):979-87, June 1999.

42. Hafner, J., et al. "Uremic Small-Artery Disease with Medical Calcification and Intimal Hyperplasia (So-called Calciphylaxis): A Complication of Chronic Renal Failure and Benefit from Parathyroidectomy," *Journal of the American Academy of Dermatology* 33(6):954-62, December 1995.

43. Chang, A., et al. "Squamous Cell Carcinoma Arising in a Nonhealing Wound and Osteomyelitis Treated with Mohs Micrographic Surgery: A Case Study," *Ostomy Wound Management* 44(4):26-30, April 1998.

44. Fishman, J.R.A., and Parker, M.G. "Malignancy and Chronic Wounds: Marjolin's Ulcer," *Journal of Burn Care Rehabilitation* 12(3):218-23, May-June 1991.

45. Lautenschlager, S., and Eichmann, A. "Differential Diagnosis of Leg Ulcers," *Current Problems in Dermatology* 27:259-70, 1999.

46. Natarajan, S., et al. "A Non-healing Ulcer Associated with Malignant Lymphoma," *Journal of Wound Care* 9(1):45-46, January 2000.

47. Newcomer, V.D., and Young Jr., E.M. "Unique Wounds and Wound Emergencies," *Dermatologic Clinics* 11(4):715-27, October 1993.

48. Smith, D.B., et al. "Brown Recluse Spider Bite: A Case Study," *Journal of Wound, Ostomy Continence Nursing* 24(3):137-43, May 1997.

49. Bates, N. "Acid and Alkali Injury," *Emergency Nursing* 7(8):21-26, December-January 2000.

50. Caccialanza, M., et al. "Results and Side Effects of Dermatologic Radiotherapy: A Retrospective Study of Irradiated Cutaneous Epithelial Neoplasms," *Journal of the American Academy of Dermatology* 41(4):589-94, October 1999.

CHAPTER 20

Wound care:
Where we were, where we are, where we're going

Where we were

Dressing wounds has traditionally been a job for nurses. Some of the earliest pictures of nurses depict young women covering the wounds of soldiers with gauze dressings. For many years, that's all we did with wounds — passively cover them using strict sterile technique to keep out debris. An essential skill was learning how to use sterile forceps to pick up and handle gauze-dressing materials. Wet-to-dry dressings were the gold standard.

We believed that turning a patient and positioning him in a 90-degree angle would relieve pressure — some patients were even secured in that position for several hours! Massaging the area around a decubitus ulcer (what we now call a *pressure ulcer*) was a common intervention. We believed that a dry wound was a good wound. Heat lamps were occasionally positioned over the local wound area to assist in this "dry healing" method. Wounds were "painted," and even soaked, in povidone-iodine solution. Scabs were considered a positive sign. Many "home inventive" remedies were developed to put in the wound, and different parts of the country had their own local favorites: sugar and bourbon, sugar and povidone-iodine, grape jelly, honey, and antacids, to name a few. "We've always done it this way," or "It works" were the yardsticks we used, rather than evidence and research findings.

Wound assessment meant looking for green or yellowish fluid and odors that indicated the presence of infection. We used a swab culture inserted into the wound drainage to assess for infection.

Wound care practices were passive. We cleaned the wound, covered it, and waited patiently as the wound healed. Because the typical hospital length of stay was long, many patients' wounds closed and healed before they were discharged.

Where we are now

A wound care revolution with emphasis on a team approach has occurred over the last five decades. The 1960s discovery of moist wound healing, coupled with advancements in wound dressing materials, has dramatically changed wound care practices. We now understand that wound healing must take place in a moist environment so that epithelial cells can migrate from the wound edges to reepithelialize, or close, the wound. This process is likened to the cells' "leap- frogging." In a dry wound, these cells have to burrow down underneath the wound bed to find a moist area upon which to move in order to migrate forward.

Wound bed preparation continues to be an important foundation for tissue rebuilding. Adequate and continuous wound debridement is needed because it removes necrotic tissue, which is a barrier to migrating cells. Enzymatic agents (selective and nonselective chemicals), autolytic (film dressings), mechanical (wet-dry dressings, whirlpool, and irrigation), and surgical/sharp are the debridement options from which clinicians can select the best method of clearing the wound bed of dead tissue and getting it ready for the rebuilding of tissue.

The way acute wounds are closed has also changed. Collagen sutures are occasionally used after cardiac catheterization, and staples have replaced sutures for closing some surgical incision wounds. Skin bonding materials are being used to "glue" wound edges back together.

Some of the solutions previously used to clean wounds (Dakin's solution, povidone-iodine, hydrogen peroxide, acetic acid) were found to kill the very fibroblast cells that were needed to allow granulation tissue repair. The pressure ulcer treatment guidelines of the Agency for Healthcare Research & Quality (AHRQ, formerly the Agency for Healthcare Policy & Research, or AHCPR) provide recommendations about which solutions are harmful and which are appropriate to use in wound care.

This new understanding of the importance of moist wound healing based on wound physiology required the development of new dressing materials. Film dressings and hydrocolloid dressings were among the first dressing materials able to maintain a moist wound-healing environment. Clinicians had to learn new application techniques and, more importantly, the clinical significance of wound fluid findings.

Our advanced understanding of wounds has also caused a revision of our view of what's "normal" in a healing wound. Clinicians needed to learn to discriminate between the normal collection of fluid under newer dressings and "pus." Similarly, we've revised our view about wound odors. Different odors occur as wound fluid interacts with different dressing materials — wounds being treated with alginate dressings, for example, may smell like "low tide."

The practice of using the same dressing material for the entire wound healing time is no longer valid. As the wound characteristics change, so too should the choice of wound dressings. For example, a deep wound with a large amount of drainage requires a highly absorbent dressing, such as a hydrofiber, alginate, or foam. As the depth and amount of drainage decreases, a hydrogel, hydrocolloid, or film dressing might be used. Over the course of healing, the treatment plan will change as the wound fills with granulation tissue and epithelialization occurs.

The notion that all wounds are alike has also changed as we've learned that understanding of the wound's etiology is essential for appropriate care. Local wound care products as well as supportive care must be individualized for the particular wound. For example, a venous ulcer may require an absorptive dressing or a hydrogel, as well as necessary compression therapy. A variety of layered bandages beyond the classic Unna boot are now used. These new schemes are replacing a 100-year-old treatment (Unna boot) with advances in minimizing edema and accelerating wound repair. Checking for ankle-brachial index (ABI) and pulses using a Doppler device has become a standard step in the total assessment of a patient with a peripheral vascular ulcer.

Pressure relief as well as an appropriate dressing must be part of the care plan for pressure ulcers. Support surfaces available as cushions, overlays, replacement mattresses, and specialty beds now exist to assist in offloading of pressure. The very way in which we position patients has changed. The Agency for Healthcare Research and Quality (AHRQ) pressure ulcer treatment guidelines recommend a 30-degree angle rather than the old 90-degree position. Massaging the periwound area is no longer a recommended practice.

Wound culturing technique is also different. Quantitative bacterial cultures obtained from wound fluid or tissue are now considered the gold standard. If a facility can't do tissue cultures, and swab technique is the only method available, the wound should be thoroughly cleaned with nonbacteriostatic saline prior to obtaining the specimen. The specimen should be obtained by rotating the end of a cotton applicator over a 1-square-centimeter surface area of the wound, with sufficient pressure to express fluid from underlying tissue. Clean technique rather than sterile can now be used in chronic wounds as per AHRQ pressure ulcer treatment guidelines.

Research and technology continue to advance the science of wound care. Research has demonstrated that acute and chronic wounds heal differently, necessitating a new approach to wound management. Wound healing options, such as negative pressure therapy (vacuum-assisted closure), are now used to interact in the wound healing process. Another example of increased understanding of the biology of wound healing and technology is the use of growth factors. Derived from a patient's own platelets or in drug form dispensed in a tube, growth factors are now used to aid in healing diabetic wounds. Research continues as to the combinations and quantities of growth factors, and when to use them, to best enhance wound healing. Yet another way technology is providing new options for wound management is in the use of bioengineered skin equivalents for healing chronic wounds. These new skin equivalents are effective in accelerating the process of reepithelialization, in decreasing scar formation, and in accelerating the healing process of chronic wounds.

Wound care is no longer the sole province of nurses; it's now a specialty practiced by physicians, podiatrists, nurses, physical therapists, and occupational therapists, to name a few. Multidisciplinary teams provide comprehensive care to patients with acute and chronic wounds in a variety of settings, including inpatient, outpatient, long-term care, and home settings. Centers specializing in wound care have been established across the country and abroad.

Instruction in the form of continuing education courses, clinical symposia, and specialized programs is available to teach clinicians the essentials as well as the advanced knowledge of managing wounds in the twenty-first century. Specialized knowledge of wound care can be demonstrated by achieving certification in wound care from the American Academy of Wound Management (AAWM) or the Wound, Ostomy, and Continence Nurses Society (WOCN). Wound care may, one day, be approved by the American Medical Association as a medical specialty.

Legal issues have also affected wound care. Lawsuits regarding lack of adequate wound management have become common. Are pressure ulcers avoidable? This question is still being debated in courtrooms around the country. Medical, nursing, and other health care experts are being used to argue for both the plaintiff and the defendant.

Regulatory guidelines may support best practices, but they don't always support reimbursement to health care facilities. Long-term care facilities and home-care agencies are required to track and improve outcomes of care in wound patients. Outcome-based quality improvement will be introduced to the acute care setting in the near future. Many health care providers are struggling with the cost of wound dressings — and the cost of high-quality care. Wound care supplies, whether routine or nonroutine, are used regularly in the home care setting. Insurers are being asked to pay for some products and procedures even though research hasn't always provided scientific proof of their effectiveness.

Where we're going

What will wound care look like in the future? Curricula in all health care disciplines will assure that graduates have the wound care essentials needed for today's practitioners. Wound care goals will change for some patient populations. For example, in acute care, minimally invasive surgeries will reduce the number of acute incision wounds that health care providers have been accustomed to seeing. We might see the day when nurses in home care are the only ones to see healed wounds and are the experts in scar management. Those working in acute care will never see a healed acute wound, because the patient will go home within a few hours or days of surgery. Laparoscopic incision sites may be the only wounds acute care providers have to treat.

Because people are living longer and many chronic illnesses lead to "skin failure," the idea that some wounds won't heal may become increasingly accurate. Patients who are dying may have wounds that can't or won't heal; for these patients, palliative wound care will replace wound closure as a goal. The idea of palliative wound care with emphasis on comfort and preventing wound deterioration rather than wound closure will require clinicians and regulatory partners to rethink wound care practices.

The standard hospital mattress will be a thing of the past. High-tech, pressure-relieving support surfaces, with special features we can't begin to imagine, will become the gold standard in the acute care setting. Bariatric care units will be added to most acute care facilities as the need to manage this rising population continues. Long-term care and home care will also be faced with managing this emerging population.

Less painful and less frequent wound cleaning and dressing change will replace present practice. Newer dressings, with antimicrobial properties that allow them to remain on the wound for seven days, are already available. Wound care products based on cell biology will be developed not just to assist in the wound healing process, but to accelerate the repair process. Wound chambers with specific antibiotic therapy may provide us with a better microenvironment in which to heal wounds.

Technology will continue to make wound care practices easier, more efficient, and less time-consuming. Will reimbursement improve to keep up with the trends in technology? Telemedicine will be integrated into every health setting. Will regulatory agencies support the financial demands of this new patient care arena? Time will give us the answers to these questions. Bonding with our patients will occur through a small monitor screen, not via the personal touch of the past. Handheld scanning devices will be used by health care providers to detect stage I pressure ulcers so that preventive measures can be implemented before the epidermis breaks down. Wound "dip sticks" will tell us the wound's pH and other characteristics and be linked to the right product to use. Just as our cars have climate control, wound products will adapt to form the appropriate environment for healing to occur. Clinicians will speak into a microphone device on their identification badges to document wound characteristics during dressing changes, and their documentation will automatically be processed to the patient's chart and the physician's office. Electronic signatures will be triggered by our fingerprints. We may consult internationally through computers and telemedicine, making our health care system borderless.

All these developments may sound farfetched, but the discipline of wound care is evolving into higher, innovative technology that we can't conceive of. Quantum leaps — in the way we think about wounds and understand healing and in technologies — will occur among health care practitioners, patients, and caregivers. The future of wound care will undoubtedly be truly amazing. We look forward in future editions to seeing when and how many of our predictions become realities.

Elizabeth and Sharon

Index

i refers to an illustration; t refers to a table; C refers to a color plate page.

i refers to an illustration; t refers to a table; C refers to a color plate page.

i refers to an illustration; t refers to a table; C refers to a color plate page.

i refers to an illustration; t refers to a table; C refers to a color plate page.

i refers to an illustration; t refers to a table; C refers to a color plate page.

i refers to an illustration; t refers to a table; C refers to a color plate page.

i refers to an illustration; t refers to a table; C refers to a color plate page.

i refers to an illustration; t refers to a table; C refers to a color plate page

i refers to an illustration; t refers to a table; C refers to a color plate page.